The Hevert Collection

PHILOSOPHY
of NATUROPATHIC
MEDICINE

In Their Own Words

The Hevert Collection

PHILOSOPHY
of NATUROPATHIC
MEDICINE

In Their Own Words

Edited by Sussanna Czeranko, ND, BBE
Foreword by Jared L. Zeff, ND

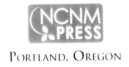

Portland, Oregon

Managing Editor: Sandra Snyder, Ph.D.
Production: Fourth Lloyd Productions, LLC.
Design: Richard Stodart

Front cover photographs: Adolf Just (left) and Louis Kuhne (right).
Back cover illustration: Louis Kuhne Sanitarium, 1899.

Published by NCNM Press
National College of Natural Medicine
049 SW Porter Street
Portland, Oregon 97201, USA
www.ncnm.edu

NCNM Press gratefully acknowledges the generous and prescient financial
support of HEVERT USA which has made possible the creation and
distribution of the *In Their Own Words* historical series.
The HEVERT COLLECTION comprises twelve historical compilations which
preserve for the healing professions significant and representational works
from contributors to the historical Benedict Lust journals.

Printed in the United States of America

ISBN: 13-digit number 978-0-9771435-3-5
10-digit number 0-9771435-3-8

Philosophy of Naturopathic Medicine is dedicated to Nature, whose immutable laws guided the historical giants of our medicine, Louis Kuhne and Adolf Just, to such a clear and profound understanding of her enduring power in healing. The voices of the past echo softly in their work, reminding us once again, as if for the first time, of the real foundation of Naturopathic Medicine.

TABLE OF CONTENTS

FOREWORD

What physicians *think* medicine is profoundly shapes what they *do*, how
they behave in doing it, and the reasons they use to justify that behavior
. . . whether conscious of it or not, every physician has an answer to what
he thinks medicine is, with real consequences for all whom he attends
. . . . The outcome is hardly trivial . . . . It dictates, after all, how we
approach patients, how we make clinical judgments.

—Pellegrino E., *Medicine, Science, Art: An Old Contro-
versy Revisited (Man and Medicine) 1979; 4.1: 43-52.*

Pellegrino captures an essential element of medical practice in his
statement; "What physicians think medicine is profoundly shapes what
they do...". All medical systems share the common essence of the desire
to aid the sick among us. Our joint calling is to ease suffering. It is not
often considered that there are different medical philosophies, with fundamentally different ideas of how to go about doing that. There is in
our culture, where one medical system is so dominant, the basic understanding that the practice of medicine is "the diagnosis and treatment of
disease". In this orthodox biomedicine mode, no other legitimate way
to think about medicine is tolerated. However, a growing recognition is
emerging, namely that there actually may be more than one way to do
this. Rarely, however, is the fundamental assumption of this philosophy
challenged. But it is a philosophy, a world view, one of several extant considerations of how one goes about thinking of illness and its remediation;
that is, of treating the sick.

An examination of this statement, "the diagnosis and treatment of
disease", demonstrates several underlying assumptions that reveal this as
a statement of philosophy rather than as a general truth. One assumption
is that there are "diseases", specific disease entities that can be identi-
fied. A second is that these "disease entities" can be treated, as if separately from the ill patient. While these assumptions are obviously true in
one sense, they confirm the standard of conventional medical system as
a disease-based system of thought. In the following pages a quite different medical philosophy appears, one that is not disease-based. What the
reader encounters here is a system of thinking that focuses upon the restoration of health, rather than on the treatment of disease. The difference
in approach and effect is profound.

If one believes that human illness is best understood as the development of the myriad of diseases from a myriad of causes, and that each
disease requires its own specific drug for correction, one's goal is the diagnosis of the disease entity, and its specific, and usually pharmaceutical,

treatment. In this philosophy some diseases have no real treatment. In other cases no curative treatment may be available, but the disease may be "suppressed" with the proper drug approach, reducing the symptomatic expression of the patient's illness. The result is not cure of the disease, but its ongoing treatment to continually attempt to reduce the symptom picture and thereby reduce the suffering of the patient.

A different understanding would lead one to practice quite differently. We read in these pages early writings of the naturopathic profession, expressing a vastly different understanding. We read here not of disease entities, but of the common basis of illness, such as abnormal composition of blood and lymph. We read how disease comes about through the violation of the laws of nature, a natural consequence of eating inappropriately and poisoning oneself thereby, or living wrongly and of thinking wrongly, so that disease is the natural consequence. We read of the developing concept of the unity of disease and the unity of cure. We read how disease is a process, and not an entity. We read of cure through the adoption of a simple diet and basic exercise program. We read of the therapeutic use of the application of water to stimulate circulation, organ function and a discharge of toxins. We read of the understanding that fever is a healing response and how to honor and work with this healing effort. We see that the treatments are not directed against a disease, but are designed to stimulate the healing reactions of the body, to reduce causes and restore normal function. The same treatments work in all the diseases, regardless of their differences, hence the "unity of cure".

As these pages develop, we come to understand a fundamentally different way of thinking, a medical philosophy that created a healing practice quite different from that which has come to dominate our culture. For example, in his essay, "Naturopathy Versus Medicine", Per Nelson, ND, writes,

> . . . the Naturopath simply assists nature in her efforts to eliminate waste material through the body's natural channels, by improving and equalizing the body fluids, and by stimulating the lungs, kidneys, bowels, and skin to normal activity, and this is the reason why naturopaths are able to cure diseases after all other systems have failed to do so.

This succinct characterization expresses the essence of the naturopathic approach, which is the expression of a philosophy that relies on the restoration of the natural process and is guided by the internal healing tendency and intelligence of the body.

I have thought about and taught naturopathic philosophy for over thirty years. What I encountered in these pages was a trove of information that we had forgotten during our scramble to restore this little profession after it had been nearly driven out of existence by the dominant medical paradigm. I am personally indebted to Dr. Czeranko for her work in reintroducing to the profession these old writings that defined our profession a century ago. It is deeply satisfying that we had re-discovered the same truths through our meager efforts. The truth of this philosophy is inherent in nature, and therefore re-discoverable. But had we had access to these writings, and had they been used to teach us and guide us, our little profession would have been a lot farther along, I believe, than it is.

Jared L. Zeff, ND
Professor of Naturopathic Medicine

PREFACE

Philosophy of Naturopathic Medicine is the second of the twelve book **Hevert Collection** entitled, *In Their Own Words*. It is the generosity of **Hevert USA** that has made this series of books possible in support of keeping our roots alive for present and future generations of Naturopaths. This volume restores to our community many important articles found in the journals published by Benedict Lust from 1900 to 1923. In those precious twenty-four years, the emerging Naturopathic profession had a lot to say about what Naturopathy was and wasn't. From 1902 and the birth of Naturopathy in New York City, the tenets of Naturopathic philosophy were being formulated by many who dared to speak out in favour of a new path to health. These early doctors wrote abundantly as they defined their new medical paradigm in a time of professional treachery and the allopathic profession stampeded to ascendancy, state by state, law by law. The early Naturopaths had much to say about the healing of diseases. Their writing reflects a profession-wide enthusiasm and passion for a medical system focused on the patient and on the planet.

While compiling this collection of articles under the heading of Philosophy, I encountered many unfamiliar names. The more I read, the more I discovered that many of these unknowns were in their own rights, men and women of immense accomplishment and stature, geniuses and giants among them on whose shoulders we stand to this day. Their gifts to our profession have been under the dustcover of time, unsung and unnoticed for the most part in the modern generation of NDs. Yet, they left behind a body of knowledge that has persisted to this day. The more I read from this abundant, rich, extensive literature, the more I am persuaded that their work is foundational, and philosophically powerful, the very basis of why we do what we do. The proof is always in the pudding! Their beliefs and convictions did not shrink in the face of deadly diseases, but instead translated into healthy patients and communities. These early practitioners of nature's healing walked their walk and showed people how to get healthy using the laws of nature.

What is the purpose of philosophy in the practice of naturopathic medicine? This question was poignantly answered by Dr. Jared Zeff in a lecture at National College of Natural Medicine to the first Naturopathic Philosophy class of the year, in September 2013. "My goal is to teach you to think like a Naturopath." (Zeff, 2013) Philosophy gives us the foundation to think naturopathically. What chaos if we were to engage in naturopathic practice while we tightly held onto some of the mechanistic views of the allopath! In choosing Naturopathic medicine, we are inherently recognizing that nature has a wisdom beyond our human comprehension. Abiding the laws of nature reinforces health.

I wish that every Naturopath in practice can find wisdom in the words of Dr. Nelson: "The Naturopath goes even further than to merely cure disease. Knowing that transgression of Nature's laws lies at the root of all human ills, he also considers it his duty to teach humanity how to follow these laws." (Nelson, 1920, 80)

So many people have their finger prints all over these pages. Without their hard work, this book would still be chugging along somewhere a thousand pages back. I am deeply grateful for the support of my colleague, Dr. Rick Severson, a gifted, dedicated librarian and archivist. His ears listened to my tales when I confronted obstacles along this journey. Dr. Severson would unclutter the path. To him, I am grateful for how he knows to convert a barrier into an opportunity, how to locate missing issues which were long felt to be lost (especially issues from 1906 and 1907). We got them, and thus the Benedict Lust journals collection at NCNM is now one spectacular, coherent and complete, unique collection. He never doubted this project for a nanosecond. His encouragement and guidance make him the rock star of naturopathic medical education library directors. I feel blessed to have a colleague who is so supportive of my work.

Behind the glossy book cover are hundreds of typed pages which were patiently transcribed by numerous, wonderful students at NCNM. In fact, there are over 800 articles typed from the Benedict Lust journals in preparation for the upcoming books. There are many more articles that are still in queue as this series emerges. I want to acknowledge every NCNM student who typed or proof read articles while navigating their intense course loads and juggling their personal lives. Huge heaps of intense gratitude to *Abendigo Reebs, Allison Brumley, Angela Carlson, Avishan Saberian, Bonita Wilcox, Delia Sewell, Derek Andre, Derrick Schull, Jennea Wood, Jennifer Samson, Joshua Corn, Katelyn Mudry, Katherine Venegas, Kimberly Kong, Kirsten Carle, Kyle Meyer, Lucy-Kate Reeve, Meagan Watts, Michelle Brown-Echerd, Natalie Paravicini, Node Smith, Olif Wojciechowski, Rachel Caplan, Renae Rogers, Rhesa Napoli, Sandy Musclow, Sarah Holloway, Tiffany Bloomingdale, Tina Dreisbach,* and to all those whom I am inadvertently missing here. I so much enjoyed working with each and every student who sacrificed scarce, precious study and leisure time for the hard work of meticulous research and transcription. As you launch yourselves into the Naturopathic profession, never forget how special and important your work has been. You have chosen a path of sacred work. You will be loved and cherished by your patients because you listen and truly care. Remember Nature!

I am especially indebted to the tireless work of *Dr. Karis Tressel* who was my diva of anti-chaos and who brought sublime organization and order to the colossal stacks of paper and minutia. Without Karis' exquisite, patient and detailed sense of clarity, I would be gray haired and frazzled. I am deeply grateful for her profound love of Nature Cure and her loving tenacity with this project.

I am very grateful for the unwavering, behind the scenes support of the Board of NCNM, Dr. Sandra Snyder, Susan Hunter, Nora Sande and Jerry Bores who understood from the beginning the importance of this project. I applaud Fourth Lloyd Productions, Nancy and Richard Stodart, my designers and coaches extraordinaire who guided me with alacrity every step of the way. Thank you both for the exquisite care that you took in every minute detail!

This book would be an historical curiosity and irrelevant to the contemporary health landscape, were it not for the thousands of Naturopaths working in their communities keeping the philosophy of our medicine alive. You took the path of nature in the health professions. Your patients know that your work and dedication are a testament that Naturopathic Medicine is as critical now as a century ago when our extraordinary naturopathic pioneers chose to walk a different path.

Lastly, I want to thank my husband, David Schleich, who typically saw the ending from the beginning and much sooner than I could. Writing takes a lot of energy and I am deeply grateful that David shares my love of history and listens to my stories with awe and deep appreciation. He always helps me find my way back to the present when I need to return from my beloved books in the NCNM archive.

You may be reading some sentences written by these early naturopaths that are a mile long, or embellished with words no longer in the current lexicon. Fear not; this is on purpose. These articles have been carefully transcribed and edited to ensure that you are taken back into time and experiencing the actual idioms, vocabulary, syntax and all. So, settle back in a comfortable chair with some green tea and enjoy these articles chosen from our pioneering elders *in their own words*.

Blessings,
Sussanna Czeranko, ND, BBE
Portland, Oregon, October 1, 2013

The physician is only the servant of nature not its teacher.

—C. Hippocrates (Lust, 1900, 17)

If an individual has not enough vitality to produce a fever and to burn and secrete the morbid matter, the same will settle down in different organs and thus cause chronic disease.

—Ludwig Staden, 1900, 100

The Naturopath goes even further than to merely cure disease. Knowing that transgression of Nature's laws lies at the root of all human ills, he also considers it his duty to teach humanity how to follow these laws.

—Nelson, 1920, 80

A doctor in the original and constantly and persistently applied meaning of the term, is first and over and above all, a TEACHER.

—M. E. Yergin, 1923, 228

If one could capture the spirit and vision of the early Naturopaths as they busied themselves molding a new paradigm for health care in America, the following words encapsulate the resolve and the philosophy which fueled their work: 'healing follows the laws of nature'. These pioneers were completely clear that nature had the power to heal. In February, 1900 Benedict Lust stated, "[the natural scientist] studies the nature of the patient and the nature of the sickness and uses natural means only." (Lust, 1900, 18) Lust insisted early and often that one must follow the laws of nature in order that nature can create health. In this volume, *Philosophy of Naturopathic Medicine*, the second in the **Hevert Collection** of twelve volumes, *In Their Own Words*, I have respectfully selected from among the hundreds of articles found in Benedict Lust's journals those which draw back to our attention the essence of what they believed, taught and practiced. The richness of their literature made the task less daunting because there was such abundance to draw from. In so many ways the pieces in this volume are the best of the best, evoking more than a century later a pervasive and persistent quality which made this labour of love less overwhelming. My respect for the courageous scholarship of our great forebears has grown these past years into deep gratitude and awe for their accomplishments during a time of severe adversity.

In the first article in this collection, Lust sets the tone. It is his often stated conviction that following nature was central to their emerging philosophy. Doctors during the early decades of the naturopathic movement witnessed with alarm the growing and dangerous reliance on medical drugs, such as the mercury based ones in calomel or vaccinations. At the same time, they also understood the related importance of treating the whole person. In this regard, Lust contends that those who "do not bother with the nature of the patient," were only prescribing "so and so many parts of some drug or other." (Lust, 1900, 17) Another area in which the early Naturopaths departed from allopathic or conventional practice was in the field of 'health' promotion. "Hygiene" was a doctrine that Lust and his colleagues adhered to, not because of the axiom of cleanliness being a virtue, but because hygiene embraced the inherent properties of health. Hygiene "recognized cleanliness as the first principle of health and [naturopaths] believed in realizing it by endeavoring to secure pure air, pure water and pure food for the people at large." (Hotz, 1900, 89)

Wilhelm Hotz defines "hygiene [as] the science of health … the first foundation of therapeutics, the science of restoring lost health, because without knowing the laws which maintain health, no physician can tell his patient the right way that leads him to health and gives him the proper advice how to regain it." (Hotz, 1900, 89) Introducing Pasteur's theories on putrefaction and microbes, Hotz considered "the microorganisms, apart from their fermentive power, as ideal watchmen of health, because their presence and action are quite often the first indication that something must be wrong, or that our body is in an abnormal state of health." Hotz introduced the concept that symptoms are not necessarily evil, but the body's attempts at restoring health.

Ludwig Staden's articles appeared early in Benedict Lust's journals. He wrote ardently about naturopathic medicine. In *The Causation of Diseases*, he addresses one of the cornerstones of naturopathic medicine, namely that "defective composition of blood" was the primary reason for disease and if only people were to "keep [their] blood pure" could health be attained. (Staden, 1900, 100)   Staden includes over eating, artificial foods and an exclusive meat diet as culprits contributing to the conditions that promote the culture and existence of bacilli that would not normally occur. Bacilli were often blamed for disease, but in fact, as Staden points out, "the bad quality of blood is responsible for [the bacteria's] existence." (Staden, 1900, 100)

While blood and morbid matter occupied the early Naturopath's theories of disease, Father Kneipp also regarded the quality of blood important. His clinical success was accomplished by taking the time to observe the patient carefully to make his assessment. "If the individual was pale and thin, he concluded that his blood was poor and of bad quality and that he lacked natural warmth." (Lust, 1900, 148) Based on this observation, the temperature of the water application would be determined including how it would be delivered.

Interpreting the symptoms that erupted during healing was also discussed and evaluated by the early pioneers. Chronic diseases had their own processes and in this early 1900 article, Lust is alluding to what eventually became known as the 'healing crisis'. He wrote that "in some diseases, pain may be actually caused by the first stages of the cure [and] these are signs of returning health." (Lust, 1900, 148) This concept, that patients may feel worse before they feel better, was a positive sign for the early Naturopaths. In fact, having symptoms during treatment actually meant that the course of cure was on track and that the patient had enough "reactive force required for the healing process." (Lust 1900, 149) The belief that healing was governed by a higher force than what science provided was held with great conviction by the early Naturopaths.

Another who stands as a foundational giant was Adolf Just. In an article, *Return to Nature*, published in 1901, Benedict Lust translated and published an excerpt from Adolf Just's book. The voice of the article is definitely Just's as he explains how the Jungborn came to be. Adolf Just, like Benedict Lust also faced a life threatening disease in which his salvation was discovering nature. Just spent time in nature and was healed. His gratitude was expressed by sharing what he learned with others. Just discloses, "I resolved to become the champion of nature, to work for her, and to point out the right way which will lead men from dreaded night to joyous light, to true health and complete happiness." (Just, 1901, 264)

In 1900, Benedict Lust had already been exposed to the works of Adolf Just and was espousing the latter's works in his journal. Just had written, *Kehrt zur Natur Zurück!* [*Return to Nature*] in Germany in 1896 which Lust began translating into English in 1900. Lust was strongly influenced by Just's work throughout his life. *Return to Nature* essentially laid the foundation for Naturopathy and would influence many future generations of Naturopathic doctors without their awareness of the work of Adolf Just. In 1900, Lust introduced Adolf Just and his philosophy that "all healing is done by nature and that science can only assist nature." (Lust, 1900, 127) Over a period of years I have come to realize that this particular article marks the beginning of the departure from Kneippism by Lust.

Just's book gave Lust a platform upon which to expand the parameters of what natural (later known as 'alternative' or 'complementary') medicine was moving towards. Just wrote his book and at the same time founded the Jungborn which was "a model institution for the true natural life, where those who wish to make arrangements for such a life at home in their own gardens can find the pattern." (Just, 1901, 264) The Jungborn model was adopted by Lust as a healing retreat center in Butler, New Jersey, and as well by Mahatma Gandhi who structured a community upon Just's principles. Just was inspired by the wonders of nature and created "a mode of life and a curative system which has nothing whatever to do with science, and in which we allow ourselves to be guided ... by the great teacher "nature" alone." (Just, 1901, 265) The Jungborn model created by Just would be replicated by Lust himself and numerous Naturopaths in America as sanitariums. Just's system of healing being based upon nature and modeled after nature was "as simple as the great teacher, nature, herself." (Just, 1901, 265)

From his study and observations of animals and nature herself, he created the 'natural bath'. Just was the first to embrace the powers of earth and water together and the result was the natural bath. He describes how in the wild "the higher land animals, especially wild boars and deer, in free nature are in the habit of lying down in small muddy swamps or pools, at first only with the abdomen, and rubbing it to and fro in the mud." (Just, 1901, 265) Just gives an account of how people can mimic such natural events by having a simple, natural bath.

Adolf Just was a deeply religious man who saw that people suffered sickness and misfortune when they departed from the laws of nature.

Lust shared this view, stating, "Men imagined that by forgetting the laws of nature they would gain powers, comforts, joys and happiness which nature did not offer." (Lust, 1900, 128) Lust adds, "The slightest diversion from the original destination must necessarily be followed by disturbances" (Lust, 1900, 128) such as dis-ease and sickness.

The secret to health and happiness according to Just and Lust was a *return to nature.* Lust notes, "After men's desertion of nature as far as their mode of living is concerned ... all sorts of ailments took hold of the body." (Lust, 1900, 128) Lust continues, "All civilized people became sick and weaker in the same proportions as their civilization was advancing until they finally were ruined." (Lust, 1900, 129) Adopting Just's methods of fresh air, light and a balanced diet lead sick people back to health. Lust exclaims, "It may sound like imaginations, but no human tongue is able to describe the joys God has prepared for those who follow his or nature's laws for nature is God's creation." (Lust, 1900, 131)

1901 was a remarkable year for Benedict Lust and his journal which was in its 5th year of publication. At age 29 he opened up the first Naturopathic College in New York City. He was riding a wave of confidence as he watched the *Natural Method of Healing* gain popularity locally and regionally. Lust was zealous to educate and inform Americans about natural healing. His journal offered a perfect vehicle to reach American households. In the early years Lust sourced some of his materials from existing authors such as Friedrich Bilz, whose colossal two volume set entitled, *The Natural Healing Method* was a rich reference. Lust relied upon Bilz and his encyclopedic knowledge of natural healing and routinely inserted excerpts from Bilz' work in *The Kneipp Water Cure Monthly.*

Bilz had established through the generosity of a grateful patient several palatial buildings constituting his German sanitarium, located in Dresden-Radebeul. Bilz's success with patients and the knowledge gained from his work, principally using Kneipp water therapies, made him confident that it was only a matter of time before this method would be acknowledged as the only natural and rational healing system. Bilz abided by the sacred "laws of life [and] how to live in order to preserve health." (Bilz, 1901, 131) Health was the ultimate wealth of a person and for the practitioners of natural healing in the early days; their message had an almost religious tone when encouraging their patients to value their health above all. Bilz remarked that people would "adopt a more reasonable and natural regimen, only when it [was] too late, and when they [had] fallen victims to their unnatural mode of life." (Bilz, 1901, 131) Like Just, Bilz believed that fresh air and natural diet were essential to create the conditions of health. Bilz advocated "sleeping with the window open" (Bilz, 1901, 131) ... [and] food and drink also have as great an influence on human health as fresh air." (Bilz, 1901, 131)

On the subject of diet, Bilz also has much to say. Not only is the kind of food eaten important, but also how the food is eaten. He states, "The chief thing is to masticate the food properly." (Bilz, 1901, 132) He reasons that in the process of digestion, "the most important element, the saliva, should be properly mixed with the food" (Bilz, 1901, 132) and secondly the teeth must grind the food until fine so that the stomach can absorb the nutrients. Bilz had a comprehensive understanding of how to live and be healthy. His work permeates the foundations of naturopathic medicine, helping to answer a persistent question attributed to Ludwig Staden in 1902, which surfaced repeatedly not only in conferences and professional gatherings, but also in the Lust journals: *What is Naturopathy?*

As part of the long, intermittent dialogue in response to that question, Staden himself began a definition by proposing two kinds of science: *pure [a priori]* and *empirical [a posteriori]* and then went on to propose that "Naturopathy in its fundamental principles [was] based upon knowledge *a priori* alone, on intuitive power." (Staden, 1902, 15) Staden attributed intuitive knowledge as the catalyst that such giants as Priessnitz, or Schroth, Rausse, Hahn, Rikli, Kneipp, Kuhne and Just sourced in the realization of the art of healing. None of these men was schooled in medicine, yet each left a huge legacy of healing knowledge that persists to this day. Staden was unequivocal that philosophy was vital and that "the soul of all sciences and Naturopathy, with their theoretical and practical tendencies of philosophy, [comprised] the soul of all methods of healing." (Staden, 1902, 15)

In the modern era, this same work has continued. The naturopathic architects of the 1989 definition at Rippling River established *six key principles,* echoing the efforts of Staden and others. Jared Zeff states, "In 1986 the definition project began at the Alderbrook convention of the AANP, the second modern era AANP [American Association of Naturopathic Physicians] conference. At the Rippling River conference in 1989, the culmination of that process was presented and unanimously passed by the AANP House of Delegates." (Zeff, 2013) Almost nine decades earlier Staden had composed *twelve key points* that he considered to be the seminal principles of Naturopathy. Some of these points we still cherish today as our Naturopathic principles, such as "the power of healing is within us. ... Naturopathy attacks always the original cause of every disease." (Staden, 1902, 16-17) In this article, the outcome of suppressive treatments of acute diseases is chronic disease, which was another basis of naturopathic philosophy of treatment, reinforcing this key principle. Staden says, "Suppressed fever diseases cause chronic diseases. Chronic diseases therefore are developed if there is insufficient vitality in the system." (Staden, 1902, 17) These twelve principles are always worth revisiting to glean an understanding of our roots and our history.

The early Naturopaths were keen observers and knew the importance of treating acute diseases with the measure of nature's laws. They also developed guidelines on how to preserve their health through dietary and lifestyle changes. We still hold diet and lifestyle modifications as core elements of naturopathic medicine. Many of the suggestions made 110 years ago are familiar to us today, such as "eat slowly and chew well ... [and] eat the fruits that are in season." (Wallace, 1902, 403) However, Leigh Wallace also emphasizes the importance of going barefoot and giving "your bare body an air or sun bath whenever you can." (Wallace, 1902, 404)

Following the suggestions given by Wallace, Lust wrote a paper to address why Naturopathy was not prospering. In some ways, Lust never missed an opportunity to air his grievances against the "regulars" who "derive their incomes from sick people and consequently are interested in mankind being sick, whereas conditions of universal health would make the profession all but superfluous." (Lust, 1903, 194) In this article, Lust explores some of the differences between allopathic and naturopathic principles by introducing some key principles that guide naturopathic practice. The first concept that Lust broaches is the *unifying cause of diseases* in the form of "foreign matter or contagious matter". (Lust, 1903, 195) The second point made by Lust is the *existence of vital force*. Lust continues, "Taking these two principles, as a basis, Naturopathy, with all its various methods of treatments, has always one end in view and one only: *to increase the vital force.*" (Lust, 1903, 195) The best treatments made "use of the elements of Nature such as light, air, heat, water, diet, recreation, exercise, magnetism, electricity and proper clothing." (Lust, 1903, 195) These elements of nature as healing tools will be repeated by many of these early Naturopaths throughout the articles found in *The Naturopath*. The elements of Nature as factors in health were commended by the Naturopaths as a preventive of disease. Lust reminds us that "the air we breathe is the most essential element to our life; we can live without food for some time, but we cannot live one minute without air." (Lust, 1904, 1)

Lust drew on his vast reading in English and German, and on his growing clinical experience to nourish his editing and writing. Lust was particularly enthralled by Adolf Just's *Return to Nature* because it provided a blueprint for a new way of understanding health and healing by adopting Nature as an ally. The first bound English edition was ready for the public June 1st, 1903 at a cost of $2.00. (Lust, 1903, Ad) Once translated, Lust would display book ads in his advertisement sections of his journals for many years to come. In *Return to Nature* were "simple truths relative to the right living." (Lust, 1903, Ad) Lust implored his readers to "Learn to draw into your own body the inexhaustible spring of youth and life and power which permeates Nature—and soon all will be well in you." (Lust, 1903, Ad)

The core philosophical paradigm of the forefathers of naturopathic medicine, then, was anchored in natural forces of nature as documented so frequently in the early literature. This belief in nature still rings as true today as in 1905 when Lust explained the phenomena of nature in the process of healing and the naturopathic principles entailed in "maintaining health and combating disease by Natural healing factors, such as Water, Light, Air, Massage, Diet, Exercise, Electricity, Hypnotism and Rest." (Lust, 1905, 176) In the article, *The Natural Method of Healing*, Lust outlines the values of each of these naturopathic modalities which were found in F. E. Bilz' book of the same name. The conviction that "physical regeneration is in the air" (Lust, 1905, 176) and that this new system would replace the drug culture of the allopaths was the message. Bilz' wrote "two handsome volumes of 1,000 pages each, 700 illustrations, 19 adjustable colored plates" (Lust, 1905, 177) that sold for a mere $7.50 in 1905.

In the early 1900's, the new adherents to Naturopathy wrote with conviction and purpose. Carl Schultz, a naturopath practicing in Los Angeles, gives an account of the origins of Naturopathy. Schultz outlines the history of the various modalities that were practiced in the context of the Medical Trust's restrictive hold on healthcare in America. He names many of the pioneers of the nature cure movement such as Jahn, Ling, Baltzer, Rausse, Munde, Thure Brandt, Just, and Palmer, who "laid down the foundation of the present 'Naturopathic School'." (Schultz, 1905, 217)

The conflicts with the emerging dominant regulars during the early years helped solidify and strengthen the convictions of the practicing naturopaths. Schultz builds on this revulsion for mercenary physicians by addressing the question of why the Medical Trust so vehemently opposed Naturopathy. He declares, "The Medical Trust opposes Naturopathy because it teaches the people how to keep well; it teaches how to raise healthy children and by this a strong healthy Nation." (Schultz, 1905, 219)

Shultz was a healer/teacher who inspired his patients as well as his colleagues. He wrote, "What a Physician needs is common sense, the gift of observance, love for his fellow men, love for Nature, the gift to understand Nature, and the ability to teach other how to live and to understand the laws of Nature." (Schultz, 1905, 218) The central message of the early Naturopaths always reverted to Nature, and Schultz was no exception. Establishing a foundation for the practice of Naturopathy was summed up succinctly in a very short list of ten life style practices targeting those suffering from tuberculosis but worthwhile for everyone.

Examples included, "avoid breathing impure air [and] walk a great deal, especially in the forests or at the seashore, and climb mountains." (Lust, 1906, 7) Respiratory health began with nasal breathing and this point was reinforced many times throughout the journals. Lust stresses, "Do not breathe through the mouth, but through the nose." (Lust, 1906, 7)

Vital force was a defining element of Naturopathy. Samuel Bloch defines for us the meaning: "*vital force is life*, they are both identical; in fact, the word 'vital' is taken from the Latin word *vita*, meaning "life." (Bloch, 1906, 256) We all know that every cell of our body operates under the influence of our vital force. "Our vital force is expended in the different activities of man's life, for instance upon all physical and mental actions, every sensation, painful or pleasant, involves an expenditure of our vital force." (Bloch, 1906, 256) He says, "the blood and nerves are the vehicles of this vital power, therefore the vitality of any organ is due to the amount and quality of blood supplied to that organ and the condition of the nerves leading to that organ." (Bloch, 1906, 257)

Nature produced foods with the greatest amount of vital force. Manufactured foods were considered devoid of life empowering nutrients and imposed an "impossibility to rebuild and reconstruct healthy cells out of dead material." (Bloch, 1906, 257) Bloch reminds us the importance of the healthy food and healthy blood. He comments, "We all know that the process of adding chemicals to the food destroys the life germ; that is, it destroys that which contains the vital force." (Bloch, 1906, 256-257) In one somewhat long winded statement, Bloch summarizes the food question:

> Health is maintained—as long as the food is of proper quality (that is foods that contain and yield the greatest amount of nutriment); as long as the production from the food is sufficient to counterbalance the expenditure; as long as all the organs perform their functions normally and unconsciously (that is, as long as the foods are properly digested and assimilated and the dead effete material eliminated); and as long as the vital force is not recklessly and criminally squandered by excesses (promiscuous sexual intercourse, alcoholism, late hours, etc.). (Bloch, 1906, 257)

Nature's role in health was undeniable for Naturopaths. For those practicing Nature Cure, its motto, "Nature alone is the true and lasting healer" (Lust, 1907, 68) was loud and clear. Nature's remedies were simple: "Air, light, exercise (gymnastics, massage), the right nourishment, dry and humid warmth in the way of water, steam and hot air baths, packs, compresses, douches." (Lust, 1907, 69) "Therapeutic medical treatment which is based on Nature or on self-power; a treatment that supports, vitalizes and leads to regeneration and health is the method of nature cure." (Lust, 1907, 69)   These healing methods sometimes had their limitations, but were often the last resort for patients. As Lust put it, "The impossible can never be expected, and conditions of sickness which have taken many years for their development, cannot be cured in a trice." (Lust, 1907, 69)

Nature Curists believed strongly in the power of nature. Lust exclaims, "As long as there is one spark of life left, and the nature physician masters his art, the patient may be restored to health, even then, when all other methods have failed." (Lust, 1907, 69)   While the nature cure treatment was "sure, thorough and without any secondary disease," (Lust, 1907, 70) that was not the case with drug therapies. "Most drugs, extracted from poisonous plants, would injure healthy bodies and are therefore not fit to cure sick people." (Lust, 1907, 69)   Lust continues in this vein, addressing drug therapies, "Drugs can never cure a disease; but may cause a new one." (Lust, 1907, 69) Drugs often left behind more symptoms and new diseases causing Naturopaths to question the integrity of a profession profiting from the distribution of poisonous substances.

The ethics of altruistic medicine were formulated from the beginnings of Naturopathy. Schultz elaborates, "A man who becomes a Physician must be a man of high moral character, a man with sympathy for suffering humanity. . . . A man who enters the profession of healing for the sake of making money will never become a good Physician." (Schultz, 1905, 218) Erieg reiterates this point in his article, *Doctors and their Exorbitant Fees.* (Erieg, 1908, 14) It was very clear to the Naturopaths that the Allopaths were charging excessive prices for their services. "The doctors for a five-minute call, and for even less time, take what most men work a whole day for, so it is seen that the poor man has burdens enough without doctors placing additional ones on his back." (Erieg, 1908. 15)

In this professional duel, drugs were definite tangibles and nature as a healing force was ephemeral and harder to define. However, Dr. C. S. Carr makes a good effort in describing nature's role in the healing process. In the first place, he writes, "what we call symptoms of disease are simply nature's efforts to restore the body to a normal condition." (Carr, 1908, 180) Carr insisted that the doctor's role was not to resist the efforts of nature, but to recognize "the high temperature and quick pulse [as] nature's struggles to rid herself of disease. To weaken these struggles is to join the disease in overcoming nature." (Carr, 1908. 180) Carr and others were clear about the need to join together with this key message.

One such zealous Naturopath, C. M. Corbin, was effusive in his enthusiasm to rally the profession. "In union there is strength" he wrote, adding, "and this old quotation can never be used to better purpose than right now in the Naturopathic movement of America." (Corbin, 1909,

769) He dared to raise his voice so others would join together "to the teaching of the great truths of Naturopathy which is to my mind the grandest work under the sun." (Corbin, 1909, 769) He throws down the gauntlet to his colleagues, challenging them with the questions, "I, for one, am going to push a little harder. Are you? I, for one, am going to live a little closer to nature's divine laws. Will you? I, for one, am willing to make greater sacrifices to my pride of personal individuality that the great whole may stand with an unbroken front which shall be as solid as 'The Rock of Gibraltar'. Are you?" (Corbin, 1909, 769)

The early Naturopaths shaped their understandings of nature for others in the profession to facilitate successful clinical practice. One such man was Henry Lindlahr who also viewed self-control as important along with a return to nature, conserving vital force, and the use of "pure foods, judicious fasting, hydrotherapy, osteopathy, massage, exercise, physical culture, light and air bath, homeopathy and simple herb remedies" (Lindlahr, 1910, 31) for the purpose of facilitating elimination of morbid matter. Lindlahr worked tirelessly to define "as precisely as possible certain words and phrases which convey meanings and ideas peculiar to our philosophy." (Lindlahr, 1910, 32) He advised "the student of Nature Cure and kindred subjects . . . to study closely these definitions and formulated principles, since they contain the pith and marrow of our philosophy and greatly facilitate its understanding." (Lindlahr, 1910, 33) Today, we can learn much from Lindlahr and his theories of chronic disease, healing crisis and nature cure principles. He, in fact, laid down the foundations of modern Naturopathic medicine with his five elements of Nature Cure: "Return to Nature . . . Elementary Medicine ... Mechanical Medicine . . . Suggestive Medicine . . . Chemical Medicine." (Lindlahr, 1910, 35) Nature cure in terms of terminology and practice had had a strong foundation in the clinical and written work of Adolf Just, but Lindlahr refined and enhanced the concepts of nature as healer.

Whereas Lindlahr in Chicago established a Nature Cure school and large clinic in Chicago, a rapidly expanding, American, urban environment, Adolf Just was taking his patients back into the forests and nature of Germany. Just explains, "In the Yungborn ... the patient [is] carried away from all the wrongs of the world and rests now in a light- and air-house, entirely in the lap of nature where balmy airs blow and the trees of the forest rustle, or who pitches his bed entirely under the open sky where his eyes are turned to the stars in fair weather." (Just, 1910, 713) Just does not understate the almost secretive, but remarkably ubiquitous power of earth medicine. He comments, "It is often surprising what great results can be had by the forceful remedies of nature, water, air, light and natural nutrition, but nothing can so much cause our admiration than the earth in its healing power." (Just, 1910, 713-714)

This understanding of the sacredness of Nature was certainly not overlooked by the early Naturopaths. The destruction of the forests was already an environmental concern and Just raised the alarm prophetically and presciently. Just states, "Man has attacked nature the most by destroying and cutting down the woods; he has caused by it conditions, and especially dangerous climatic and aerial changes, which are to-day very detrimental to man and to beast." (Just, 1910, 716) The wonders of the forests and the healing power of earth, water, fire and air were very precious to Adolf Just and the early Naturopaths.

Even as these elements and facets of naturopathic medicine evolved, there was a common thread that held the fabric of naturopathy together. It was the strong belief that there was "really but one cause of physical disease, and that [was] the 'violation of the natural laws of our being'." (Buell, 1910, 454) In his *Social Health and Personal Health*, C. Buell addresses the practices of medical doctors naming "symptoms and trying to find ways of suppressing them" (Buell, 1910, 454), while not addressing the true causes of disease. Buell, as president of the Minnesota Health League, was concerned about the failures to identify the true causes of illness especially in the social sphere. He cited manifestations of social disease as "lack of employment for willing workers ... sky-scraping tenements ... labor unions and strikes for the workers, etc. The hardships faced by people working in difficult jobs." (Buell, 1910, 455) Buell was impassioned about addressing the social injustices and writes, "Unjust laws lie at the bottom of all social disorder ... [and] creating and maintaining unequal opportunities among men constitute the only real social disease." (Buell, 1910, 455)

Buell offers an exit to these social evils and that is to give people a chance to "return to nature and live a free, pure, healthy, natural life." (Buell, 1910, 456) He contends that most of the social evils are man-made and need to be discarded so that Nature will then cure the social disease very quickly. He emphasizes, "Each man, woman and child has just as much right to be in the world as any other man, woman or child; and that the bounties of Nature the air, the sunshine, the water, the soil ... are as much for one as for another." (Buell, 1910, 456) Lust and his colleagues concurred. For example, Lust himself had embodied in the 'Yungborn' health resorts accessibility to Nature and Nature Cure for all.

Many Naturopaths established these health resorts in remote areas where all of the elements of Nature Cure could be practiced. In the 1911 article, *J. Austin Shaw Explains Yungborn Nature Cure,* Shaw describes his visit to Benedict Lust's Yungborn located in the Ramapo Mountains near Butler, New Jersey. The 'Yungborn' was the name of a health resort or sanitarium first named and established by Adolf Just. At the Yungborn, visitors would participate in sun baths, air baths, nature walks and live in 'Air cottages' and eat nutritious vegetarian fare. Shaw outlines with a flourish, such daily activities during his stay at Lust's Yungborn.

Another vocal advocate of Nature Cure was an MD who lived in an urban environment of Buffalo, New York. John W. Hodge was a fearless, tireless and notable spokesman against compulsory vaccinations. In his 1911 article, *Preventative Medicine*, Hodge recounts the superstitious beliefs of disease that existed in the past. At one time, "Doctors in those days declared: 'Cold water in fever is certain death.' 'Do not give the patient a drop.' 'Give a dose of calomel and a teaspoonful of warm water.'" (Hodge, 1911, 712) Hodge, like his Germanic colleagues, excelled at long, convoluted sentences, an example of which follows here in which he describes the progression of hygienic practices:

> Owing largely to the advances made in hygiene and in sanitary science, and to the discovery and application of the homeopathic law of cure with its mild medicines, single remedy, small dose, and brilliant results, the harsh and drastic modes of treatment which were common half a century ago, have been dropped one after another by the profession until now the instinctive calls of nature are being more and more heeded by the medical practitioner, and the profession as a whole is daily approximating nearer and nearer to the constructive art of healing which takes more cognizance of sanitation and hygienic living, and far less account of poisonous drugs. Calomel and bloodletting have had their day. (Hodge, 1911, 712)

Hodge continues with this theme of preventative medicine: "Prevention is far more logical than cure in the philosophy of medicine. . . . It is apparent to the scientific hygienist that preventive medicine is destined to become the medicine of the enlightened future." (Hodge, 1911, 713) Today, as allopathic medicine finally embraces this notion, MDs are now accepting and monetizing preventative medicine, although often expressed in elaborate webs of laboratory testing and invasive procedures to prevent disease. Ironically this branding or preventative medical practice has come to be known as 'Integrative Medicine'.

One of the branches of this recent Integrative Medicine framework is Environmental Medicine. One of the first mentions of environmental mismanagement in any medical system was raised by Hodge decades before biomedicine took up the torch. In his district, Niagara Falls, the population experienced "hundreds of deaths from typhoid fever" (Hodge, 1911, 714) which he correlated to the sewage and pollution entering the Niagara River. He was quick to offer a reason, "The corner stone of modern society is self-interest and in its service we do not identify our neighbor's with our own, but rather sacrifice our neighbor's life that our own selfish interests may the better thrive." (Hodge, 1911, 714)

While Hodge was outraged by careless activities producing unnecessary pollution of the Niagara River, A. A. Erz was fuming over the working conditions of those who labored in match factories. "The poor victims are the scantily paid, ignorant tools of the greedy instigators of this unhuman [sic] industry, resulting in a most cruel affliction known as 'phossy jaw' or phosphorous necrosis of the jaw bone. . . . The insidious poison finally attacks the teeth and gums, gradually afflicting the covering of the jawbone, inevitably inducing a process of slow decay in the bone itself." (Erz, 1912, 423) The disfigurement and painful symptoms of phosphorous necrosis and "all the terrible physical and mental suffering implied in the production of white phosphorous—tipped matches is a needless horror. . . . The United States is the only important civilized country where this barbaric industry still prevails to the extent that some 4,000 match workers must ever be exposed." (Erz, 1912, 424) Currently, Naturopaths are bringing to the attention of their patients and communities the dangers of environmental toxins and body burden. Erz, in this article written over a century ago, was on the forefront of raising consciousness around environmental medicine and questioned the role and integrity of public Health Boards and their inspectors who did nothing to alleviate the suffering of the workers. Erz appeals to his colleagues, "Stop using any poisonous white phosphorous matches, known as 'palor' or 'lucifer' matches and get all your friends to join the protest and the boycott." (Erz, 1912, 425)

Just as these magnificent pioneers called attention to environmental degradation, so too they worked to understand the disease process and these efforts quickly espoused many theories on health and disease. The fascination with bacteriology was in finding new bugs, but Arnold Ehret focused on diet, as a quite different cause for disease: eating the wrong and unnatural foods and over eating. Ehret, the author of *The Mucusless Diet*, shares his notion that people get sick "as soon as the introduction of mucus by means of 'artificial food', fat meat, bread, potatoes, farinaceous products, rice, milk, etc." (Ehret, 1912, 167) He explains, "First of all I maintain in all diseases without exception there exists a tendency by the organism to secrete mucus and in the case of a more advanced stage—pus (decomposed blood)." (Ehret, 1912, 167) The 'mucusless diet' has found its place in Naturopathy ever since in that we are quite familiar with which foods constitutes mucus forming ones. Ehret followed a fruit based diet excluding all mucus forming foods and "attained a degree of health which is simply not imaginable nowadays." (Ehret, 1912, 168) In his opinion, fruit was the only food that was truly mucusless and "everything prepared by man or supposedly improved by him is evil." (Ehret, 1912, 169)

Ehret's contributions to Naturopathic dietary knowledge have had enduring appeal. Another less familiar Naturopath, Helen Sayr Gray, lived in Portland, Oregon. She wrote with wit and intelligence and published a derisive booklet, *In Justice to Thomas and Tabby*, in which she exposed the medical superstitions of the 20th century. Two MD's, CB Reed and W McClure, found 'dangerous germs' on cat's whiskers and urged, "the extermination of cats as a menace to health." (Gray, 1912, 501) Her argument was simple: "Germs are everywhere. Why should cats' whiskers be an exception to the rule? If Thomas and Tabby could retaliate and examine doctors' whiskers, doubtless as many—or more—virulent varieties of germs would be found nestling there. [Doctor's beards] harbor not merely four deadly varieties, but 47. Doctors are a menace to public health, for they disseminate germs quite as much as do cats." (Gray, 1912, 502) Her satirical solution: Therefore, exterminate the doctors." (Gray, 1912, 502)

Gray had strong opinions about germ theory. She comments, "The belief of the medical profession that contagion and infection pass from one human being to another—from a sick man to a healthy man—is an old superstition unworthy of this age. Disease will not go from person to person, unless they are in physical condition that renders them susceptible." (Gray, 1912, 505) Gray voiced the differing point of view between the Allopaths who gripped tightly to the germ theory and the Naturopaths advocated that germs could not thrive in healthy conditions. Gray insisted that "so-called contagious and infectious diseases are self-limited. If it were not for this self-limitation, the world would be depopulated every time an epidemic of a severe character succeeds in getting a start." (Gray, 1912, 505)

Not only did the early Naturopaths not join their Allopathic counterpart's intractable belief in germs, but they also did not share their scientific viewpoints in the realm of psychology. In fact, unlike the Allopaths, the Naturopaths firmly believed that "psychology ought, more than any other subject, be studied by all physicians, since without its knowledge their practice degenerates into mere guess-work and chance-intuitions." (Erz, 1913, 81) Erz reasoned, "Medicine is lacking the knowledge of the true science of life which explains the nature and measure of life, and what is beneficial to it and what injurious. In Erz' view, life was the union of body, mind and soul" (Erz, 1913, 82) and formed the basis of "health [which] is but the result of perfect co-relation of the physical, mental and spiritual forces." (Erz, 1913, 85) The early naturopaths believed strongly that "without the higher knowledge of the constitution of man in his triune nature, modern science was yet groping in the dark." (Erz, 1913, 82)

In this regard, the Naturopaths of this early period stood firmly on their beliefs that body mind medicine had validity. Unquestionably, they observed, "emotions of fear, worry, anger greatly interfere with the serous secretions, and produce chemical changes of a deleterious character, impairing other functions." (Erz, 1913, 84) The 'regulars' were quick to discredit the body mind component of health as "a mere humbug and [to] call any drugless healing system an outright fraud; while today, medicine tries to adopt the very same ideas and names of the once tabooed methods."

This story sounds familiar to the contemporary naturopathic physician, in a healthcare landscape where the Integrative Medical movement assimilates everything in its path. Erz saw the 'regulars' as incapable of becoming drugless practitioners. From his perspective, they were "utterly unfit to comprehend any system of natural healing, and [were] hardly ever capable of practicing anything else in the line of healing methods, but medicine." Erz continues, "[the 'regular'] will usually make a very poor drugless healer, as no matter how hard he may try to unlearn the ingrained habit of drugging people, and of looking at disease from the materialistic medical standpoint." (Erz, 1913, 83) Even after one hundred years, these sentiments still stand.

An important principle throughout these debates and one that has guided naturopathic practice has been to address the cause of disease. In the article, *Remove the Cause*, Fred Kaessmann counsels his fellow colleagues, "Before you try to remove the symptoms, REMOVE THE CAUSE." (Kaessmann, 1913, 159) Naturopaths recognized that the temptation to give patients temporary symptomatic relief without treating the cause meant not taking the time "to learn WHY they were sick." (Kaessmann, 1913, 158) Kaessmann encouraged his colleagues to "be sure to point out to the patient the reason for his ailment—and also be sure to explain what it may lead to—AND WHY." (Kaessmann, 1913, 159)

In fact, there is some basis in recognizing that Kaessman's therapeutic model of *treat the cause* contributed to a core principle of contemporary Naturopathic medicine. In the following article, *Symptomatic Treatment a Waste of Effort and Time*, Carl Strueh adds another familiar principle that Naturopaths hold dear to their heart, the *vis medicatrix naturae*. Strueh presents his own words of counsel:

> We can suppress most any symptom by means of a remedy, we can produce sleep in a person suffering from chronic insomnia by a dose of veronal, we can cause an evacuation of the bowels in chronic constipation by a laxative, . . . we can quiet a neurasthenic by means of a sedative, we can lessen the frequency of convulsions in an epileptic by administering bromides, we can relieve chronic headaches by a dose of aspirin. But we do not cure in this manner. (Strueh, 1913, 170)

Strueh admonished his colleagues to abstain from symptomatic treatment and instead "to go to the root of the evil". He continues, "Disease is not ordained by providence but is the logical result of our irrational way of living." (Strueh, 1913, 170) Early and contemporary Naturopaths would both add that a spoon of medicine could hardly eradicate our lifestyle follies. Strueh and his contemporaries understood well the "*Vis medicatrix naturae*, i.e., the inborn natural healing power which exists in every living body: it is the power which in health as well as sickness, directs the action of every organ and cell of the body." (Strueh, 1913, 170) Strueh closes his article by emphasizing the importance of individualized treatments which "conform with the condition of each individual patient, [for this] is the art of the physician." (Strueh, 1913, 171)

In the following year, 1914, the New York Society of Naturopathy wrote a brief in their pursuit of regulation. Carl Strueh submitted Brief 7 in an attempt to define Naturopathy and this he did by introducing the naturopathic concepts of 'vital force' and '*vis medicatrix naturae*'. It may have been a bit presumptuous for him to start with a bold attack on all other medical methods; he does state his position on the virtues of nature healing opposed to drugs. "The vigor of the patient's vitality being the deciding factor in the cure of disease, it follows that any kind of treatment having a healthful, invigorating influence, will improve the chances of recovery, while any sort of treatment which is apt to diminish the patient's vitality, will naturally accomplish the contrary." (Strueh, 1914, 254) Strueh does not mince words and declares openly, "For this reason the superiority of Naturopathy over the drug-method is undisputable." (Strueh, 1914, 254)

In this article, Strueh explores the limits and benefits of drugs. It is quite easy to see how the Naturopathic profession at the time struggled to find its place in a world that was inexorably changing. Drugs were inching forward quickly and making treatment easy with a pill for each disease. However, "the physician practicing Naturopathy must be well able to individualize, i. e., apply the treatment according to the conditions existing in every individual case." (Strueh, 1914, 257) Strueh reminds us once again, "We must not treat sicknesses, but sick people." (Strueh, 1914, 257)

Naturopaths early in their professional formation held high ideals and espoused a strong ethical framework for the profession that they were building. For example, in June, 1913, Benedict Lust began the discussion of medical ethics. In *Principles of Ethics*, Lust adopted a draft acquired from the International Alliance of Physicians and Surgeons of a code of ethical principles for his Naturopathic colleagues to consider. Implementing ethical standards within the Naturopathic profession was, in his view, a very high priority. In this article, the duties of physicians to their patients and to other professionals were outlined. The notion of patient confidentiality, a key ethical dimension for a healing profession, was addressed early in Naturopathy. Lust wrote, "The obligation of secrecy extends beyond the period of professional services." (Lust, 1913, 377) As well, professional services were discussed. "Physicians should not, as a general rule, undertake the treatment of themselves nor of members of their families."

While the Naturopathic profession was expanding the discussion of Medical Ethics, Edward Earle Purinton was seeking a definition for 'Nature Cure' itself. He wrote a contentious article, *Efficiency in Drugless Healing, Standardizing the Nature Cure* in March, 1915. In his survey of Nature Cure, he could not find two doctors who would agree on what it was. The plethora of dietary plans and schools made it impossible to determine how diets and food could cure when each system contradicted another. "The editor of this magazine believes in sane fasting, in thorough mastication, in wholly natural foods. The editor of another health journal ... maintains we do not eat enough, calls Fletcherism rank folly, and declares white flour bread a much better food than whole wheat! Now where is the truth?" (Purinton, 1915, 143)

Purinton asks, "Does Nature Cure properly include osteopathy, or chiropractic, or mechano-therapy, or none of them?" (Purinton, 1915, 143) To Purinton, the practice and diagnostic methods of the Nature Cure practitioners were eclectic and "wild and irrational". (Purinton, 1915, 146) Purinton was astute enough to realize that the Naturopathic movement needed to professionalize itself in order to be taken seriously. His counsel to the emerging Naturopathic profession was as follows:

> Nothing can be legalized that has not been standardized. Hence, the first step for drugless physicians to take is to decide among themselves what the Nature Cure is and what it is not, why it deserves legal recognition, and how its practice should be safely regulated. (Purinton, 1915, 147)

In a rebuttal letter to the profession, William Freeman Havard attempted to answer the questions raised by Purinton. Havard pointed out that when the various medical systems are surveyed, what was fairly accurate and certain is the agreement that the knowledge of the clinical sciences such as anatomy, physiology, pathology are undisputable and that "granting an accurate diagnosis, failure is due entirely to the misapplication of therapeutic measures." (Havard, 1915, 211)

Havard also wades into the rhetorical questions of "what is disease and what is a symptom?" (Havard, 1915, 212) In answering these questions, he outlines his theories of balance between positive and negative in terms of health and disease and absorption and elimination. His definition of Nature Cure is simply, "the employment of every method which is in accord with the natural physiological action of the body in order to bring about the complete elimination of disease." (Havard, 1915, 212) Later in the same article he explains how to do Nature Cure so that the doctor can "increase the patient's power of resistance, increase elimination by opening up all channels designed to carry off waste products, increase oxygenation and circulation of the blood, prescribe mainly eliminating foods and give the body its required rest." (Havard, 1915, 213)

Havard reacted to Purinton's view that Nature Cure's undeserving approval by the lawmakers was "premature, and has failed simply as all things premature and rash deserve to fail." (Purinton, 1915, 147) Rather than seek sanctions from government for medical practices, he felt that individual doctors need to take full responsibility for their actions. Havard argued, "Legalizing a profession shifts nine tenths of the responsibility upon the State and absolves the individual from risk. The Physician feels at liberty to experiment upon his patients knowing that even in the event of the patient's death he will not be held in the slightest degree responsible." (Havard, 1915, 212)

Havard opposed Purinton's ideas that Nature Cure was "wild and [involved] irrational conflict of theory." (Purinton, 1915, 146) In fact, he embraced the diversity of natural therapeutics as long as there were "some law and principle to guide the healing of disease." (Havard, 1915, 253) He was sure that eclecticism in drugless therapy would adhere to common principles. He contends, "As the body follows laws of operation in health and as disease is caused by the reaction of these laws, so there must be some law and principle to guide the healing of disease." The tendency to create systems to categorize disease resulted in what we call today 'cookbook therapy'. Havard felt that lumping everyone into systems ignored "the fact that no two individuals are alike in all respects [and that it] had been overlooked in the construction of 'systems'." (Havard, 1915, 253) He continues, "Medicine has always treated the disease, never the patient." (Havard, 1915, 253) By respecting the law that no two individuals are alike, "Eclecticism teaches us to know all and to use judgments and reason in selecting that which will be most effective in producing the best results in any individual case." (Havard, 1915, 253)

Purinton's article raised some commentary from Havard and soon Lust followed with his own responses. Lust was dismayed by Purinton's uninformed comments and wrote an open letter to The Naturopath readership. Lust states, "You have not yet the inside consciousness and are not familiar with the therapeutic possibilities of drugless methods, therefore you are no judge to give a final comparison of the two systems, Naturopathic and Medical." (Lust, 1915, 538) Purinton was viewed by other Naturopaths as not living up to Naturopathic principles. Lust continues, "Dr. Carl Schultz, Dr. Lindlahr, Dr. Strueh, and others have expressed themselves in recent letters to me that in your efficiency articles you are not bringing out strongly enough the Naturopathic Physician's superior methods, intuitive powers, unselfishness and love for the sick." (Lust, 1915, 538) Lust's disappointment with Purinton did not end in banishment from further publications but did set the record straight for his position.

While Lust raises the preeminence of Naturopathic therapeutics, Howard Tunison points out the versatility of naturopathic care without the reliance upon patent drugs. "Qualified Naturopaths, however, do not place exclusive reliance upon any one natural healing branch. They are eclectic (liberal and selective) in their choice of drugless methods of treatment." (Tunison, 1916, 372) Tunison, like many of his colleagues believed that drugs were not essential in the treatments of acute and chronic diseases that Naturopaths faced.

Exploring the nature of disease and drugless therapy, Tunison presents his definitions of what disease is and how to restore health. The quality of blood determined health and disease. He says, "Good health can be restored by eliminating or getting rid of blood waste material; by improving assimilation and by supplying natural wholesome nourishment." (Tunison, 1916, 372) Tunison continues on the topic of bad blood, "An unhealthy mortal … who is on the verge of being 'sick,' has a blood-stream which is very much befouled with waste or 'garbage'." (Tunison, 1916, 373-374) He provides a comprehensive list of drugless healing systems which can aid in restoring health and supporting the *Vis*.

The early Naturopaths knew that the *Vis* was vital for the healing process, and that this principle of 'life force' extended to the environment in which the body lived. For this reason the early Naturopaths saw much vulnerability to health, for example, with the use of chemicals to clean up or "purify the lake water … by the use of alum, chlorine, and other poisonous chemicals." (Muckley, 1917, 335) Ferdinand Muckley's 1917 article is significant in that it is one of the earliest Naturopathic accounts of environmental toxicity related to health outcomes. Our notion that Environmental Medicine is a contemporary phenomenon is quite erroneous. Muckley's observation was that these toxic chemicals introduced into a public water system elicited "catarrhal condition of the mucous membrane [and] in men, acute and chronic stomach and bowel troubles prevail, while in women, goiter and other throat gland troubles predominate, even girls of ten being subject to these afflictions." (Muckley, 1917, 335) Also of note is that cancer was associated with the symptoms of related stomach and bowel troubles. "The stomach and bowel troubles that affect the male residents of the Lake Erie region are so severe that every tenth individual dies from cancer of the stomach, bowels, or rectum." (Muckley, 1917, 335)

The interests of Naturopaths were not limited to the physical factors promoting health but, as referenced earlier in the work of White (1909) and Gulick (1909), also included mental health.

Another bedrock of the Naturopathic medical system evolved when emotions and mental development were included within the naturopathic definition of health. In the 21st century, we face the claws of stress daily; a century ago, stress would show up as "mental depression [or] grief, anxiety, discontent, remorse, guilt, distrust [which] all tend to break down the life forces, and invite decay and death." (White, 1909, 697) The importance of sound mind and spirit was included in the naturopathic dialogue about health. Dr. Gulick expresses the significance of thoughts and health, "We are just beginning to understand the part that good thinking holds in good health. Our thoughts are just as real part of us as are our bodies." (Gulick, 1909, 697)

Edward Earle Purinton was well versed in mental culture and wrote prolifically on the subject. He contributes an article on *Affirmations* that he defines as "a mental exercise which, when sufficiently repeated, strengthens the good, and crowds out the injurious thoughts." (Purinton, 1918, 33) He provides several examples of affirmations, such as, "I am growing each day in health, strength and power." (Purinton, 1918, 33) Another Mental Culturist who was prolific and considerably successful in delivering her message of mental science was Helen Wilmans. Benedict Lust had created space for a column, *Home Course in Mental Science* and published each month a lesson from Wilman's work. Lust was excited about this inclusion in *Herald of Health and Naturopath*. With his exuberance, he announces, "We take pleasure in announcing that we have secured the rights to publish the Twenty Lesson Course in Mental Science by the founder of Mental Science, the late Helen Wilmans, of Seabreeze, Fla." (Lust, 1918, 168) In lesson one, Wilmans presents her philosophy of unlimited 'Life Principle'. In her explanations of the esoteric realms of omnipresence, and the Life Principle, she states, "We are manifestations of the unchanging Life Principle; of the Universal Spirit of Being; the inextinguishable I AM." (Wilmans, 1918, 170) The article explores her perceptions of the laws of attraction and the universal laws that were the basis of Mental Science.

Louis Kuhne was another early Naturopath who contributed immensely to early naturopathic concepts and philosophy, most particularly concerning the cause of disease and morbid matter. Benedict Lust published frequently excerpts from Kuhne's *The New Science of Healing* (first published in 1891) which mirrored the philosophical viewpoints of the emerging American Naturopathic profession. In fact, Lust had translated and re-published Kuhne's book and renamed the book, *Neo-*

Naturopathy, The New Science of Healing in 1917. The significance of Kuhne's scientific findings is that he was the first to recognize the unity of all diseases and made the conclusion that there is only one cause of disease and also only one disease with many different manifestations, depending which organ is affected. According to Kuhne, the cause of disease "can be traced back to encumbrance of the system with foreign matter [morbid matter]." (Kuhne, 1917, 337)

Kuhne states, "All the various forms of disease are, as we have seen, only efforts of the body to recover health." (Kuhne, 1917, 337) He cautioned against using suppressive treatments that the orthodox medical doctors practice. "Disease if repressed or rendered latent, leads slowly but surely to severe and wholly incurable conditions of health." (Kuhne, 1917, 337) These words of Kuhne bring to mind the message of many of the early Naturopaths and in particular, Henry Lindlahr.

Kuhne's premise that "there is no disease without fever, and no fever without disease" (Kuhne, 1917, 354) is the correlate to why people have cold extremities and hot heads. Hot head and fever are not hard to comprehend, but cold extremities do not make sense one may contend. Yet, Kuhne explains that the head fever has the same origins as cold feet. He continues, "Fever [or] fermentation this [morbid] matter is transported from the abdomen into the remotest parts of the body. Some is deposited in these remote points, that is, in the head, feet and hands." (Kuhne, 1917, 355) Lindlahr followed in the footsteps of Kuhne and based his own theories of nature cure and the unity of disease upon the work of Kuhne. In the writings of Kuhne, we can recognize many of Lindlahr's core concepts which Lindlahr used as a basis of his publications and teachings.

Lindlahr concurs with Kuhne's theory that the accumulation of morbid matter in the body "endanger[s] health and life, then the organism reacts to these disease conditions through acute healing efforts in the form of inflammation and fever." (Lindlahr, 1918, 123) The fever was pivotal in the recognition and cure of both acute and chronic diseases. Lindlahr explains the need to not suppress the fever. He continues,

> These inflammatory processes, if properly treated and assisted, are therefore always constructive, that is, purifying and healing of nature, always run their course through the same five stages of inflammation, and if allowed to do so, always result in effecting better conditions; that is, they leave the system purer and more normal than before they started their salutary work of house-cleaning. (Lindlahr, 1918, 123)

Lindlahr proudly declared that "the unity of disease and cure, as taught in Nature Cure Philosophy with the greatest possible efficiency in the treatment of all acute disease, is undoubtedly the most valuable contribution of Nature Cure to medical science." (Lindlahr, 1918, 123) While acute symptoms were suppressed by the Allopaths, driving the poisons deeper into the body, Lindlahr counters with:

> Nature Cure, on the other hand, through natural methods of living . . . builds up the blood, purifies the system, adjusts the mechanical lesions, harmonizes the mental and emotional conditions so that the organism can once more arouse itself to a cleansing, healing effort in the various forms of acute elimination. (Lindlahr, 1918, 126)

The question that Lindlahr poses was top of mind for these early naturopathic professionals. He asks, "Is it not clear that the very 'treatment' of the symptoms makes the cure an impossibility?" (Lindlahr, 1918, 126) The suppression resulting from symptomatic treatments was obviously to the Naturopaths, not the answer to health. In an editorial, Havard continues in the same vain, arguing, "Acute diseases, such as typhoid, smallpox and the host of other healing crises, are but the outbreak of accumulations of morbid matter." (Havard, 1918, 419)

The polarity between Allopaths and Naturopaths was accentuated by their unique stance on what accounts for disease; on one side: germs and vaccinations, and on the other morbid matter and improved sanitation. "Medicine persists in looking upon every disease manifestation as a separate entity in itself, and with their germ mania rampant at present, they turn a dead eye on basic causes." (Havard, 1918, 419) The importance of changing the internal conditions to support health varied greatly with medicine's concern "only with the counteraction of symptoms and the suppression of nature's curative efforts. Cure is entirely different process from counteraction." (Havard, 1918, 420)

Wigelsworth weighed in on this medical debate by eloquently presenting the gist of what acute diseases really are. He pronounced, "All acute diseases are eliminating crises." (Wigelsworth, 1918, 731) His explanation did not differ from his colleagues. In his view, acute diseases do not occur without a cause but come on "to cleanse a body laden with morbid matter accumulated through changes in structure which interfere with functional activities, wrong living, inherited tendencies, or any one of a dozen or two other causes." (Wigelsworth, 1918, 731-732) Wigelsworth is only repeating what many other writers in the *Naturopath and Herald of Health* had been saying. In summing up acute and chronic disease, he wrote, "acute disease is a beneficial thing when correctly treated, for it is an effort on the part of Nature to throw off that which goes to cause chronic disease. It's the 'Safety Valve'." (Wigelsworth, 1918, 732) Like Havard and others, Wigelsworth was clear on how to treat chronic disease. "Chronic disease must be treated to bring it to an active eliminating stage, or it can never be cured." (Wigelsworth, 1918, 732)

At the 22nd Annual Convention of the American Naturopathic Association, held on June 6-8, 1918 at Hotel Winton, Cleveland, Ohio, Havard addressed the topic of rational healing and continued this discussion of acute and chronic diseases. Havard was trained in mechano-neural therapy or neuropathy and found that when he employed these effective tools he discovered that "inevitably the [patient] who was being treated for some chronic condition would develop in the course of his treatment an acute condition." (Havard, 1919, 272) Havard shared Wigelsworth's conclusion but also he found his training as a neuropath inadequate and delved into other medical systems, but still he was "thoroughly discouraged and disheartened." (Havard, 1919, 272)

After much study, he "came to the conclusion there were definite laws regarding the health or the normal operation of the body, and I came to conclusion there must be definite laws regarding the unnatural operation of the body or the operation which took place during the process of disease." (Havard, 1919, 273) With these convictions coupled with two chance encounters (one, the reading of Kuhne's *New Science of Healing* and second, meeting with Dr Henry Lindlahr) Havard saw the answers laid out before him. He asserts, "I could now explain scientifically, in accordance with our knowledge of anatomy, physiology and pathology every step in the process of disease and every step that is necessary to be taken towards the cure of disease." (Havard, 1919, 273)

Havard points out that practitioners of physiological therapeutics combine all of the physical methods of therapy used in Nature Cure and proceed to treat the symptoms. "While the nature curist has a plan in mind, and he employs these various methods of treatment with the idea of producing two effects . . . he [then] leaves the rest to nature." (Havard, 1919, 273) He reinforces the importance of letting nature do her work. Havard explains, "The best thing you can do in your treatment of any acute disease is first to get rid of the idea of trying to counteract symptoms and nurse the case." (Havard, 1919, 427) The first element of rational treatment in his view was "to produce greater elimination . . . [and] raising the individual's power of resistance to a point of establishing a reaction." (Havard, 1919, 273-274)

The germ theory, which was dictating the medical paradigm of the early and even current Allopaths, reinforced the creation of pharmaceutical centered treatments. The use of drugs to establish health countered everything that Naturopaths believed in. Havard and others knew that if the body was strong and the *vis medicatrix* was strong, disease would not prevail. If the system of medicine was so advanced, Havard insisted, why were so many people suffering? Nelson, another Naturopath from Hartford, Connecticut, who like Havard questioned the validity and wisdom of serum therapy, writes,

> We can readily grasp the reason why practically all of the research work conducted in medical circles today is concentrated on the discovery and production of serums or antitoxins that will kill off these germs, and, as shown during the recent influenza epidemic, they have succeeded in this respect so remarkably well, that not only the lives of the germs, but in many instances also the lives of the patients were taken." (Nelson, 1920, 79)

Knowing the nature of health and disease was core to the Naturopathic philosophy. Nelson comments, "Acute diseases are simply Nature's way of expelling poisonous waste matter from the system, and [because] chronic diseases are caused by the sealing up in the body of these same substances, it is easily reasoned out that elimination" (Nelson, 1920, 80) must be essential to treatment. Nelson contends that Naturopaths supported Nature and its effects to eliminate these waste materials but also that "the Naturopath goes even further than to merely cure disease. Knowing that transgression of Nature's Laws lies at the root of all human ills, he also considers it his duty to teach humanity how to follow these laws." (Nelson, 1920, 80)

Naturopathic trust in the *Vis* came also in the form of Mind Medicine in the sense that "the Mind **can** and **does** heal all diseases." (Dickenson, 1920, 140) The power of thought in the realm of disease is not foreign even today. We can accept that our minds can influence our body and much research in orthodox medicine currently has validated this. "Constructive, harmonious, optimistic thinking strengthens the heart, stomach and other organs, makes the blood circulate more freely, helps in assimilation and excretion and makes the body young and supple." (Dickenson, 1920, 142)

Today, we do not have any doubts that thought can influence our disease state, yet a hundred years ago, those who believed and practiced *Mind over Body* faced incrimination. One such person was Helen Wilmans. Dickenson recounts:

> Helen Wilmans, called the 'mother of mental science', in her long fight with the post-office department and government officials who tried to send her to prison for healing without medicine, proved in court that she had healed persons in her presence and persons at a distance simply by the power of thought. (Dickenson, 1920, 141)

The early Naturopaths faced criticisms from all directions. Lust, in an editorial, addresses a comment published in a medical journal, *Review of Reviews*, mocking the Naturopathic principle of 'immutable laws of nature'. The idea of 'nature' seemed to cause a reaction among his medical contemporaries. Lust wrote this response to demystify nature's immutable laws. He provides a primary law of life, and extrapolates the law to living cells, "Every cell in the human body will function perfectly provided its environment remains congenial to it; i.e., provided it receives the proper quantity and quality of food material and oxygen, has its waste products removed promptly, it is not injured by exposure to extremes of temperature, or by violence." He continues, this is "a state of health." (Lust, 1921, 162) Lust asks a rhetorical question: can this law be broken? Of course it can. He contemplates many examples of this question of the possibility of immutable laws.

Nature had many ways to express the violation of its immutable laws and pain was one of those expressions. Carlos Brandt viewed pain as "an admirable warning of nature; a means to preserve life." (Brandt, 1921, 373) Brandt describes further, "When man begins to detach himself from his natural environments; that is when he begins to transgress the law of the conservation of life, he begins to clog his body with foreign matter." (Brandt, 1921, 373) Brandt continues on the subject of disease and defines acute disease as a curative crisis in which "foreign matter, clogging the body, is removed." (Brandt, 1921, 374) Acute diseases express symptoms that are essentially the body's efforts to free from the body foreign matter. These symptoms should never be suppressed. Pain and disease have much in common; both are reminders from nature to listen to our bodies and correct the faulty habits that we indulge in.

Lust's 1921 editorial was actually in response to the next article written by Herbert Shelton. Shelton was disappointed by the dismal succession of medical wonders. He saw the litany of new therapies come in vogue with favorable reports inducing other practitioners to follow suit. Shelton states, "Yet in the space of a few short years the boasted remedy has lost its virtue; the disease no longer yields to its power while its place is supplied by some new remedy, which, like its predecessor, runs through the same career of expectation, success and disappointment." (Shelton, 1921, 283) Although, the above citation was directed at the shortcomings of the Allopathic fixation of finding the one drug cures, Shelton was attributing similar characteristics to the 'Nature Curist' or 'Naturopath' who was searching for a 'conglomeration of therapeutic measures' and loses "sight of those great laws of Nature upon which we first [built]." (Shelton, 1921, 283)

Our profession can be accused even today of chasing after many available gadgets and exotic equipment with which to fill our offices. In this regard, Shelton relates a story:

> The head of an institution where I was employed, said to me once in conversation: "Now there's electricity," pointing to his machine, "it may not do any good. I don't know. Anyway it works on the mind." And this, I

think accounts for its popularity. "It works on the mind." It furnishes an excellent means of entertaining the patient." (Shelton, 1921, 285)

While Shelton was disillusioned with the gullibility of his Naturopathic colleagues in identifying with fads and gizmos, Lust was equally concerned by the public's reliance on drugs even when "their experience gives them usually, if not always, unsatisfactory and often fatal results." (Lust, 1922, 5) Lust declares:

> Over-eating, the lack of exercise, the excessive use of tobacco, excessive eating of meat and starchy foods . . . seem to be . . . the underlying troubles the drugs are supposed to cure, but, which at the very best, only temporarily relieve or suppress the disease and gradually lead to the degeneration of the tissue and to premature death. (Lust, 1922, 5)

In his view, rather than become therapeutic agents, these drug interventions posed more health problems which proved to be powerful agents of destruction. The effect that drugs had on small children was a particular worry and was often raised by the early Naturopaths. Rather than use drugs for the treatment of fevers for example, "mothers very often use cooling medicines for their babies." (Lust, 1922, 5) Lust offers common sense suggestions to incorporate cool water as a therapeutic agent for such fevers. "Cool abdominal packs give excellent results in fever." (Lust, 1922, 6)

Natural alternatives to the increasingly pervasive use of harmful drugs to treat a fever, whether in a child or not, constituted an opposing method, one health promoting and the other, a potentially dangerous chemical. Lust found the practices of the Allopaths an "utter failure to teach natural and rational disease prevention" (Lust, 1922, 583) and contributed, he thought, to the cause of social unrest and moral degeneration.

It is easy to detect in this remarkable early literature the incremental alarm of the Naturopaths who watched the Allopaths systematically dominate by targeting "every department of life in America, Federal, State, Municipal, Army and Navy, Educational, Church, Home and finally the individual." Lust goes on to declare, "They have prostituted our Public School system, our educational and health boards, and they are claiming the right over the child even before it is born." (Lust, 1922, 584) Lust opposed the control that Allopathic medicine had on American people and believed medical freedom was an inherent right. He continues, "In the year 1896 its founders wrote in its constitution that every citizen of the United States must have the choice of his method of healing and the free right of his body and mind and every doctor should have the free exercise of his profession [parity of all methods of healing]." (Lust, 1922, 584)

A Proclamation was drafted for the 26th Annual Convention of the

NY and NJ State Societies of Naturopaths. In this illuminating document, Benedict Lust wrote with great clarity about the essence of Naturopathy in its applications. With a 26 year record, the American Naturopathic Association [ANA] had as its objective, teaching and practicing the natural method of living. Lust writes, "The [ANA] is a union for the mutual advancement of non-drug physicians and other progressive men and women of the United States and Canada who not only lead the natural life themselves but who employ and teach non-drug methods of therapeutics and disease prevention." (Lust, 1922, 583) He lists the six major health variables which stand as the foundation in Naturopathy. "These essentials are air, light, water, food, physical culture [or exercise] and mind" (Lust, 1922, 583) which constitutes the foundation of the therapies offered, such as "atmospheric cure, the light cure, the water cure, the diet cure, the earth (clay) cure, the work cure, and the mind cure." (Lust, 1922, 583) The adjunctive therapies or the minor therapies included Mechanotherapy, psychotherapy, electrotherapy, physiotherapy [hydrotherapy and nature cure], phytotherapy, biochemistry, orificial and bloodless surgery. (Lust, 1922, 583) As we can see by these two lists, currently, we have inverted the primary therapies with the adjunctives.

Lust was outraged by the Medical Trusts which systematically and forcefully dominated medicine in America. He described the burden of Naturopathy and the term, Naturopath, as being a form of 'protest', its very name . . .

> coined in the days of persecution when the New York County Medical Association arrested and fined with heavy money sentences and long prison terms the noble pioneers and humanitarian characters that stood up as representatives of the rational healing art and for the rights of the people. (Lust, 1922, 584)

The primary focus of the Naturopath was "essentially [to be] a teacher in his locality and his mission is rather to prevent than to cure disease." (Lust, 1922, 584) When the etymology of the words, doctor and physician were analyzed by Dr Yergin, during this period, predetermined that "the term doctor means first and over and above all other things, a TEACHER." (Yergin, 1923, 227) He adds, "The word PHYSICIAN is from the Greek *physis*, nature; and the terminal which means a student or philosopher,—one who studies and works according to the laws of nature." (Yergin, 1923, 227) Yergin counsels, that "this is the high calling to which all naturopathic doctors and physicians are called." (Yergin, 1923, 228)

The early Naturopaths took that high calling to heart. Herbert Shelton cites Dr Lahn in saying "the highest aim of the physician is make himself dispensable." (Shelton, 1923, 541) In such a natural medical system, the doctor instructs his patients to be independent and take care of themselves. Shelton continues "all disease is an outgrowth of a common fundamental cause—toxemia." (Shelton, 1923, 541) Shelton, who took a great interest in Tilden's work and Nature Cure adopted very high ideals in his own philosophy. In this article, *The Functions of a Health School*, he reminded his colleagues that "In our HEALTH SCHOOL the patient learns why he was sick, how he got well and how to stay well." (Shelton, 1923, 542) And most important, "we teach [our patients] self-reliance." (Shelton, 1923, 542)

Sussanna Czeranko, ND, BBE

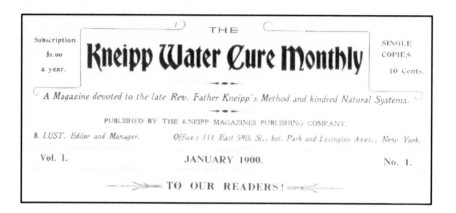

THE
Kneipp Water Cure Monthly

Subscription $1.00 a year.

SINGLE COPIES 10 Cents.

A Magazine devoted to the late Rev. Father Kneipp's Method and kindred Natural Systems.

PUBLISHED BY THE KNEIPP MAGAZINES PUBLISHING COMPANY.

B. LUST, *Editor and Manager.*

Office: 111 East 59th St., bet. Park and Lexington Aves., New York.

Vol. 1.   JANUARY 1900.   No. 1.

TO OUR READERS!

Masthead for the first English edition of *The Kneipp Water Cure Monthly* Magazine.

THE NATURAL TREATMENT AND MEDICINE

by Benedict Lust

The Kneipp Water Cure Monthly, I(2), 17-18. (1900)

Medicus naturae minister non magister.

Already 400 years B. C. Hippocrates said: "The physician is only the servant of nature not its teacher," and more than 2000 years after him Professor Dr. med. Rudolf Virchow in Berlin said: "It is the task of medical science to remove all causes which obstruct the normal discharge of vital functions. Therefore medical science should become public property."

But there would be no gain for mankind, if the medical science of to-day would be public property. People already swallow poisons enough with the aid of physicians and ruin their systems quick enough as it is. *Natura sanat, medicus curat,* "nature heals, the physician cures," said the same Hippocrates and he was right. The physician or any human being can only assist nature, as long as nature is strong enough to perform the process of healing. Where one's nature does not possess strength enough for the process of healing, all assisting, all cures will be of no avail, while drugs under all circumstances will hasten the end.

The physicians of to-day call their science physiological medicine, that is a science which recognizes the laws of nature and is guided by these laws. Is that really done by those learned gentlemen? No, the physician does not bother much with the nature of the patient, he only prescribes so and so many parts of some drug or other.

He knows his drugs will stop this or this ailment, but that the drug will produce other evils does not concern him. Should other ailments arise, he will prescribe other drugs until all the drugs have done their work and no more drugs are needed, for the patient will be killed by the drugs.

There is one little case which happened lately and shows very plain the difference between the effects of a natural treatment and a treatment by medical science. A baby-boy of nine months was teething very hard, besides that he had a cold, whooping-cough and a very high fever. Of course the mother consulted a druggist who had studied medical science and got his diploma as physician. Some medicines were given but had a very bad effect. The child became very restless and for three nights mother, father and baby were up all night. During the fourth night the father who has read Kneipp's books and other works on natural healing got tired of giving the medicine. He was fully convinced that the child would soon be killed by the drugs and that the mother would get sick too for she could not stand the strain much longer. He had read in one of his books, that a short packing would quiet the child, reduce the fever, and produce sleep. A natural treatment was suggested by him the first day, but the mother would not allow the application of a cold water-packing, she was sure that such a thing was humbug and would, if not kill, but surely hurt the baby. Her belief in the drugs was shaken during the fourth night. She consented to the application of the packing. A soft towel was put into cold water, wrung out and put around the body of the baby and a dry heavy piece of wool put over the wet towel. In two minutes the baby was quiet and to the greatest delight of mother and father smiled, turned over on one side and was, after the restlessness of four days and three nights, fast asleep in five minutes. The mother fell asleep too, while the father watched the child for some time to find that after one hour the fever was gone. In the morning the child awoke at the usual hour. His health was improved greatly. The mother of course did not think much of drugs any more.

The physician learns this or this drug will cure that or that sickness. He does not know why, he is taught, that the drug will do it and that satisfies him. They experimented with their drugs on animals and drew their conclusions, but of what value are those experiments? The difference between man and animal from a physiological standpoint is so great, that all such conclusions are valueless.

For green-sickness and anaemia physicians prescribe iron-preparations. Iron is a very important component part of the human organism, but iron-preparations taken as medicine will never supply this organism with the necessary amount of iron, for the stomach will not be able to digest it, on the contrary, these preparations will irritate digestion and cause loss of appetite and constipation. The origin of the sickness has to be removed and the sickness will disappear. In cases of green-sickness and anaemia the organs of digestion produce poor or very little blood, therefore digestion ought to be aided and the whole organism ought to be strengthened to overcome the sickness. As soon as these organs do their work in the natural way, good blood will be produced and this blood will contain all the iron nature wants it to contain; as soon as these organs work properly all the blood necessary will be produced.

Space does not permit us to go more into details, but the terrible effects of opium-, morphium-, quinine- or mercury-preparations, to cite an instance, are too well known. Medical science of the old school knows no other means or does not want to know the simple and natural means of healing. The natural scientist does not experiment with drugs on the human system. He knows, that nature has provided for everything. He allows nature to take its own course and only assists nature. He studies the nature of the patient and the nature of the sickness and uses natural means only.

Cleanliness—The First Principle Of Hygiene

by Wilhelm Hotz, M.D.

Director, Sanitarium, *Bad Finkenmühle*, near Mellenbach i. Thür., Germany.

The Kneipp Water Cure Monthly, I(6), 89-90. (1900)

Hygiene, the science of health, is undoubtedly the first foundation of therapeutics, the science of restoring lost health, because without knowing the laws which maintain health, no physician can tell his patient the right way that leads him to health and give him the proper advice how to regain it. Hence disease, as we call lost health, must be in one or the other way the consequence of departure from the natural path of life, or, in other words, disease is the indication of the loss of the vital equilibrium; its symptoms are the manifestation of the vital force to regain the normal state.

By studying such abnormal conditions and the way by which nature is seeking to lead the organism back to the prior state of health, we will find out not only the proper way of cure, but learn also how to keep up our health, i.e., the principles of hygiene.

Hygiene is as old as the history of mankind. Its highest development has always been found in the most civilized countries, to-day as well as several thousand years ago, not because they have the highest civilization—nothing in the world develops without necessity, its motive power—but because the more a people has advanced in so-called civilization the more are the natural laws of life usually neglected, so that it may be doubted whether the high development of science, technics and industries of the modern world is really the result of mental progression, or is not rather the necessary effect of reduced vitality and lessened resistance to morbific influences, according to the law of self-preservation. Such facts induced man to find means to preserve his species and to study the laws of health to that end.

Hygiene is therefore as old as the history of mankind, but wherever we find sanitary measures, in ancient or modern times, they always relate directly or indirectly to cleanliness. To-day we admire the magnificent structures that have been built many thousand years ago by the old Egyptians only for the purpose of securing a pure and abundant water supply. Greeks and Romans built luxurious bathing houses for the public use, knowing already that proper care of the body is a potent factor in preventing disease. Had not Hippocrates already taught that prophylaxis is the best part of the science of medicine?

The first hygienic measures in regard to personal health which man recognized are physical cleanliness and abundant exercise. Soon after followed the acknowledgment of moderation in eating, drinking and general manner of living. From the individual experience in relation to personal health resulted, in larger communities, the public health, viz.: general sanitary measures, as, for instance, the regulation of water supply and the securing of pure food by the erection and supervision of public slaughter-houses and bakeries, the disposal of the dead and of the excreta, etc. Hence the more the human family developed their faculties in the direction of modern civilization, the more new measures and precautions have been found necessary to protect public health, till finally the whole affair became a matter of government supervision. In brief: All hygienists, from the ancient Egyptians down to the modern scientists, recognized cleanliness as the first principle of health and believed in realizing it by endeavoring to secure pure air, pure water and pure food for the people at large.

The notion, however, of what cleanliness means, its correct definition, was never perfectly clear or the same to every body, because the effect of the contrary condition is also not always alike. The man of a good constitution who can stand great extremes, for instance, offers a stronger resistance to injurious surroundings and stands in less need to take care for his physical welfare than a man of more delicate constitution; his idea about cleanliness in regard to his body, food and surroundings, will therefore be not as clear and exact; consequently the conception of pure or impure is a matter of individual agreement, so long as no certain scientific definition can be given of it. Such a definition can not yet be given in every respect, but it can be very evidently and without doubt in regard to septic materials.

Pasteur, the late French scientist, discovered that all putrefaction is caused by microbes. Other scientists found that in almost all diseases microbes are present, that disease is consequently a process of putrefaction started by certain microörganisms which found their way into our system. But the action (or better), the existence of said microörganisms is fortunately limited, as well as of other living organisms and depends on suitable food; without the proper nutritive elements they are not able to exist beyond a certain length of time, or at least not to propagate themselves. Since Pasteur's discovery we know that no putrefaction of organic matter can take place without the presence of microbes; we know further that all microbes need organic material as a first condition of their existence and that dead organic substance is a more suitable soil for them than living organisms, because the latter offer a natural resistance to all noxious influences. So we find microbes most numerous wherever dead organic matter exists—the primary enemy of health. Hence the quick and complete destroying of all dead organic matter, which is and can not be well protected from putrefaction, would be the best method of preventing the spreading of pathogenic microbes, those species which we have chiefly to deal with in health and disease. If microbes were necessary in nature's economy to decompose all dead organic matter in order to set free the latent energy which is stored up in all the higher compounds the organic world represents, it would be different; such seems not to be the case, however, since there are other much more efficacious factors by which dead organic matter can be reduced into single inorganic elements, than by the mediation of organisms, and which force would be better to that end than fire? Why do we not make use of the same wherever it is advisable, instead of allowing the ground on which we live to be soiled by waste and refuse of organic nature of every kind? Why is it that, in contradiction to our modern progress and our knowledge about the origin of disease, we still let the ground get infected by following the old method of burying corpses of men and animals and letting nature take care of them by the way of the most slow and unwholesome process we know of, the action of putrefaction, the same one which we know to be the starting point of almost all diseases? I consider the microörganisms, apart from their fermentive power, as ideal watchmen of health, because their presence and action is quite often the first indication that something must be wrong, or that our body is in an abnormal state of health. Without the prompt action of microbes on diseased tissue it would be extremely difficult to discover the lesion and its origin soon enough to prevent further injury to the system. I can not believe that the pathogenic microbes are the direct cause of disease, but rather think that about in the same way as pure chemical poisons affect the system, disease is originated either by toxic materials, as the products of our own metabolism, poisoned air, impure food and bad surroundings, or as in cases of inoculation of specific microbes by their products of metabolism. If this view, as given above, should prove to be correct the hygienist has only to deal with poisonous or non-poisonous substances man is liable to come in connection with; while he should consider all the pathogenic, saprophytic and fermentive microörganisms as useful agents and as our natural guardians which protect us from disease. So the deductions from the bacteriologic propositions point again to cleanliness as the first factor to maintain our health.

But not bacteriologic researches alone and their practical demonstrations show the truth of cleanliness as the first principle in hygiene; still more is this assertion proven by the study and observations made on the human body under circumstances of great sensitiveness to all unfavorable influences.

In cases of direct injuries and wounds, for instance, where the natural protective organs are entirely excluded from action, we notice the influence of any infectious matter first of all in the most marked way. Thereupon is based, as you know, the aseptic method in surgery. The least carelessness in this respect may be followed by ill effects and shows evidently how careful we ought to be in introducing foreign substances into our system.

Next to the effect of direct infections by wounds, we notice a high sensitiveness of the system to all kinds of impure influences in case of disease. The first thing nature tries to do in case of disease usually is to clean the system from foreign substances and to prevent further supply. Such symptoms as loss of appetite, nausea, vomiting, diarrhea, profuse sweat, etc., tell us very distinctly in what way the body will regain its normal state, and also where the origin of the abnormal condition lies. In nine out of ten cases I am sure that the cause can be traced to carelessness in regard to cleanliness, that there is a lack somewhere, either in reference to cleansing, dressing and general surroundings of the body, or that the internal system has been neglected, the secretory and excretory organs are out of order; so that the poisonous products of metabolism cause a kind of auto-intoxication; but as I said, the practice of cleanliness alone may prevent at least nine out of ten cases of disease.

The first and most important advice, therefore, the physician gives to the sick refers to general hygienic measures based upon good ventilation of the sick room, pure and easily digestible food and proper care of the body. What the physician does and the only thing he can do for the sick is certainly to assist nature in its efforts to restore health, and, as far as the symptoms indicate the need of the system, the physician has to be only a true student of nature in order to be also a successful physician. Is the surgeon who uses the scalpel to remove or to reach the diseased part, doing more than assisting nature in its endeavor to get the pus and impure matter out of the system? No; both medical practitioner and surgeon correspond in so doing to the first principle of hygiene.

Cleanliness in every respect is a vital question in infancy. Nothing, I believe, is more fatal for the newborn than neglect nursing, insufficient cleansing and impure food. The immensely high death rate, especially among the lower class of people, is certainly due to the carelessness with which children are nursed and left to themselves, growing up in filth and fed on improper food, more like animals than like human beings. Indeed, there is still a great field for action for the physician, where he can realize the simplest hygienic measures without having to fear that the health of the people will reach such high state, and the people itself will become so well educated that every one may be able to be his or her own physician while the practitioner will have to starve. No matter how far off that time may be, it would certainly be better and more honorable for the profession than is our age of progressive physical degeneration where almost every one believes himself to be able to act as his own adviser in illness, but in his ignorance swallows drugs and so-called patent medicines in astonishing quantities, according to his fallible judgment instead of following the natural laws of hygiene, or in case of disease calling for a competent physician.

I think the more man progresses in regard to general civilization and special culture of mind, the more stress he must lay on general health, if he does not want to endanger all that he has gained through pain and difficulties of every kind for centuries past. And if experience and science clearly teach us that cleanliness in its fullest extent is the first principle in hygiene, as I have tried to prove, then we should strive not only to acknowledge, but still more to apply this axiom of health in all respects. The deeper we go into this matter the more we realize the great truth there is in the well known quotation: "Cleanliness is next to godliness".

Hygiene, the science of health, is undoubtedly the first foundation of therapeutics, the science of restoring lost health, because without knowing the laws which maintain health, no physician can tell his patient the right way that leads him to health and give him the proper advice how to regain it.

I consider the microörganisms, apart from their fermentive power, as ideal watchmen of health, because their presence and action is quite often the first indication that something must be wrong, or that our body is in an abnormal state of health.

The first thing nature tries to do in case of disease usually is to clean the system from foreign substances and to prevent further supply.

THE CAUSATION OF DISEASES

by Ludwig Staden, Naturarzt

The Kneipp Water Cure Monthly, 1(6), 100. (1900)

The principal physiological cause of all diseases is found in the blood, which causation we call dysaemia or defective composition of the blood. This is the root of all ailments, we therefore may say, it exists only one disease, which manifests itself in different forms. The reason of this defective condition of the blood will easily be discovered in the unnatural and effeminating mode of life. Nowadays everybody eats more than he can digest and principally eats food which is artificially prepared, consequently harder digestible than food in its natural state. The most essential food is meat, and such an exclusive meat diet causes a more accelerated change of matter, which we try to balance through alcohol; meat and alcohol are the ruin of the individual and national health, they are the causes of luxury, effemination and degeneration.

An exclusive meat diet produces a surplus of uric acid, which neutralizes the natron of the blood and prevents it to absorb the carbonic acid, one of the greatest self-poisons and enemies of vitality; all processes of life suffer considerably under this abnormal quality of the blood. This is the reason why Dr. Alex. Haig, physician of the Metropolitan Hospital of London, looks upon uric acid as a fundamental causation of disease and he is right in so far. Blood which contains too much carbonic acid is especially qualified for the culture and the existence of bacilli, in pure blood such germs would never settle, which proves that not the bacilli can be the cause of disease but only the bad quality of the blood is responsible for their existence. Bacilli are foreign or morbid matter in the blood. If the vitality of the individual is strong enough, the presence of such foreign bodies causes fever, the organism endeavors to get rid of them under a higher pressure of temperature, which again proves that a fever is a healing and the most natural purifying process. If an individual has not enough vitality to produce a fever and to burn and secrete the morbid matter, the same will settle down in different organs and thus cause chronic disease, or if a natural healing process like fever gets disturbed or suppressed by medicines, i. e., chinnia, antipyrin, etc., the same result will take place. A great many of chronic diseases are the result of acute diseases, supposed to be cured (!) by medicine; for instance many eye- and ear-troubles after the grip, measles, scarlet fever, etc.

If the blood contains too much uric acid, the crystals of uric acid accumulate in the muscles and joints and produce those painful diseases called gout and rheumatism; also sulphuric acid frees itself from

the flesh and tissues which destroys the red corpuscles, the support-
ers of oxygen. No wonder that the change of matter becomes entirely
abnormal and effects proportionally the nervous system and the mental
powers. Lassitude, physical, intellectual and moral weakness, loss of will
power take hold of the patient and he becomes dissatisfied with himself
and the whole world, a condition which often develops into perfect nervous prostration. The excessive quantities of meat and in connection with
these alcoholic liquors cannot be assimilated entirely, the surplus remains
in the body and fat and obesity are the results, the sugar in the muscles
cannot be absorbed through lack of oxygen and that fearful disease diabetes appears. The use of alcohol is the ruin of the red corpuscles more
or less, the dissection of drunkards shows a white color of the lungs, the
great lack of oxygen made it impossible to purify the venous blood in the
lungs, the function of the heart became heavier day by day and the finale
was apoplexy.

All people who suffer from dysaemia of the blood are tormented by a
great thirst, because nature tries to attenuate the dysaemic blood, but this
thirst induces the sufferer to overflow his tissues with fluid, they become
flabby and stagnative and can be compared with a swamp. Tissues in such
a condition are the most qualified places to cultivate bacilli and in times of
epidemics like cholera, typhoid fever, yellow fever, etc., individuals of such
a disposition form the majority of the victims. If one intends to harden
and regenerate people, one must ask them to abstain from drinking too
much water and other fluids, this was the theory of Johannes Schroth,
who performed so many wonderful and phenomenal cures, among which
the celebrated cure of the Prince William of Wurttemberg. His method is
known among the natural methods of healing as the Cure of Regeneration. At this occasion the great abuse of table salt may be mentioned,
which also causes great thirst. Mineral salt, which is not one with organic
matter, can never be assimilated by the process of changing matter, it will
always be secreted again, especially by the kidneys or it remains in the
body as foreign matter and thus causes disease, a special form of disease
caused by the abuse of salt is the scorbute. It is absolutely unnecessary to
use table salt, we get all the necessary nutritious salts in abundance from
the vegetable kingdom, where these salts are in organic form and therefore can be assimilated by the system.

Every man with common sense will understand what he has to do in
order to avoid the original causes of disease, which can be given in the
few words "keep your blood pure". Add to simple, non-stimulating diet
the use of plenty of fresh air, sunlight and especially airy, well ventilated
bed-rooms, cleanliness, hardening of the body by cold water and assist
nature in the process of secreting foreign matter with steam baths and
packings occasionally, light clothing covering the body equally, harmoni-

ous exercise and rest, and pure thoughts, and you will have a guarantee of health, which is far more valuable and surer than all medicines in the world.

The principal physiological cause of all diseases is found in the blood, which causation we call dysaemia or defective composition of the blood. This is the root of all ailments, we therefore may say, it exists only one disease, which manifests itself in different forms.

Bacilli are foreign or morbid matter in the blood, if the vitality of the individual is strong enough, the presence of such foreign bodies causes fever, the organism endeavors to get rid of them under a higher pressure of temperature, which again proves that a fever is a healing and the most natural purifying process.

Just And His Method

by Benedict Lust

The Kneipp Water Cure Monthly, I(8), 128-131. (1900)

The 19th century can claim that its last decades have brought many and many blessings to mankind. The science of natural healing has been studied by many and even by medical men who have come to the conclusion that all healing is done by nature and that science can only assist nature.

Christ preached his gospel of love 19 centuries ago and healed the sick and wounded. His teachings and his deeds were the cause of all the hatred of his enemies, but in spite of this hatred Christ's teachings have conquered the world and triumphed in the end as truth always will triumph over lie. The victory which the gospel of love has won over its enemies makes us hope that the gospel of truth preached by the apostles of natural healing will triumph too in the end. There have been many such apostles of natural healing, they too, like the apostles of the gospel of love had to suffer from ignorance and hatred but the sick and wounded who have been cured are the best proof of the righteousness of their cause and their intentions.

Among the apostles of natural healing who have won name and fame during the last two decades of the 19th century there is one who by his "war-cry" *Return to Nature* has called the attention of the whole Christian world to his method and to the fact that something must be done to save mankind from utter ruin. People may not believe it but without a stop being put to it in time, the ways of living are so far from what they ought to be that a few centuries more of such unnatural living would have made our race a race of weaklings constantly troubled by all sorts of ailments.

Return to Nature is Just's war-cry and this war-cry has found many followers and is gaining more every day. This method is well worth to be studied, for it has saved the life of many a sufferer who was given up as incurable by physicians. Just has established a sanitarium in Eckerthal in the Harz Mountains where patients are treated according to the rules of his method. Just calls his sanitarium the Jungborn or the "Well of Youth" and as strange as it may sound to the outsider who knows of nothing of the healing power of nature, all the patients who ever visited the Jungborn uphold his method and are united in declaring this sanitarium in those German mountains a genuine well of youth.

Experience has been Just's teacher. After years of terrible physical and mental suffering which brought him so near to death's door that he was about to give up all hope, the enlightening ideas came to his mind, ideas destined to save Just and thousands and thousands of his fellow sufferers. Just is not only a healer but a philosopher as well and has based his methods upon philosophical reasoning which is as interesting as it is sound.

God is love. Out of mere love God created the world and men and out of mere love God preserves the world and men. Men were the crown of the creation, the last work done during the seven days of creation. The good, beautiful and noble only could result from the creation of God's love, almightiness and supreme wisdom. Nothing bad, no pain, no sickness, no need or misery could come from God's love. Everything was created perfect, the world was a paradise. Even men were without faults on body and soul, without sickness, without sin and without misfortune. The earth produced food for men and animals spontaneously. Men knew their food by instinct and taste like all other beings and did not need any clothing like the animals did not need any. Originally men led a life free from hard work, worry or apprehension. To enjoy true happiness was the only purpose of men's existence who were the favorites of God.

God has given sense to men, so that they may understand their coherence to God, his almightiness and supreme wisdom, that they may esteem his love and stand higher morally and physically than the animals. The gift of sense gave men a certain liberty of action which animals were lacking. Animals are forced by nature to adhere to their mode of living; animals do not know and cannot manufacture artificial food nor are they able to make artificial cloth for themselves. Men only were able to part from nature's rules and soon used this power but not to their advantage. As stated above, nature, or what is the same instinct, tells us what is destined to be the food of men or animals. Each animal knows its food and does not try to partake of any other. Men's instinct done the same, but men were not satisfied with those foods destined for them by nature. They used artificial means to make tasty those foods which in a natural state did not agree with their nature.

MEN PARTOOK OF THE FORBIDDEN FRUIT. Men imagined that by forgetting the laws of nature they would gain powers, comforts, joys and happiness which nature did not offer. Sense, the gift of heaven, became the curse of men.

All life in the great universe, where every little part is connected with another like the wheels in a clock, can only be a sound and happy one as long as it is in harmony with the rest. The slightest diversion from the original destination must necessarily be followed by disturbances, pains and misery. Men's organs, especially the organs of digestion were prepared to digest only such food as nature had destined for men, that is such foods which were spontaneously produced by nature for men.

The taste of such foods in their natural state was pleasant to men and agreed with their systems. As soon as men commenced to prepare foods artificially, and partake of foods which did not agree with men in their raw state, substances got into men's systems which were bound to make them weak and miserable. The organs of digestion of course were not able to digest such foods properly or what is very often the case could not digest them at all. By and by foreign substances and matters were formed in the stomach which in a fluid or solid state or in form of gas went through the whole system, producing heat which always becomes very dangerous to the organism. The development of the body was disturbed by these foreign matters in a high degree and the human body originally beautiful in every respect became ugly and was subjected to spells of weakness, all sorts of ailments and an early death.

After the first step which led away from nature others followed. With the change of food men's nature changed. They felt the cold for they had lost their natural protection against it. They invented the artificial protection against the influences and changes of temperature— the clothing. These again reduced the natural warmth of the body, for after the body was covered by clothing, light and air, the producers and preservers of life, partly lost their beneficial influence upon it. Men are the highest specimens of light-air-beings. Nature of God (as you will, the name has got nothing to do with it, the power is there all the same who we do not understand) has created men without a covering of hair for the only purpose to give the soul, the highest light-air—creation, the means to exist by direct contact with light and air. The pores were given to our skin to absorb light and air as well as to secrete all what is impure. Next to the artificial food the artificial unnatural clothing is responsible for the degeneration of the body. As said before all powers in or of the universe produce perfectness by harmonious action. The unnatural, artificial food produces changes which interfere in serious ways with the welfare of the human being. Artificial cloth made matters worse. The loss of the beneficial direct influence of light and air upon the body again made digestion worse and assisted the formation of substances foreign to the system of men.

As everything in the universe, body and soul of men are in close connection and coherence. The body carries or covers the soul or life while the soul gives life or movement or strength in the body. Every incident in or accident to the body at once affects the soul or vice versa every impression upon the soul has its affect upon the body in a favorably or unfavorably way according to circumstances.

After men's desertion of nature as far as their mode of living is concerned (for luckily altogether they are not able to free themselves from it or the human race would disappear forever) all sorts of ailments took hold

STUDY THIS FACE!

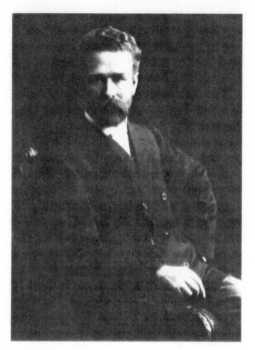

It is that of Adolph Just.

No better index exists for h.s "Return to Nature" teachings.

Gentle, simple, earnest. sincere. hopeful—with an abundant faith in Self and the assurance of experience to back it—wouldn't you like your physician to be such a men as this?

He has suffered deeply—you can tell that by the look of understanding.

But he has also triumphed nobly—from conquest alone comes such an expression of sane contentment.

Doesn't the spirit of this teacher appeals to you?

Don't you want his secret of victorious living?

Remember he was given up to die by the foremost specialists in Europe. But no man with a great message ever dies until he has voiced it—his soul won't let him. This man's message is that of Self-regeneration. He has proved its marvelous power— years ago people ceased calling it a dream. You can prove it too. No matter what your disease, whether of body, mind or soul, there's the record of other worse ones cured speedily and lastingly by "Return to Nature" methods. Send for Adolph Just's book. Do it to-day. If you should decide, after a fair trial, that you'd rather have the $1.50, I'll return it instantly.

Meanwhile, believe absolutely in your potential perfection. You were born to be strong, sweet, beautiful, wise, joyous, opulent, lovable. If you fall short, it's because you've stopped growing. "RETURN TO NATURE" helps you grow up into Your Self.

Benedict . Lust,

124 EAST 59th STREET,   **NEW YORK CITY.**

Advertisement for Adolf Just's book, *Return To Nature*.

of the body according to their location in the body. Men got diseases of the lungs and nerves, eruptions of all kinds, men became blind and deaf, even paralyzed and got the gout. But by these diseases, ailments of the body, the soul is influenced. Stupidity, clouding of the mind, irksomeness, sorrow, discontendness [sic], dissatisfaction, melancholy, vice and crime followed. The happiness of men was destroyed, they experienced need and misery and early, too early death. Death as a consequence of some disease or other became the rule not final painless dissolution without any trouble to mind or soul as nature wanted it.

The voice of the people is the voice of God and the people in general have not lost the feeling that there have been better days before the fall of men before they ate of the forbidden fruit and forgot the laws of nature. Folk-lore in all parts of the globe tells about the same story but the best and most sacred of all is told in the bible in a beautiful and very convincing way.

After the Paradise of health and happiness was lost, it was not more than natural that men would try to blame others or look for reasons outside of their ownself. Finally people were under the impression that a part of their misery was a natural consequence of the rules of nature. This idea again was the foundation for new troubles. Here is an instance: Clothing and apartments in which people live to-day keep light, air, warmth and cold from the body, these powers consequently cannot exercise their natural influence upon the body. Digestion is first affected and hampered with. Foreign substances begin to accumulate in the body. As soon as all superfluous clothing is removed and in such a state light, water and air touch the body a change is brought about at once. These powerful remedies of nature commence at once to remove all these foreign substances. The whole system is set to work to accomplish this and the poor human being is under the impression that a cold is contracted. Here again men interfere with nature. Instead of letting nature have its course they interfere with nature and keep those foreign substances in their bodies by means of drugs which again make matters worse. Men do not want to know and understand the beneficial effects of nature's ways and means. Men are too much inclined to consider nature an enemy on the look-out to hurt or harm them, while just the opposite is the case.

The fear of getting cold is too much settled in the people and asks and receives too many victims daily. Men out of mere fear of cold, close their bodies up against light and air and weaken their systems more and more. In this way alone an enormous number come to an early death lamented by relations and friends.

Bacteria have frightened many and do so to-day, but bacteria will be found wherever there is fermentation of decomposition of foreign matter in nature. Men who partake of natural hygienic food only and allow water, light and air to cleanse their systems will have no trouble with bacteria. The bodies of such men would not offer any chance of formation or existence to bacteria just as much as men who keep their bodies clean are not bothered by vermin of any kind.

Sickness, etc. and early death are not considered by men as a natural consequence of their unnatural mode of living. He who insists that by regular baths, light, air and a natural diet he will be able to prevent an early death is considered either a fool or a sinner against God's will. There even are men who believe that God sends sickness to better men and that all sorts of misery serve God to attain his wisest purposes.

In this way men make a caricature of God's love and wisdom.

In many ways men tried to regain the lost Paradise—health and happiness. They made sacrifices to God, brewed magic potions, tried to find the philosopher's stone, etc., etc., and hoped in this way to get healed from all sufferings of body and soul. All those physicians, law-makers, teachers, etc., who hope to heal the ailments of the body and save the soul in any other way then by a complete return to nature are like the Danaides, the daughters of Danaus, who tried to fill a barrel, the bottom of which was full of holes.

As long as men lived according to the laws of nature they were satisfied and contented. They did not ask in which way their happiness was produced, they were satisfied to be happy until the tempter said; "You will know what is good and bad" or better according to the original text of the bible; "What is hurtful and useful?" A craving for knowledge took hold of men. They wanted to know how life worked in their bodies and what the power of nature is. One cut open the dead to study the formation of the human body and its organs. One analyzed the food and observed the effects of the different elements upon another to find and manufacture remedies and foods for suffering humanity. One studied the laws of the spiritual life of men to form illusions. Men are still hard at work to find the truth, but all their work is in vain, nature does not give away the secret of life.

Practically all these great discoveries of science have done very little to produce true happiness. All civilized people became sick and weaker in the same proportions as their civilization was advancing until they finally were ruined. And to-day while science and civilization are in their flourishing times, men themselves are in misery. Sickness and misfortune have taken hold of them, vice and crime are on the increase, the lunatic asylums are not large enough for the many unfortunates and suicide is an every day's occurrence. Where shall help come from? There is only one way and that is: "RETURN TO NATURE."

But what does Just mean by a "Return to Nature"? That is easy to explain. Return to a natural diet, allow water, light and air to influence your system and all ailments will disappear, as well as all misfortune and discontent. Do no expect anything from the masses, but start for yourself a natural mode of living.

Originally men were without clothing and got their nourishment or food from nature. Nature provided men with everything they needed and they were truly happy. Of course, it is impossible for one generation to return at once to a genuine natural mode of living. But this genuine natural mode of living we may employ as a means of healing and strengthening the sick and the weak.

Just employs as healing factors first:

THE BATH

All animals and birds take a bath once in a while. It is therefore right to take it for granted that nature provided the bath for men just as well. But what kind of a bath should men take? The full-bath which covers the whole body from the neck down is not a natural one for men. The bath was taken by men according to their instinct, but we have lost this instinct during the long time mankind did not live according to the rules of nature. Just has discovered a bath with a sort of a self-massage treatment which has proven wonderfully effective. For all particulars about this bath we have to refer our readers to Just's book, *Return to Nature*.

Next to importance as healing factors in Just's methods are:

LIGHT AND AIR, IN HIS JUNGBORN

Men are the highest specimens of light-air-beings. Their life depends upon pure air and light. Water may strengthen their health and refresh their systems, but light and air are for men the principal life producers and preservers. The best air for men is the air of the woods, full of fragrance of trees and herbs. In his Jungborn Just offers all opportunities for a genuine return to nature. His patients live in what he calls light-air-houses. These little buildings are built of wood entirely and are erected under the trees of two beautiful parks, one for ladies and one for gentlemen. On all sides of these houses there are plenty windows and air valves, which may be opened or shut according to circumstances and in order to enable the inhabitant to regulate the fresh air supply. The arrangements enable patients to be in direct contact with light or air all the time, to take sun- and air-baths whenever they choose to or be with little or no dress all day. These parks offer at the same time all facilities for Just's bath and the best and surest way for a return to nature.

Plants and animals fade away in the dark and gain life when brought into light. The same takes place with the human body which also fades away in the darkness of clothing and gains new life when brought into direct contact with light and air. A great and wonderful change takes place in the whole organism. Digestion improves at once and all organs start an effective process of healing.

THE TERRESTRIAL CURRENT

The terrestrial current or the terrestrial power too is made use of by Just. Men and animals are according to Just nothing but moving plants, plants which in consequence of a higher development were able to free themselves from the ground. But all the same they receive their strength and refreshment from the ground. For this reason Just advocates walking barefooted and resting on the bare ground in order to give to the patient the full benefit of the terrestrial current. As a proof of the correctness of this idea Just points out that all animals who live in the forests for instance remove all leaves, shrubs even snow to rest upon the bare ground, to be in direct contact with it. Just has found that the influence of the terrestrial current is a wonderful healing factor. Walking barefooted and resting upon the bare ground created new activity even in the dullest patients.

THE DIET

The diet is another important factor in the Just cure. According to Just only nuts, berries and fruit are the natural foods for men and nutmeat should be the principal one. Men were satisfied with such a natural diet until they discovered the way to make a fire. From that moment they commenced to experiment with everything and cook anything even such products which their natural instinct told them not to be proper foods for them. They cooked meat, vegetables, potatoes, beans, made bread, alcoholic beverages and medicines. An ancient folklore tells us that in heaven Prometheus stole a fire and brought it to men. The possession of fire was considered such a dangerous one by the Gods that they fastened Prometheus to the Kaucasus Mountains and send vultures to tear the liver out of him. His liver was growing all the time so that the vultures could come back and punish the fire-thief over and over again. The enormity of the punishment serves to show the enormity of the crime and harm done to mankind.

The knowledge of fire enabled men to bring foreign substance into their system by partaken of unnatural food. Such food is bound to produce ulcers, eruptions, fever and other states of ill health or disease. Medical science removes these external and visible signs of disease by the application of salves and other medicines. But as soon as they are removed they appear again and a new application of remedies becomes a necessity.

Of course, it would be impossible for men to return to a natural diet at once. One should start with a mixed diet of nuts and milk. That this is right is proven by the habit of a young mammalia which do not give up their mother's breast milk until their stomach is fully used to the food destined for them by nature. It seems to Just that this is the only way to make the disordered stomach of the human being of civilization fit for nature's genuine foods. Just advices to drink the milk raw or sour, he also recommends a little cheese with some white or gluten bread. In case a patient cannot chew nuts on account of bad teeth he recommends plenty of milk as a substitute for nuts and a fat producer. Just's experience has taught him that patients who followed his advices in this respect in a short time did not long for any other kind of food, felt well and improved constantly.

The natural diet stops the formation of foreign matters at once. The organs of digestion are eased and work in a normal way, while the body instead of being fed on foreign substances gets what it needs to prosper and grow. Consequently all organs work easier and produce their own warmth, freshness, strength and activity. Real happiness takes possession of the whole being. In Just's sanitarium nuts, almonds, berries, apples, pears, cherries, plums, figs, dates, bananas and apricots or oranges and milk form the principal diet. The milk was produced by cows fed on the herbs of the Harz Mountains. These herbs in connection with the pure mountain air made the cows as sound and healthy as they possibly could be, their milk too, was in consequence of the pure food they got, a very healthy and pure food for men. In exceptional cases Just allows a mixed diet of meat and vegetables. Just's whole system is built upon nature's laws in the same way as it is Just's most earnest endeavor to bring back men to nature's simple mode of living and to enable every human being to be his or her own physician. The Jungborn therefore is not so much a sanitarium as an institute of study of nature's wants and nature's means of healing. In this sanitarium one does not entrust one's most valuable property, one's health, to the care of men who are liable to make mistakes easy, every patient is taught to observe his own nature and act accordingly. It is the principal object of the Jungborn to live up to what its name promises to wit: To provide men with new strength and activity for the battles and enjoyments of life. Liberty and health are the most valuable properties of men, nobody is therefore persuaded in the Jungborn sanitarium to make use of the whole system at once. Every opportunity is offered to the patient to return to nature but he is allowed to use his own judgment in regard to the use of the baths, light and air, the terrestrial current and the diet. In cases where parents for instance wish that the applications are controlled by the management such is done.

Nature has had its reasons to give the freedom of action to men, even when at present men use this freedom to their disadvantage. It is very likely that after years of sorrow, ailment and misfortune men will return to natural ways of living and be the more happy after all. This time may be far off, but the sooner and the more men return to nature the better it will be for them. All cannot return to nature at once, for not all are in the position to make the change without any trouble to themselves. The organs of digestion have to become used to a natural diet. As soon as that is done the battle is won. Every one has to be his or her own judge and his or her own physician, for every one can only judge for one's self. The animals which live in a natural way are never sick and whenever we meet a sick animal we may rest assured that this sickness is men's work who either destroyed the forest in which the animal lived, or poisoned the air or water, etc., etc. Hunters often have occasion to look in astonishment at wounds splendidly healed which were inflicted by their bullets. Men are superior to animals in every respect. An animal would not be able to stand the unnatural life men lead. The strong constitution of men only kept mankind in existence otherwise men would have disappeared from this globe long ago. As soon as men will return to nature altogether, as soon as men will perform the necessary water applications in the only natural way, as soon as they will allow light and air to regulate the movements of the organs of digestion and act upon the whole system, as soon as they will allow the terrestrial current to run through the body and as soon as they will follow their own natural instinct in regard to the selection of their food, men will be better, wiser and healthier. Cures will be more effectful than now, for they will be natural. There is only one sickness and one remedy. Men's desertion of nature caused all diseases whatever they may be, consequently there is only one remedy the return to nature which will heal all ailments, as long as there is strength enough left in the body to assist nature. No understanding is left to men in what close coherence body and soul are. As soon as the body is freed from all ailments the soul becomes free too, and no more vices will torment body and soul. Men will enjoy the greatest and true happiness.

It may sound strange to men that a natural treatment of diseases should be followed by such great and beneficial results. It may sound like imaginations, but no human tongue is able to describe the joys God has prepared for those who follow his or nature's laws for nature is God's creation. But nevertheless, when in the spring time the sun sends its warm rays through the atmosphere, giving light and life to all beings, when high up in the azure blue of the sky the lark sings its sweetest songs, when the nightingale in the rosebush sends its melodies direct to our heart, when in forest and field millions and millions of flowers greet us, when the deer with elegance and ease takes all hindrances, when everything in nature's wide, wide kingdom is healthy, beautiful and happy, then the anticipation of the true happiness of a natural mode of living overcomes the sickly poor wretch called man.

Many peoples claiming a certain kind of civilization have disappeared.

May be the time has not come yet for men to be truly happy. Never before in the history of men we have heard of so many and so earnest labors to bringing men back to nature.

To-day the majority of men believe in artificial means of healing, but we fully believe that practical physicians who would like to help suffering humanity and who have been often enough disappointed by these artificial remedies know very well that only nature can cure. It is in many and many cases not so much the fault of the physician who most always knows better but the fault of the patient who wants prescriptions and medicines to satisfy his own self. As soon as people in general will demand that physicians must resort to natural means of healing only they will do so and we are sure will do so with great delight.

We cannot conclude this item without giving space to the wording of the testimonial of Dr. Santaetsrath (member of a German Board of Health). C. Franke recommended Ad. Just's Jungborn to the German government which is strict in all matter pertaining to the health of its subjects. Dr. Franke wrote:

> Since thousands of years it is a fact known to medical science that light, air, water and a well regulated fruit-diet are the most important factors of healing which are at the disposal of men. Most every physician uses water and certain forms of diet as means of healing, but for centuries men in general as well as physicians forgot the value of these natural means of healing until Vincenz Priessnitz and Sebastian Kneipp aroused humanity by their wonderful cures.
>
> Pure air is only known and valued by the rich of to-day, I am sorry to say who only are in the position to leave the cities for a certain length of time every year and refresh body and soul in the pure mountain air. If one visits the sleeping apartments of the poor one is impressed by the fact that they have to do without this *pabulum vitae* this "life food" commonly called pure air.
>
> The influence of light and air are very little used now-a-days as healing factors in opposition to the ways of the ancient Greek who not only were far advanced in the arts but made ample use of these natural means of healing. I must say that this is so to the direct loss of all suffers, for the important part which the organs of respiration have to perform in most every power of healing is known too well.
>
> As every one of these factors of natural healing in itself is sure to bring about beneficial results, it will be easily understood that the success must be a real great one when all of them are brought into action. The beneficial result of an united action of light, air and water upon the human system was experienced by Mr. Just personally who suffered from nervousness and weakness for years. His system has made a strong healthy man out of him and it is his wish to give the benefit of his experience to his fellow-men who have to suffer because they do not know how to heal their ailments.

Mr. Just has selected a place well fitted to all requirements of his system and if he is not hampered with I am sure that his sanitarium will become a blessing to suffering humanity and will serve as a means to demonstrate to all classes the value of light, air and water as healing factors.

The science of natural healing has been studied by many and even by medical men who have come to the conclusion that all healing is done by nature and that science can only assist nature.

Men's organs, especially the organs of digestion were prepared to digest only such food as nature had destined for men, that is such foods which were spontaneously produced by nature for men.

Men and animals are according to Just nothing but moving plants, plants which in consequence of a higher development were able to free themselves from the ground. But all the same they receive their strength and refreshment from the ground.

Since thousands of years it is a fact known to medical science that light, air, water and a well regulated fruit-diet are the most important factors of healing which are at the disposal of men.

The Kneipp Cure, II

by Benedict Lust

The Kneipp Water Cure Monthly, I(9), 148-149. (1900)

As Father Kneipp never examined a patient by auscultation or percussion, and yet achieved such remarkable results in the cure of diseases, it is worthwhile to enquire how he arrived at his diagnoses, and yet arranged his plans for treatment.

1. His first look at a patient, which, owing to the number of sufferers whom he had to look at, was a very keen one—generally enabled him to form an opinion of the case. If the individual was pale and thin, he concluded that his blood was poor and of bad quality, and that he lacked natural warmth. His first object then was to stimulate their appetite and circulation, which he accomplished for the most part by partial washings or affusions; local applications and packs being in such cases inappropriate. If the lack of natural warmth was very marked, cold applications were preceded by warm ones, such as steaming of that part of the body which was immediately afterward to receive a cold affusion. As a consequence of the improved appetite and circulation which followed that treatment, the supply of blood and natural warmth were increased, and the whole system was roused to greater action

2. In the case of corpulent persons, his attention was directed to augmenting the excretions; an object which must be pursued with caution if the heart of the patient is affected, as is frequently the case in corpulency in a greater or less degree. Although the physician rejects water entirely in cases of heart complaint, Kneipp was of a wholly opposite opinion. He said to himself: "A well-ordered circulation is beneficial to the sufferer from heart complaint, and that can only be attained by the proper employment of water. By knee, thigh and back affusions, for instance, the blood is drawn downward from the weak heart, which is thereby entirely relieved. At the same time the warmth of the blood is better distributed, and the natural strength of the patient is increased, so that it becomes impossible to proceed to upper, or even full affusions."

3. Out of every hundred persons ninety are nervous. Therefore must be graduations of treatment in every case. With most patients, the mild applications come first; a beginning being made with the feet; walking bare-footed in the house, or street when the sun shines. In that way the circulation of the blood in the feet is enlivened, and it is then possible to proceed with the stronger applications. When nervous pains and spasms

call for relief, warm applications are prescribed. In some diseases, pain may be actually caused by the first stages of the cure; but these are but signs of returning health, for it is not to be expected that a circulation which has been irregular for years can be brought into good order without a slight revolution, of which such pains are the best proof. In this way the slight attacks of cough, or pain in the back increase, or cessation of the regular functions, may occur at the beginning of the cure. All such symptoms are, as a rule, so many proofs that the patient will certainly recover. Indeed, if they are altogether absent in chronic cases, the course of the cure is general unsatisfactory, from the want in the patient of the reactive force required for the healing process. It is to be regretted that some invalids allow themselves to be frightened by these symptoms into changing their method of treatment for some other which removes them still further from the desired goal of recovery. Upon such and similar natural and reasonable grounds Kneipp based his plans of treatment.

Sad to say, it was not permitted to the great Samaritan at Woerishofen to continue his work as long as—in the interest of the spread of his doctrine of the Natural Method of Healing, and of suffering humanity could have been desired. A malignant malady, an insidious formation on the bladder, carried off the hale and vigorous old man in the course of six months. He died on the 17th of June, 1897, deeply mourned by the many thousands whom he had succoured, as well as by all friends and followers of the natural healing art.

Honor to his memory!

FUNDAMENTAL RULES

The following are fundamental rules and maxims which should be born in mind in the application of the Kneipp affusions, bath, etc.

The shorter the application the better its effect.

The colder the water, the shorter must be the time of its employment; and the greater will the reaction be. Weak patients must, nevertheless, begin with water of a moderate temperature; at first 66°, cooler after a time, down to 59° and 55°, and at last quite cold. The body must be as warm as possible before the application of cold water. If there is a lack of natural warmth, the first applications must be warm.

There should be no drying of the body by artificial means, after the use of water; but the clothes should be put on quickly, and, in order to help [assist a] reaction, exercise should be taken, rapidly at first and slower by degrees. If there is no reaction, or if the patient is very weak, the warmth of bed should be sought.

Hardening the body is the best means of preserving the general health, and of protection against attacks of disease.

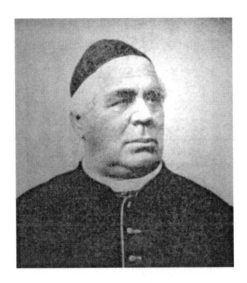

Father Sebastian Kniepp.

As Father Kneipp never examined a patient by auscultation or percussion, and yet achieved such remarkable results in the cure of diseases, it is worthwhile to enquire how he arrived at his diagnoses, and yet arranged his plans for treatment.

In some diseases, pain may be actually caused by the first stages of the cure; but these are but signs of returning health.

The colder the water, the shorter must be the time of its employment; and the greater will the reaction be.

DECLARATION OF PRINCIPLES

by Benedict Lust
The Kneipp Water Cure Monthly, (1900), 1(11), 193.

We believe in the universe and in its laws.

We affirm it to be the part of wisdom not to attempt to change those laws, but rather to investigate and obey them.

We know that by and through obedience to the laws of nature, we find our only salvation from disease, weakness, poverty and degradation.

We declare that the enlightened reason and the educated conscience are our highest guides; and that it is our duty to follow and practice righteousness.

We affirm that all men are equal in the right to think, to speak, to labor and to live; and that it behooves us, as members of the common brotherhood, to do our utmost for the promotion of the general welfare.

We know that selfishness and hate are wrong and degrading; and that we are both happier and nobler when we live for the higher ideals of justice and good-will.

We believe that it is our duty, as rational beings, to do what we can to secure the peaceable overthrow of superstition and the establishment in its stead of the reason which is the surest guide to, and guarantee of, the blessings of true civilization.

1901

How To Protect Oneself Against Disease And Illness
F. E. Bilz

Return To Nature
Adolf Just

THE BILZ BOOK

A Golden Guide to Health, Strength, Happiness and Old Age

A COUNSELLOR TO THE SICK—A GUIDE TO THE HEALTHY

25 Gold Medals and Diplomas. Translated into 18 different languages. Enormous sale of nearly 3,000,000 copies

These are the strongest arguments in Favor of the Bilz Book

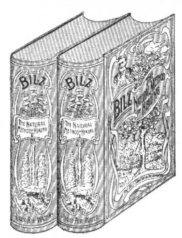

HEALTH IS WEALTH

The BILZ BOOK is the greatest Encyclopædia, which shows you the only correct and reasonable way of treating all Diseases at *Home without Medicine*, and teaches in the clearest possible manner how you can *protect yourself* and your family *against Disease*. If you are thoroughly healthy, you are able to work and earn money whereby to maintain and keep yourself, your wife and children in Happiness and Comfort, but if you—the Breadwinner—become ill, *your Family is then in danger of* starving and becoming ill also.

Sorrow, disease, distress, pain and grief then reign in your Family, instead of Happiness, Joy and Health, and the danger for the Family becomes more serious, when the Breadwinner's illness gets worse and worse, and his state at the end hopeless.

You can ward off this misery and terror from you and your Family if you live in accordance with the rules of the great BILZ DOCTOR BOOK.

NATURE, THE GREAT HEALER

All diseases may be cured by natural self treatment

The Famous BILZ BOOK

Exhaustively and exclusively describes the wonderful methods developed and inaugurated by the celebrated F. E. BILZ of the famous Bilz Sanatorium

What the Bilz Book Teaches

The Bilz Book scarcely needs an introduction to the American public, for its fame in many lands has caused it to be widely spoken of here.

The Bilz Book teaches no complicated doctrine —no intricate formula—it simply consists of a wise, thoughtful and lucid expression of the Natural Method of Healing, so successfully practised for so many years by the eminent F. E. BILZ.

The adherents of this method of healing number millions—high and low, rich and poor. It is efficacious for all—economical for all. It teaches you how to utilize God's good gifts for your preservation and health. *The Ingredients are free*—the advantages open to all.

The Bilz Book is a wonderful compilation of over 2,000 pages. It describes minutely the best method of cure for every disease and ailment of humanity. *The Bilz Book is the Doctor in the Home.* You simply turn to its pages, and then, as thousands of others have done, you cure yourself.

The greatest tribute to this treatment lies in the fact that many eminent medical men treat their patients according to its methods. *With the aid of the Bilz Book you can treat yourself.*

Advertisement for Friedrich Eduard Bilz's book, *Natural Method of Healing*.

How To Protect Oneself Against Disease And Illness

by F. E. Bilz

The Kneipp Water Cure Monthly, II(5), 131-134. (1901)

Of all laws, regulations or rules, the law of life, how to live, in order to preserve health, is that which everyone should hold to be the most serious and sacred,—the one which should be the most punctually observed. In it the happiness or unhappiness of mankind roots and culminates. Wealth and possession, reputation and honor, all these gifts of fortune are equally insipid to the sick man. A disconsolate, painful condition of mind and body smothers every joy and nips every hope of pleasure in the bud. Be it therefore accepted as an axiom, that the first and most earnest endeavor of each one of us should be to keep the body, and so also the mind (for sound, fresh intellect can abide only in a sound body), as healthy as possible. At present, that duty does not appear to be admitted, for if we look around us at mankind today, we find, unhappily, the reverse. Men begin to take thought for themselves, and to adopt a more reasonable and natural regimen, only when it is too late, and when they have fallen victims to their unnatural mode of life.

The great and grievous offences which people commit against themselves and their health, and to which the numerous diseases of the present generations are traceable, are mainly due to the following:

First, present conditions do not permit a man to enjoy his natural and full measure of health, because they never give him the opportunity of learning precisely how he ought to live, in order to keep his health.

Secondly, the material condition of individuals is generally so unfavorable that it is impossible for them to keep their health; sometimes because of work of an over-fatiguing kind carried on too long, and perhaps in vitiated air, as is so frequently the case in our industrial establishments; sometimes because of poverty and destitution.

Thirdly, the great indifference and carelessness which prevails and which is the principal cause of all.

It is always, however, the unfavorable circumstances of each individual, which have made and kept him indifferent to a question of such high importance.

Let us examine the causes of the numerous diseases, or of the unhealthiness of the human race, more closely. Let us look first at the living, sleeping, and work-rooms, in order to discover whether that most precious and necessary of human possessions, healthy air, is there to be had. What a shudder passes through us, as we find the air everywhere impure, often thoroughly vitiated. In bedrooms, for instance, in which four or even more people sleep, and which are scarcely large enough to contain the beds and other furniture, not a window will be opened the whole night through, although the whole of the oxygen is consumed in a few hours. Yet more—many people will not once open a window in the daytime, and when anyone accustomed to and fond of fresh air enters such a bedroom, the choking atmosphere literally throws him back. It is not only necessary that a window should be kept open, but a means of ventilation for carrying off the vitiated air should be provided, in order to make room for pure air to come in.

The state of things in living-rooms and in work-rooms appears to be almost as bad. It may, therefore, be taken for granted that the greater number of modern diseases are thus engendered. It may be assumed with equal certainty that until adequate ventilation in living, sleeping, and work-rooms is secured by legislation—until it is universally understood that fresh air is not injurious to sleepers—until, in fact, legislation compels the supply of fresh air alike to the sleeping and to the waking,—and until everyone feels the absolute necessity of open-air exercise for several hours daily, the race will remain unhealthy, and die premature and unnatural deaths.

SLEEPING WITH A WINDOW OPEN

This is of the greatest importance because the breathing is most regular and deep during sleep, and consequently the air, which surrounds a sleeper, is the most utilized. If people cannot bear sleeping with a window open, they must learn to bear it. This can be managed in the following way: If you are an enlightened person and free from all prejudice as to fresh air being injurious to a sleeper, open a part of the window, and do so, even if the air blows directly in upon you. As a precaution on the first night, tie a cloth or handkerchief round your neck. If you are very delicate, open the window only a little at first, and then more and more on succeeding evenings, or move your couch near and nearer to the window. If your unnatural mode of life has so thoroughly disused you to fresh air that you cannot bear a breath of it, and consequently you get a swollen cheek or an inflamed throat, or find it difficult to swallow, do not be down-hearted,—the small trouble can be set right before nightfall if you employ natural means to that end. You may afterwards adopt precautions, but never leave off observing this beneficent rule of life, for you must learn to bear the effect of fresh air by night as well as by day. Fresh air is worth more than money. Pure air and cold water, these two indispensable gifts are essentially necessary for the physical welfare of man, and should be supplied without stint even to the poorest, if they appreciate and respect it. Mankind seems at present to value those possessions only which can be bought with money.

Food and drink also have as great an influence on human health as fresh air, but before the present generation can and will cease from the many misuses and excesses which are indulged in, in this department of human economy, they must be taught clearly what foods and beverages are suitable and what are injurious to man. Most men are, unfortunately, quite in the dark on this subject, without expert knowledge and full of mistaken prejudices. People could very often secure for themselves far greater enjoyment and nourish their bodies better than they now do and that at the same or even less cost. The simple rule of varying the diet, and of preparing only just so much food as is required for a meal, will secure both enjoyment and economy.

In this regard, I consider it absolutely necessary that full and clear instruction on this highly important subject should be given to all classes, even to school-children. All the instruction at present given in the schools is entirely fruitless, so long as no attention is paid to the solution of such highly important questions as these—how a man should live, what he should eat and drink, how he should sleep and clothe himself, in what manner and by what means the adult and the child alike may harden the constitution, how long they should take exercise in the open air, how necessary are baths, gymnastics, swimming, leaping, etc., in order that health may be preserved. I cannot help thinking that our legislation leaves much to be desired, in that it takes no account, or insufficient account of such momentous questions.

"Man is the product of his circumstances," that is the theme of the first part of my other book, *The Solution of the Social Question.* The present generation is, in the same sense, the product of existing conditions or existing want of rightful conditions, and is indeed still uninstructed in the most essential principles of human economy—is not trusted with them. Let us try, then, to enlighten mankind on this subject, and to ensure for all fairly suitable conditions of life; due efforts will then be made to escape out of the darkness.

THE IMPORTANCE OF TRANQUIL SLEEP

Fresh air and natural diet are not the only essential conditions of health. There are others, for instance, regular and deep sleep. In this respect the greatest regularity should be observed. Everyone should retire to rest at a fixed hour on all days alike (the animals, guided by instinct, do so), and all the surroundings of the sleeper be quiet and undisturbed, as if themselves in slumber, as wood and field, birds and other creatures sleep. If men will follow all the other rules and indications which hygienic science puts before them for observance, they will no longer toss about for hours before they can go to sleep, as so often happens now, when on getting up in the morning they find themselves more worn out than they felt when they went to bed the night before.

Under present circumstances—when, on Sundays and holidays, noises, music and singing continue through half the night, if not all night, or when, before and after midnight, wheeled traffic prevents sleep—a proper night's rest is not to be had, and one is inclined then to shut the window and breathe impure air rather than to suffer from disturbed sleep. The proposals put forward in my book provide for all men having sufficient time for their pleasures and business during the day. The people who have lived to the greatest age and kept their health have always observed regular hours of sleep as one of their ordinary rules of life.

The crying of children, which so often disturbs the sleep of their elders, would be less often heard under such improved conditions as I advocate, because the children would be more healthy, owing to their being more naturally brought up. Further, instead of worry and anxiety, a man should have only joy and peace of mind,—that and much more is necessary to him in order that he may keep his health.

WHEN, HOW, AND WHAT SHALL A MAN EAT AND DRINK?

On this question I wish to make a few remarks.

1. As to "when" he shall eat. He will do his best to eat three times a day, in order to give the stomach rest between whiles.* His evening meal should not be too late or too abundant, because the nerves of the stomach and brain are in close connection, and if the stomach is not at rest the brain will also be kept in activity; thus the rest will be disturbed by dreams, and consequently less strengthening than it ought to be. The same disturbing effect will be produced if the mind is overstrained by work shortly before bedtime, by reading or hard thinking, discussions, political business, etc. Mental excitement of that kind draws an excessive supply of blood to the brain, and the sleep will be rendered less refreshing by disturbing dreams.

2. "How" shall a man eat? The chief thing is to masticate the food properly, for two reasons: First, because in the process of digestion that most important element, the saliva, should be properly mixed with the food; and secondly, because the teeth must do their part in grinding the food finely before it is passed on to the stomach. Only in that way can the food be reduced, in the stomach, to the required consistency of pulp (chime), in which it should leave that organ. In order to be able to supply the stomach with food in a properly comminuted state, one must have good teeth, a condition which is too seldom fulfilled in the present generation.

---

* Whiles is a common 19th century word meaning while.

If the teeth are to be kept sound, they must be frequently cleaned, and neither food nor drink should be taken hot. Taking food or drink hot spoils the teeth, and is extremely injurious to the gullet and stomach. People should be most particular not to take warm and cold food or drink directly after one another, as by doing so they will very soon destroy the enamel of the teeth (their natural protective coating), and the teeth will then certainly decay. Soup and soft food should be taken only in moderate quantity: bread should not be softened, but eaten rather hard. The teeth are there for the purpose of chewing, and they should be made to do their work. Teeth which are not allowed to do their work will go bad.

It may be remarked here that, under favorable circumstances, the teeth may be kept sound to the very end of life. It has been proved that diseases of the teeth, like other forms of disease, are transmitted and inherited through some taint in the juices of the body, and that, consequently, they cannot be completely cured in one generation. It may be held with equal certainty that toothache will no longer be known when people come to have a sound mixture of the alimentary fluids, and therefore, a sound set of teeth. Among the animals, which live in a state of nature, we scarcely ever find diseased teeth as we find them among mankind.

Further, there is an old proverb. "When the food tastes best, leave off eating"—("Always leave off hungry"). That precept contains much wisdom, and is well worth attention in relation to the present unnatural conditions. From a purely natural point of view, the precept may appear superfluous, since it is not to be believed that nature, otherwise so wise in her arrangements, would give human beings the appetite for more food and drink than their organism requires or can bear without discomfort. If today it be unfortunately true that human beings have an abnormal appetite, and therefore consume a greater quantity of food than the organism can bear, we must regard that state of things as against nature, and not as due to her economy. If we watch birds and other animals, we shall never observe that they suffer discomfort after a meal, even though it be a full one.

In spite of the prevailing prejudice against going to rest with a full stomach, I advise everyone, who can do so, to lie down at full length for half or three-quarters of an hour after the principal meal of the day, because when the limbs are at rest, the circulation of the blood is more fully at the disposal of the stomach, which can then better fulfill its digestive functions. I also strongly recommend the practice of taking a few deep breaths in the garden or open air after the meal, in order that the blood may be adequately supplied with oxygen, which is very necessary to digestion.

3. "What" shall a man eat and drink? In the main that which is easily digestible and free from all injurious constituents. Thus only can he continue in really sound health. Among non-injurious, easily digestible foods are to be classed all the fruits, which the earth produces and ripens, e.g., wheat, from which the nutritious and palatable whole-meal bread is made. Whole-meal bread, made of wheat or rye, is nutritious and wholesome for human beings, because the bran contains the gluten which lies immediately under the husk of the corn, and which, in addition to its other beneficial qualities, is highly phosphoric. Phosphorus is of great importance, particularly for the brain. "Without phosphorus there would be no thought," writes Moleschott. That principal foodstuff, the gluten, must not be eliminated from the flour; it is especially indispensable for the body and for the mind.

It is a matter for serious complaint that so important an aliment as whole-meal wheaten bread is not universally known. Vegetables, green and leguminous, potatoes, etc., should also be eaten. I recommend fruits and berries as most particularly necessary to man; if, in these days of overstrained exertion, they are not sufficient of themselves to keep the body in full strength, it is by no means proved that they did not, in primeval times, form the only food of man. Our primeval ancestors lived in warmer and more fertile lands than ours, where fruits are found to this day—such as bread-fruit, dates, melons, figs, etc.—on which mankind lived exclusively. The over-exertion of the present day is unnatural and self-imposed. The law of nature demands only half the amount of work, and, consequently, food less solid and less rich in nutritive material. The professional "fasters"—Dr. Tanner, Succi, and others—have shown us that a human being requires very little nourishment, in order to exist. Fruit should come on the table every day because of its refreshing and health-giving properties. How a sufficient supply of fruit is obtained is shown in my book, *The Solution of the Social Question.*

I come now to speak of meat, and my first word must be, to beg everyone to regard it only as an auxiliary or supplementary article of diet. Meat is stimulating and, therefore, injurious to the system. The fact that is forbidden by doctors to fever patients should lead to the conclusion that it is a food of a character which cannot be entirely commended. Nourishment which is injurious to the sick must also be more injurious than useful to the healthy, although the latter do not at once discover its advantages. The nutritive value, also, of meat is far less than is commonly supposed, there being more nutritive material in a pound of whole-meal bread, made of wheat or other cereals, or in a pound of leguminous seeds, than in a pound of beef.

Very mistaken notions prevail on this point. Most people think that, if they want to maintain their health and strength, they must consume a great deal of meat—the only food, they believe, capable of keeping their vital force up to the mark.

The excessive use of meat is, therefore, much to be deprecated. Natural foods, on the other hands, fully and entirely satisfy the sense of taste, produce a feeling of comfort, gratify mankind, and make them strong and vigorous in body and mind. The contrary is the case with the non-natural foods and beverages and rejuvenating process, puts on new life and excites our admiration, so the natural foods exercise a refreshing and re-animating influence and charm upon the human organism, and are not followed by reaction, as is the case with beer, spirits, coffee, tea, meat, and tobacco.

Spices stimulate the stomach powerfully to increased activity, and unless the quantity used is increased, the organs in question become visibly relaxed. The more and the longer people indulge in unnatural enjoyments or dainties of this kind, the more unnatural will they become in body and mind. Is it then to be wondered at when a sudden change from a non-natural to a natural diet does not at once suit the body? Once must also remember in such cases the power of habit.

An experience of discomfort of shorter or longer duration, but certain to pass off, will be followed, if a natural mode of life be perseveringly carried out, by a state of physical health which the individual has, perhaps, never before known.

Spices, as above stated, are injurious; therefore, I advise everyone to be as sparing as possible in the use of them. He who has accustomed himself to highly-spiced and salted dishes or foods, has not done well or wisely for himself, and had better lay aside the bad habit. Non-irritating eatables are as palatable to people who are accustomed to them as sharply pungent preparations of food to those who indulge in such things. Every product of the earth is provided by nature with its own savor,—fruit, berries of various kinds, potatoes, the cereals and other products of the soil, for instance; then water, milk, etc., ... all can be enjoyed by man without seasoning of any kind. Only a modern use in the preparation of foods and drinks has made the addition of spices and seasoning necessary.

If I now proceed to answer the questions, "What should people drink?"—the reader will not expect me to recommend to him anything which will do him harm. My object is not to rid people by force of the many failings and bad habits which, by degrees, have become their pet propensities, but to save others from falling into similar ways. Those who will not or cannot leave off injurious habits, in spite of the clearest proofs of their harmfulness, must carry them to the grave. My wish is to guard and save their children.

First and foremost, I cannot recommend beer, spirits, wines, coffee, Chinese (or Indian) tea, etc. If these cannot be altogether avoided under existing circumstances, their use should be restricted within the narrowest possible limits. The drink most suitable is fresh spring water, and of that one may drink almost more than is required to quench the thirst. If people cannot bear cold water in its natural state, they are sick, and will continue to be so until cold water comes to agree with them. If people would learn how to make it agree with them, let them proceed as follows: At first drink only a little, about as much as a doctor would prescribe if it were medicine; that is to say, a spoonful every hour, in order that the stomach may warm it; otherwise its effect, instead of being beneficial, will be injurious. By degrees the quantity should be increased, until an ordinary draught of cold water can be taken without inconvenience. People with whom cold water and fresh air do not agree are dried-up plants.

[This article is an excerpt taken from F. E. Bilz's *The Natural Method of Healing.* —Ed.]

From a purely natural point of view, the precept may appear superfluous, since it is not to be believed that nature, otherwise so wise in her arrangements, would give human beings the appetite for more food and drink than their organism requires or can bear without discomfort.

Return To Nature
Jungborn, Stapelburg, Harz, Germany

by Adolf Just

Translated from the German by B. Lust
The Kneipp Water Cure Monthly, II(10), 264-267. (1901)

II. The Voices Of Nature

The more man sets his face again towards nature, the more his conscience and instinct will re-awaken within him, and the more acute will his organs of sense become. He is still surrounded by many happy creatures; children and especially animals, who have preserved these higher guides of life and from whom he can learn the true course in all emergencies.

If man, therefore, has gained sufficient power of resistance to the seductions of science, he may easily be led by the hand of nature, and will then surely soon recover health and true happiness. He will no longer be tossed about upon the ocean of life, like a ship without a rudder, destined to be dashed to pieces against rocks and reefs.

The Jungborn

When, after a long, long search I came from error to truth, from night to light, from disease to health, I was seized by a great desire to impart my experiences to my fellowmen and to let them profit by them.

I determined to place the strength and vigor which I had but just regained, entirely at the disposal of the great cause. I resolved to become the champion of nature, to work for her, and to point out the right way which will lead men from dreaded night to joyous light, to true health and complete happiness—those purblind and deluded men who no longer understand nature and who abuse her marvelous goodness to their own destruction. The mere thought of devoting my life entirely to nature and her great truths was indeed blessedness.

I soon began to write this book.

But I also founded the place called Jungborn, in the Harz, between Isenburg and Hartzburg. This is, first of all, a model institution for the true natural life, where those who with to make arrangements for such a life at home in their own gardens can find the pattern. It was also meant to show, from the start, how the most intimate communion with nature can be re-established, and at the same time to demonstrate in practice how easy and what a blessing such communion is.

In the meantime the Jungborn has fulfilled its purpose completely.

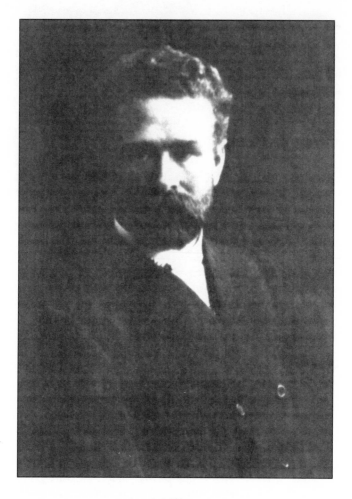

Adolf Just.

After its pattern many have already made the requisite arrangements in their own homes or gardens.

Other similar institutions are coming into life.

The Jungborn has now also practically demonstrated the correctness of the return to nature method, and its significance for the welfare and salvation of man.

For the rest it has always been my aim to show how we can lead a natural life at home, under ordinary circumstances, and establish a relationship with nature, for in this way alone can my book be of service to the masses.

It was necessary to mention the Jungborn here, as I shall have occasion to refer to it.

A detailed description of the Jungborn and its arrangements will be found at the end of this volume.

THE NATURAL BATH

Within the last century great and gifted men have taken up the nature cure method. Their genius led them to the ways of nature. Priessnitz, Schroth, Graham, Rausse, Rikli, Kneipp, Kuhne, Densmore, Trall and others have already achieved great things, and have won for themselves immortal honor, for from darkness they penetrated into light.

But these men have by no means been fully and clearly conscious that they must allow instinct alone to lead them, and they have not strictly and carefully followed the other voices of nature, which I have often mentioned. They have not sufficiently studied the ways of children and animals, those beings who still possess the true guides of life in a higher degree than the adults of modern civilization. They have considered with sufficient care many of the contrivances and intentions of nature. Therefore their systems and teachings have not been perfect, they have contained mistakes and errors. The systems have now partly been forgotten, and in the course of time will be entirely swallowed up in the seat of oblivion.

After mankind had deviated from nature for thousands and thousands of years, it is very evident that they can only gradually regain a true insight as to which are their duties toward nature and her laws.

All the men who have hitherto built up the nature cure methods are deserving of our highest praise. We must by no means heap reproaches upon them and accuse them, because their systems are faulty and because they did not yet reach a complete natural method.

The nature cure method has evidently inspired the most serious and largest movement that civilized mankind has yet seen. It concerns itself with the health of the individual, that greatest of worldly possessions upon which such an infinite amount of well-being and happiness depends, and which is the only possible safety and redemption from all misery and evils—from final ruin. Therefore we may not remain silent or conceal anything concerning any person, but must above all things keep our eye upon the great cause, and subjugate everything, every other interest and every person to this cause.

From this point of view I shall not hesitate to uncover the mistakes of former nature cure methods, of the old vegetarianism, etc. But in doing so I do not wish to hurt any one.

I shall now advance a mode of life and a curative system which has nothing whatever to do with science, and in which we allow ourselves to be guided, as I have frequently stated before, by the great teacher "nature," alone. Thus at last a beautiful, bright morning sun will rise from dark chaos, which mankind will greet with joy.

We now have a simple nature-cure system, as simple as the great teacher, nature, herself. This nature-cure system is the same for all diseases, and all cases, even as the origin of all diseases has but one cause, an unnatural mode of life, and there exists a unity in all the laws of nature and in all her manifestations. All the former nature-cure methods will gradually dissolve in this one true nature system.

In this method there is nothing to be learned in the usual sense of the word, every one who has but freed himself from the spell of modern wisdom and science can apply it. Through it men become free from all dependency and slavery to the entire fraternity of physicians, doctors of medicine as well as nature doctors.

Nature does not err, therefore in her the errors and contradictions which are now keeping so many away from the nature-cure methods, do not exist.

The invalid who allows himself to be guided entirely by the hand of nature is led gently, without severity and distressing deprivations, much more gently, and more pleasantly, quickly, and more surely than by the former nature-cure methods, back to health, strength, and vital energy unto a fresh, green meadow full of flowers and sunshine. And above all, the severest and most desperate diseases, in the presence of which the ordinary nature doctor is helpless, loosen their grip and drop off before Nature.

The true nature-cure system penetrates with its healing power into the innermost recesses of the mind and soul. Dark veils are lifted from the mind; even the soul participates in the healing balm. Man is released from vice and crime, hatred, envy, and malevolence. Peace, joy, brotherly love, happiness once more take up their abode in the breasts of the unhappy beings of to-day.

Now at last the morning of a new spring dawns for humanity; paradise is regained.

As I have said before, I once fled from the error and confusion, the strife and dissensions of man to nature. Here alone I found rest, peace, and truth.

When in the present century mankind instinctively turned their faces once more toward nature, it became evident to them that all diseases had their origin in impure matter in the blood, in the body,—in disease or foreign matter. On the basis of this correct discernment people, in treating the sick, soon refrained from exercising the devil with Beelzebub by introducing more foreign matter and poison into the body, as medical science does by drugs, medicines, etc. They sought rather to cleanse the sick body of its foreign matter, and that, indeed, with but one natural remedy, with water.

In this respect the peasant Vincent Priessnitz was the pioneer. He is therefore to be considered as the real founder of the present nature-cure method.

The nature-cure method was in the beginning only a water-cure method, and only water-cure institutions were at first established.

Therefore it was my first endeavor to obtain from nature herself directions for the right use of water applications.

In my endeavors I did not observe that an inner voice directed me to a special use of water—namely the instinct.

But I learned from foresters that the animals of free nature which follow only their instinct, take a bath according to definite rules.

I began to observe them and reached the following conclusions:

The natural bath does not consist in jumping into the river and taking a full bath. **The Full Bath Taken In The River Or In The Bath Tub Is Contrary To Nature.**

Land animals not only take no full baths, they are actually afraid of them. One need only to throw an animal (especially a monkey) into the water and see how eagerly it makes for the shore. To other water applications also animals submit only under compulsion and most unwillingly.[1]

On the other hand, the higher land animals (mammalia), especially wild boars and deer, in free nature (in the forest), are in the habit of lying down in small muddy swamps or pools, at first only with the abdomen, and rubbing it to and fro in the mud.

Hereupon the animals rise and generally sit for awhile with their posterior, their anus, in the mud. After awhile they roll in the mud for a moment with their whole body, and then rub themselves against the earth, trees, and other objects. Hunters call this bathing of the animals "wallowing".

The birds, on the other hand, go to brooks or springs, and by immersing their necks throw water over their bodies by means of the hollow that is formed between the neck and the trunk, and by splashing themselves with their wings. Then they rub or scrub their body with their head and bill and their wing-elbows, if I may so call the wing joint which corresponds to the human elbow.

It has always been vainly asked why it is, for instance, that the stag, the king of our forests, this beautiful, otherwise so cleanly animal, that carefully avoids soiling his lair, and in many other respects shows himself most cleanly, can lie down in such muddy water to bath, while birds will bath only in clear water.

I am of the opinion that mammals bathe in the mud only because they can thus rub and scrub the abdomen and the sexual organs, which they could not do in clear running water with a hard bottom.

Birds, on the other hand, because they are built differently and can rub themselves with several limbs, do not require the mud for the purpose of rubbing and scrubbing.

The explanation that the mud is required because it enables the mammals to rub themselves, is considered a most plausible one by all foresters, too.

We see, then, that the more highly developed animals bathe.[2]

The roe, the chamois, etc., do not bathe, probably because these species have been placed by nature upon high mountainous and rocky regions where water is not always to be had. Neither do beasts of prey bathe. It is likewise quite evident why they do not bathe. The bath has a quieting influence, but beasts of prey cannot allow themselves to be quieted, they must be bloodthirsty and wild, their place in nature requires it, otherwise they would lack the incentive and the capacity to win their prey. It is the meat diet that develops these bloodthirsty cravings.[3]

There is no reason, however, why man, the highest creature, should not bathe. It must rather be assumed that nature prescribes a bath for the preservation and strengthening of his highest physical and spiritual powers.

Men have, indeed, always had an instinctive longing for baths, and even if the inner voice no longer plainly indicates the right kind of bath, every one still feels a need to cool the abdomen, the anus, and the sexual organs by means of water.

Thus we see that animals bathe in different ways according to the construction of their bodies. Mammals take their baths in a different way than birds.

Now whoever has carefully watched animals at their bath and has observed the pains they take to rub or cool the sexual organs in the mud (or water), easily takes the hint of nature and comes to see what the natural bath for man ought to be, especially when he attempts to take a bath in the open air where no artificial apparatus or other aids are to be found.

I shall now proceed to describe the natural bath. Since most people must, for the present, take their bath in a room, and have not always an opportunity to bathe in the open air they must naturally have a basin or tub. It may be any sort of basin or but in which a person can comfortably sit with his knees drawn up.

The following cuts show tubs that can now be procured in the market.

The bather sits down in the tub which contains naturally cold water, about three and a half inches (8 cm.) deep, so that the seat, the feet,

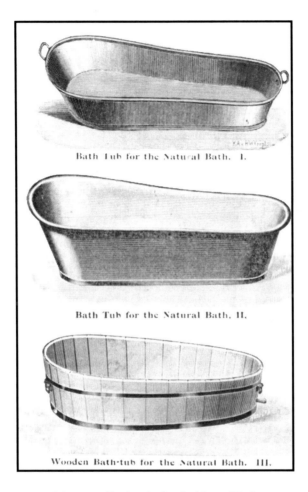

Bath Tub for the Natural Bath. I.

Bath Tub for the Natural Bath. II.

Wooden Bath-tub for the Natural Bath. III.

Selection of bath-tubs for the Natural Bath.

and the sexual organs are for the most part in the water. Only the seat and the feet touch the bottom of the tub, while the knees are quite aways above the water.

The knees are now spread apart, and the water is vigorously dashed over the abdomen with the hollow of the hand. The throwing of the water is flowed by a brisk rubbing of the abdomen in the middle, on both sides, and all over with one or both hands. After this alternating process has been carried on awhile, the woman rubs the region of the groins and the external part of the sexual organs with the open hand under water (the sexual organs are supposed to be submerged). The man also rubs the region of the groins, the testicles, and the dam (the region between the sexual organs and the anus) with the open hand, under water. Hereupon the entire body is rapidly washed with the bare hands. A second person can assist in rapidly washing the body. Then the body is rubbed with the bare open hands (not with a towel or flesh-brush) until it is completely dry. The body ought never to be dried with a towel after a bath. The rubbing with the hands can be done by the bather himself. This is at the same time a beneficial bodily exercise. But the rubbing can also be done profitably by a second person. I shall return to this further on.[4]

Notes

1. Individual exceptions which occur among domestic animals that already lead unnatural lives, prove nothing to the contrary.
2. It cannot be called a bath if our domestic dog goes into the water on a very warm day.
3. It is easy to see how beasts become bloodthirsty through a meat diet.
4. The bath of the sexual organs, after the manner indicated, is very important, especially for woman; it is especially effective and healing in cases of sexual excitement and irritation.

The more man sets his face again towards nature, the more his conscience and instinct will re-awaken within him, and the more acute will his organs of sense become. . . . The Jungborn has now also practically demonstrated the correctness of the return to nature method, and its significance for the welfare and salvation of man. . . . This nature-cure system is the same for all diseases, and all cases, even as the origin of all diseases has but one cause, an unnatural mode of life, and there exists a unity in all the laws of nature and in all her manifestations.

1902

WHAT IS NATUROPATHY?
LUDWIG STADEN, NATUROPATH

—·—

GENERAL RULES FOR THE
PHYSICAL REGENERATION OF MAN NOTICE
C. LEIGH HUNT WALLACE

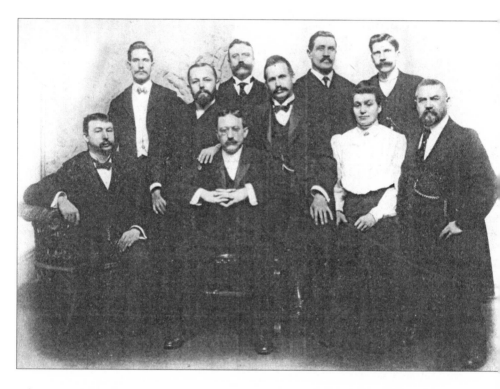

Charter Members of the American Naturopathic Society, established in 1896, which formed the nucleus for the American Naturopathic Association.

What Is Naturopathy?

by Ludwig Staden, Naturopath

The Naturopath and Herald of Health, III(1), 15-18. (1902)

Everybody knows what Allopathy and Homeopathy is, but very few people know what Naturopathy means.

There are two kinds of sciences: absolute, or pure, and empirical science. If a sentence has absolute general legality and lawfulness, its perceptive faculties are absolute, pure of *a priori*, that means its perception is free and independent of experience on the contrary of perception and knowledge borrowed from experience which is empirical or *a posteriori*. Reason is the power which offers us the principles of knowledge *a priori*; it is the highest power in man if in harmony with the conscience. Anything that is founded on knowledge *a priori* is absolute eternal truth, and anything that is based on knowledge *a posteriori* is subject to change. It has a beginning and has an end and consequently cannot be an eternal truth but is subject to error. Matter is changeable and therefore the study of matter is empirical. Materialism never produces eternal truth. Tyndall in his preface to his Belfast address says, "The continuity between molecular processes and the phenomena of consciousness is the rock upon which materialism must inevitably split whenever it pretends to be a complete philosophy of the human mind." Medical science based on materialism therefore causes us thousands of disappointments; it is knowledge *a posteriori* borrowed from experience; is continuously changing, and is without stability in its perceptions and self-reliance without one absolute eternal truth.

Naturopathy in its fundamental principles is based upon knowledge *a priori* alone, on intuitive power. Its postulate is the principle of the great philosopher Plato, "Unity in variety, and variety in unity." This is the cardinal point in Naturopathy, which entitles it to recognize actually only one disease and to explain the apparent diversity of forms and symptoms. How could it otherwise be possible that a man like Priessnitz, the originator of Naturopathy, who could not write nor read, was able to perform such wonderful cures that his name became known all over the world? Or did Johannes Schroth, Rausse, Theo. Hahn, Arnold Rickli, Father Kneipp, L. Kuhne or A. Just ever study the science of medicine? No, each one simply was a genius in the art of healing. What else could have made these men and many others true physicians, but the intuitive knowledge, the knowledge *a priori*, the knowledge from within.

The great philosopher Schopenhauer says that empirical science without philosophical tendencies equalizes a face without eyes; I used to compare it to a beautiful marble statue without life. Philosophy is the soul of all sciences, and Naturopathy, with its theoretical and practical tendencies of philosophy, is the soul of all methods of healing. It is a method and is none; it is a method because it stands on incontestable eternal laws; it cannot be so classed because the healing factors are infinite. Nature is its alma mater; nature which is the unbound, boundless book, Goethe says, offering us on all its pages true values. "Nature never deceives but revenges inexorably every trial to deceive her." Nature is the best teacher we have, Cicero says: If we will always follow Nature as our leader we will never go wrong. No doubt that there is always an empirical scientific part in Naturopathy and this part is also of importance. Experience will always be man's first teacher; all the practical modes of treatment in curing disease in Naturopathy are the result of experience, but they never will be an objectionably uniform method; for this is the point where intuition and experience are united. The true Naturopath will always treat individually; he is treating the person, not the case. Each person is differently constituted, consequently every case must be different; that means forms and symptoms which are dependent on the condition of the person. Being at bottom only one disease the naturopath knows that all diseases are curable, but not in all individual patients. The latter is impossible because all power of healing is within ourselves, and if a patient has wasted his spare vitality almost entirely; if he himself gives himself up, then there is no power in this world that can cure him. It is only himself, and himself alone who can cure himself, and everybody has to work out his own salvation physically, morally, intellectually and spiritually. "That what you sow you will reap." There is no higher truth, no higher law that this universal law of cause and effect. What beautiful, incomparable, peerless words these are; what a phenomenal high truth, if man would only comprehend them this world would be a paradise. Everything in this world is based on action and reaction, and what else can disease be, than the reaction of an action which caused disease; and what else can cause disease but sin against the laws of nature. Wholesale sinning causes epidemics besides other contagious diseases, as we can notice in times of war. There are two kinds of original causes of all diseases: the psychological cause, which begins with our thought, and the physiological cause, which Naturopathy explains as disturbed "change of matter". You must always take into consideration that Naturopathy has two explanations for disease: a psychical and a physical or a philosophical and an empirical. The Naturopath therefore stands on both knowledges: a priori and a posteriori; on intuitive power first, and on experience second. The way to avoid errors is to get at the truth of the matter, which is to be found between them. Throughout the universe as man knows it; both the psychical and the physical are real and interrelated. This is the wonderful combination that no other method of healing can produce.

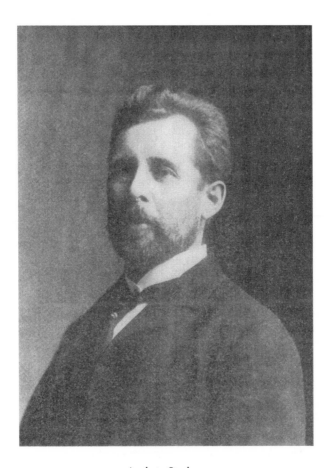

Ludwig Staden.

Medical science stands only upon abstract intellect, without perception *a priori*, without philosophical tendencies. Then there are Mental and Christian Science standing on psychological knowledge alone, not recognizing a body, which cannot be right, as we cannot deny matter; there are the common Water-cure, Massage-cure, Physical Culture, Osteopathy standing on empirical knowledge influenced unconsciously by knowledge *a priori*; and there remains Naturopathy comprising in itself the great discoveries of medical science in regard to anatomy, physiology and pathology as far as our common sense needs them, combining the immense influences of the power of the mind, also all the practical natural treatments of Hydrotherapy, Massotherapy, Heliotherapy, Physical Culture, Osteopathy, etc., etc.

Let us now recapitulate in brief the essence of Naturopathy.

1. It is the method of healing all diseases without medicines, drugs, poisons, and almost without any operations.

2. It is based on the highest scientific principles: (a) on the harmony of our perceptive faculties with the physiological and psychological laws of nature; it stands on reason, conscience and experience. (b) The change of matter functioning normal or abnormal is the standard of physical health or disease. All physical life is based upon the change of matter of the cell or upon the vibration within the cell. The vibrative process in the cell being disturbed more or less must be the physical cause of all disease and this is the problem which has to be solved in healing disease.

3. The power of healing is within us; Nature only, Nature alone, solves the problem; man presses the button, nature does the rest.

4. Naturopathy knows that there is but one disturbance which manifests itself in different forms, symptoms, and names.

5. Being but one disturbance or disease, there can be but one original cause; this is divided into a psychical and a physical one; the first is the impure thought; the second the disturbed vibrative process in the cell, as mentioned above. The occasional causes are infinite just as the symptoms and forms are.

6. The most important differences of form and symptoms in disease that Naturopathy recognizes are acute and chronic disease.

7. Naturopathy's materia medica consists of the principal elements which are derived from nature: light, air, water, heat and clay, beside non-stimulating diet, exercise and rest, electricity, magnetism and massage calisthenics, physical culture, mental culture, etc., etc.

8. Naturopathy attacks always the original cause of every disease. The human body being an organism containing thousands of nerves, blood vessels, etc., which are all most intimately connected, Naturopathy consequently is always treating the entire body.

9. It looks upon the fever as the greatest natural healing process, which should never be suppressed by poisons like quinine, antipyrin, etc., but should be guarded like a wild fire. No healing method has ever had such as immense success in treating fever diseases as Naturopathy. Suppressed fever diseases cause chronic disease. Chronic diseases therefore are developed if there is insufficient vitality in the system; if nature is healing a chronic disease it always produces a crisis of a more or less acute form, which may be repeated several times and finally finishes up with a fever. The fever is the sick man's greatest friend.

10. In the action and reaction of extreme heat and cold Naturopathy finds the greatest physical power to correct the inharmonious change of matter.

11. The food question is divided into a raw food diet consisting of fruits, berries and nuts of all kinds, besides such vegetables and cereals that can be eaten raw, and in a cooked food diet, based on the saline vegetarian theory of Dr. H. Lahmann, Dresden.

12. Stimulating and nerve-irritating food of any kind is entirely eschewed by strict Naturopathy, especially alcohol in any form, coffee and tea, meat, beef, juice, beef extract, vinegar, spices, etc., etc.

The above are the principal points and they will be sufficient to give anyone endowed with common intelligence a correct idea of the principles of Naturopathy. One important item, however, I have still to explain: the question of a diploma in Naturopathy.

There is no school or college of Naturopathy; and indeed, for the man who feels the desire in himself to become a true Naturopath, there need not be any such, as the intuitive power is the foundation stone on which Naturopathy has been built and this intuitive power is the crown of all knowledge and capacity of healing. But his power cannot be got by abstract learning; cannot be given by any diploma; it has to be discovered in ourselves by perception alone. Enlightenment is what you need; understand nature and you can assist natural healing in the only true way.

This of course will not satisfy the ignorant masses nor the legal authorities; and it is for this reason that we ought to have legally authorized colleges—and we will have them in a short time to come.

The true Naturopath will always treat individually; he is treating the person, not the case.

The power of healing is within us; Nature only, Nature alone, solves the problem.

It looks upon the fever as the greatest natural healing process, which should never be suppressed by poisons.

GENERAL RULES FOR THE PHYSICAL REGENERATION OF MAN NOTICE

by C. Leigh Hunt Wallace

The Naturopath and Herald of Health, III(10), 403-405. (1902)

D are to be wise!

Abstain from:—Fish, flesh, fowl, and dishes prepared from them; alcohol, tobacco, and all intoxicants; mineral water; fermented foods; mineral salt, and salted foods; from preserved foods unless sterilized by cooking only; baking powders, vinegars, and pickles; sour milk and unripe or decomposing fruits; uncooked dry fruits (except absolutely fresh and sound), or wormy fruits, and most manufactured foods— unless it is known that they are unadulterated and innocuously prepared; from artificially isolated food elements, and from artificial food compounds; tea drawn for longer than three minutes, black or boiled coffee, or coffee made from coffee-beans that are not under or pale-roasted, or chicory used as an adulterant; unboiled milk, or unboiled water. Do not eat fruit skins unless they are washed or scalded, as worms' eggs are frequently lodged on them, neither allow fruit peelings or fly-blown banana skins, to remain on the plate you are eating off, as microscopic maggots, and maggots' eggs, are likely to adhere to your bread and butter, or other food.

Abstain from drugs of every description, whether in the form of sleeping or other draughts; pills, castor oil, cod liver oil, pick-me-ups, tonics, jujubes, lozenges, etc.; or for outward applications, as lard, ointments, vaseline, acetic acid, blisters, arsenic, zinc, or other mineral solutions; medicated soaps, face powders, hypodermic or medicinal injections; hair dyes, lotions, etc.; or, as inhalations—smelling salts, iodine, sulphur, or other corrosive vapours; or pastilles, or medicated waters for bathing, etc.

When faint for food take a nutrient, not a stimulant.

Never eat idly or between meals.

As a rule never eat less than two nor more than three meals daily.

Never eat when over-fatigued, but rest till actual exhaustion is relieved and a sense of hunger is expressed.

"Eat slowly and chew well," reducing all food to a liquid, as nothing that is not soluble can be assimilated. Have artificial teeth if your own are useless or lost. Be moderate in quantity, and particular in the quality of all food. Remember that every grain of food taken has its mission for good or evil upon the organism.

Observe regularity in eating, drinking and sleeping.

Keep all food covered from air germs and dust, moths and other insects, also from being fly-blown, or contaminated by vermin, and never buy food that has been exposed for sale.

Eat the fruits that are in season.

Cook all food upon the scientific principles introduced and taught by Mrs. Wallace. These enjoin that all vegetables shall be conservatively cooked, that is, stewed or baked in their own juices or served with the water in which they are cooked in the form of sauce or gravy.

Cook all food digestively, that is, so thoroughly that it is easy of assimilation and, in the case of foods containing starch, considerably dextrinized.

Employ waterless cookery whenever possible, that is, cook fruits and vegetables in their own juices, or in the juices of other vegetables or fruits, thus using only organic, instead of inorganic water.

When water is used for cooking purposes, let it be either distilled or boiled.

Use china-ware for cooking fruits or acid vegetables.

Supply the fluids needed by the body as much as possible with the organic waters got from fruits and vegetables. Drink boiled water when you cannot get distilled.

Have all water cisterns kept covered, and cleaned out at fixed periods, three months being the longest. See that the water for flushing the drain-pipes is not in any way connected with water used for food purposes. Let the water which has been standing in lead or other pipes all night, or for any lengthened period, be drawn off before any is taken for drinking, or cooking purposes.

Take bodily rest for bodily fatigue, and conserve your strength wisely.

Learn to sleep on your back, with limbs straight and muscles relaxed, also without a pillow if it is possible to do so in comfort; otherwise lie one half of the night on one side, and the other half on the other. Learn to sleep with your mouth closed.

Sleep as many hours as you find necessary to completely recuperate your strength, and, as near as possible, take half of these hours before and half after midnight.

Accustom yourself to arise from your bed as soon as you feel perfectly rested and refreshed. Avoid artificial light as much as possible.

Insist upon the bowels having at least one full and free action daily. Regulate this by diet and exercise.

Wash or bathe the body at least every twenty-four hours in cold, warm, or hot water, according to your condition of health; bathe the whole body, including the head, in hot water at least once a week.

Give your bare body an air or sun bath whenever you can.

Clothe in undyed all-wool, all-over-porous materials, whether for underclothing or linings, using colored stuffs only for upper and outer garments. Have all underclothing washed at least once weekly, and oftener, if subject to odorous or excessive action of the skin. Do not sleep in any clothing worn during the day. At night hang all day-clothing up (outside the sleeping apartment if the room is small or crowded, and it is convenient to do so), where they will get well aired, separately, and turned inside out; do not wear garters, waist bands, or corsets; have boots made to fit the feet, with wide soles and broad, flat heels; do not wear mackintoshes or starched clothing; have waistcoat linings of wool; wear a combination garment first; have each petticoat made with bodice and skirt in one; also the dress foundation as in the princess-robe form. The rule is to choose and fashion your clothing that it retains the greatest possible amount of heat with the least possible weight. Regulate the amount according to health and weather temperature. Avoid black or dark shades for clothing or drapery. An average from 4 to 7 pounds in warm weather, and 7 to 10 in cold should be sufficient.

Go barefoot when it is safe to do so, or wear sandals when convenient and the feet can be kept comfortably warm.

Furnish the sleeping apartment with single beds, with wire or spring lath frames, upon which place a horsehair, wool or woven wire mattress. Do not have a feather bed on this. Let all night-clothing and bed covering (except, perhaps, the sheets) be all wool, and light in weight; do not use close heavy cotton quilts, eider down, or fur rugs; have windows open night and day and protect from draughts by screens, and from cold by head coverings; do not have gas, lamp, candle, or night-light burning in your sleeping room, nor standing soiled water. Keep drinking-water covered.

Systematically exercise every muscle in the body daily; but do not produce a sensation of exhaustion or weakness. Practice deep breathing, and always through the nostrils, with closed mouth. Stand or sit erect with chest raised, shoulders back and abdomen drawn in. Walk several miles daily, but never to exhaustion.

Live in the open sunny air as much as possible.

Avoid the lung-poison air of crowds in confined places.

Employ yourself from six to eight hours daily in some useful and non-injurious occupation.

[This article is an excerpt taken from a different journal entitled *The Herald of Health*. —Ed.]

1903

What Hinders The Propagation Of Naturopathy?
Benedict Lust

—··—

Return To Nature
Benedict Lust

An advertisement placed by Benedict Lust.

What Hinders The Propagation Of Naturopathy?

by Benedict Lust

The Naturopath and Herald of Health, IV(7), 194-195. (1903)

Many medical scientists consider Naturopathy plainly as quackery and not a few medical authorities feel strongly inclined to condemn it. It is difficult to explain why Naturopathy does not find acknowledgement but even contradiction from the medical profession. The latter has gone so far in certain cases that some of its representatives who have become convinced of the superiority of Naturopathy and have become converted to it, have been expelled from medical societies, under the pretense that they did not understand to maintain the honor of the medical profession.

As, however, more and more followers of the profession continue to become Naturopaths this affords the best proof that the value of Naturopathy is recognized by the more progressive members of the medical profession. It is therefore all the more astonishing that so much should be done by medical authorities, especially of the higher class, to oppose Naturopathy, as being charlatanism. It is not difficult to draw unpleasant conclusions from such conduct.

The opposition developed against the development of Naturopathy is not dictated by conscientious considerations, but by material interests. If all physicians set themselves in earnest to prevent all diseases they would have to starve as well as the druggists; therefore, as a class we can hardly expect them to extend the hand of friendship to Naturopathy.

Physicians derive their incomes from sick people and consequently are interested in mankind being sick, whereas conditions of universal health would make the profession all but superfluous.

In these material interests, there we find the reason why everything possible is done by medical authorities to obstruct the victorious propagation of Naturopathy throughout the world.

And while we would be slow to say that physicians intentionally prolong diseases and neglect to take measures for their prevention, in many cases we believe they do these things almost unconsciously. It is a well-known fact, by the way, that, as in other professions, one physician often envies another, and the results of envy, found in the middle Ages, appropriate public expression in the saying, *Medicus medico luppissimus*, which means, "Physicians are the greatest wolves toward physicians."

Looking at things from this standpoint the Chinese, for instance, seem to be wiser than we, because they pay their physicians only as long as they are well, and when they fall ill the salary is suspended till the patient recovers. In that country the disciples of Aesculapius have consequently the greatest interest in seeing their patients in permanent health.

If we now ask how best to resist the hostile influence of medical science against Naturopathy, there is only one reply, and that is, "Appeal to the masses!" The sick have no interest in the prosperity of the medical profession, as such; what they want is to recover in the best and quickest way possible.

Let us leave the controversial question between medical science and Naturopathy to the public; the people will not be long in finding out which system should receive the preference, as the importance of the various methods can be rightly valued only by the sick. Our duty is to make the public thoroughly acquainted with all the principles that capabilities of Naturopathy, so that is may form its own judgment. The purpose of this article is to illustrate this in an objective manner.

GENERAL PRINCIPLES OF NATUROPATHY

Naturopathy is based on principles that are easily grasped, among which are:

Most diseases, (practically all), no matter how different their symptoms may be, arise from the same primary cause.

This cause is "foreign substance or contagious matter," which has accumulated in the body owing to disturbance of its functions, especially that of digestion. Of course external or internal injuries, caused by accidents, etc., are exceptions to this rule. Now, Nature has provided that the body always endeavors to throw off all foreign matter thus accumulated, through the natural channels, and in cases where the body possesses the necessary strength this work will always be done without disturbance and will be successfully accomplished without assistance.

But the case is different if the body does not possess the necessary strength. Then the body must necessarily suffer, because it finds itself unable to expel the elements causing disease, and it becomes diseased.

An important principle of Naturopathy is to develop the so-called vital force of the body. It takes the right standpoint by saying that the body became diseased only because it did not possess sufficient vital force, to drive out the foreign matter. If we succeed in increasing its strength, then it will be better able to take up its interrupted work and will become master of the disease. In other words, if we increase the vital force, we put the body in a fit condition to successfully resist disease.

Taking these two principles as a basis, Naturopathy, with all its various methods of treatments, has always one end in view and one only: *to increase the vital force.*

Now, as in the vast majority of cases, the prime cause of disease is a departure from the manner of living intended by Nature, it is not difficult to find the correct way in which we should deal with it.

If, for instance, a man is ill because he has eaten too much, it is only reasonable that in order to get well again he should restrict his diet; if sickness has been caused by living too long in bad and unhealthy surroundings, a visit to a place where he can get plenty of good fresh air, and take sufficient physical exercise will suffice to restore him to health.

Thus Naturopathy always and in every case only follows good sense, and gives treatment only by the use of the elements of Nature such as light, air, heat, water, diet, recreation, exercise, magnetism, electricity and proper clothing.

The opposition developed against the development of Naturopathy is not dictated by conscientious considerations, but by material interests.

Nature has provided that the body always endeavors to throw off all foreign matter thus accumulated, through the natural channels, and in cases where the body possesses the necessary strength this work will always be done without disturbance and will be successfully accomplished without assistance.

Naturopathy, with all its various methods of treatments, has always one end in view and one only: to increase the vital force.

Benedict Lust offered a money back guarantee for dissatisfied readers of *Return to Nature* and subscription discounts.

RETURN TO NATURE!

by Benedict Lust
The Naturopath and Herald of Health, (1903), IV(7), advertisement.

FRIEND:

ARE YOU a broken-hearted man or woman, weary with yourself and with life, nervous, fretful, easily discouraged? Do you know that you share this condition with thousands, and what it means? Do you know that it is you who are sick and not the world you live in which is bad? And do you know that you can be cured, that your disease can be overcome and eradicated by the simplest of means? That as well as being a sick, tired man or woman, you might now be full of energy and power, overflowing with life? You might as well.

RETURN TO NATURE!

That is the whole secret. Learn the simple truths relative to the right living. Learn to draw into your own body the inexhaustible spring of youth and life and power which permeates Nature—and soon all will be well with you. And you might as well learn one other little thing—namely: To shun as you would the pest that always growing host of quacks, electric belt men and other imposters of their kind, who flood the newspapers from one end of the land to the other with their shameless advertisements. *These men are the ghouls of modern business life! They feast on the sick and the dying!* In our magazine, the *Naturopath*, we may in the future find room to make some startling disclosures to the public relative to the doings of these men. Meanwhile we advise that you shun them.

RETURN TO NATURE!

You would wish to learn the secret of youth and happiness. We all would. And if you would learn to overcome your disease and troubles by simple, natural means, you may write us. We advocate nothing of which we are not positive, nothing which we have not demonstrated to ourselves and through ourselves is the truth. Our methods and means are as simple as they are sure.

RETURN TO NATURE!

It is the name of the famous German Naturopath, Adolf Just, which has recently startled the old world. In plain, simple language, which everybody can comprehend, the master tells of the causes of human scourge, disease, and how it may be overcome in almost every instance by self treatment. We have just rendered a translation of this great work in the English language. It is now in press and will be ready for the public about

June 1ˢᵗ. Orders are streaming in. The first edition will probably be sold out before it leaves the printer, and if you desire to have the book among the first, place your order now. The work will then be sent to you as soon as it comes from the press.

Meanwhile you might interest yourself in learning something about us and our work. To this end send for our literature, sample copy of our magazine, *The Naturopath*, and prospectus of our beautiful Sanitarium, "The Youngborn"* at Bellevue, Butler, N.J. We know that you will be our friend as soon as you learn to know us and our work.

To encourage the weak; to raise the sick; to lift the veil of ignorance with its resulting harvest of misery and disease from off the face of the world. That is the goal for which we are contending.

We stand for humanity.

The price of *Return to Nature*, Volume 1, English or German, bound, will $2.00, stiff paper $1.50. Price of Volume 2, English or German, bound, in cloth, $1.75, stiff paper, $1.25. Sent postpaid on receipt of price. Address orders to:

Benedict Lust
111 E. 59ᵗʰ St. New York.

---

* Benedict Lust used two spellings interchangeably for Yungborn/Youngborn.

1904

NATUROPATHY
BENEDICT LUST

—.—

SAYINGS
ELLA WHEELER WILCOX

I could say it in two words, "Be Kind".

Kindness is the keynote to happiness, your own and that of others around you.

Kindness covers charity and all the other virtues of human relations.

It is the foundation of the Golden Rule.

It is the manifestation of universal love.

It is priceless yet costs nothing.

Before it enemies turn friends.

Because of it, burdens become lightened, joy replaces sadness, tears of sorrow dry upon the cheek, gloom fades into cheer, the sun of a brighter day dispells the mists of agony, fear and doubt.

Kindness, the great panacea for the world's troubles! Yet how it is withheld!

But holding it neither profits the one nor the other.

How can we improve on the words of One, "Love thy neighbor as thyself"?

What philosophy of life or selfishness can equal it?

We will ever remember a great writer who has recently passed on for these lines,

> *So many gods, so many creeds,*
> *So many paths that wind and wind,*
> *When all this sad world needs,*
> *Is just the art of being kind.*
>
> *—Ella Wheeler Wilcox.*

Be Kind—Ella Wheeler Wilcox.

NATUROPATHY

by Benedict Lust

The Naturopath and Herald of Health, V(1), 1-3. (1904)

LIGHT

The importance of light is undervalued by most people. Everybody, no doubt, is aware that plants which are deprived of light remain thoroughly white and pine away, while in sunlight they retain their beautiful green color. It is a similar case with the man who gets little or no outdoor exercise; he becomes pale and sickly, and will only gain healthy color by living much out-of-doors, in the sun.

Look at the different aspect which the field laborer presents who is exposed to the rays of the sun the whole day! His skin, as far as the rays of the sun have touched it, is heavily browned, his eyes glisten and his whole appearance denotes energy and good health.

Sunlight has the wonderful power, too, of destroying all microorganisms, bacteria, etc., dangerous to the human organism. This alone should sufficiently demonstrate the high value of sunlight and how important it is that we frequently expose ourselves to the sun.

The greatest regard for good health should naturally make us have our living-rooms as sunny as possible, so as to allow the very most light obtainable to enter them. Those whose business compels them to sit very much should never fail to utilize every free moment for exercise taken out-of-doors and in the sun, as this is the only antidote for the consequences of sitting in close rooms.

Take the typical Englishman as an example. He understands making use of every free moment by strengthening his body in out-door sports, while many of our "home-birds" prefer to take their "recreation" in barrooms reeking with tobacco smoke. No human being can live under such conditions for any length of time without becoming ill. Light is used as a curative agent in sunbaths and light-air baths.

AIR

Air is just as important to the body as light. It consists of seventy-seven parts of nitrogen and twenty-three parts of oxygen. The air we breathe is the most essential element to our life; we can live without food for some time, but we cannot live one minute without air.

Only healthy, oxygen-containing air, however, furnishes us with the elements we need most for the support of our body.

It is, therefore, of greatest importance, particularly in the cities, to bear in mind that our living- and bed-rooms must always be supplied with good air. Frequent ventilation by open windows is the best way to obtain a good circulation of air. It is not absolutely necessary to have the whole window wide open in order to ventilate the room sufficiently. This is, of course, a good thing to do in summer time, but in winter it suffices to open the windows a few inches in order to promote ventilation, and on the other hand not to allow the temperature to cool off too much. People who cannot open their bed-room windows at night, or who do not care to do so, may keep the windows in the adjoining room open and leave the door to their bed-room ajar.

The quantity of air we need for breathing purposes is so large that, in our average-sized living- and bed-rooms, it will be spoiled within an hour if proper ventilation is not provided. It cannot be impressed too earnestly how important it is for our health that we should continually have fresh air. There is much room for improvement in this respect, particularly in schools. Children should there be taught the necessity of having fresh air in the school-rooms instead of having them be afraid of every little draught and making them believe that it is dangerous. It is really ridiculous, and from the standpoint of common sense incomprehensible that so many even educated and sensible people are so opposed to the opening of windows. They would rather sit in close, smoke-filled rooms than allow the opening of a window, even a little way. In all questions of hygiene man is still a most wonderfully narrow-minded creature.

REST

Every human being needs much rest. We require nearly half of our life for sleep. During sleep our body works most actively internally for its rebuilding up. Sleep is the time when digestion is promoted most actively. If a man works too hard and too long and has not sufficient rest he will become ill. Light disturbances, such as headaches, etc., are very often entirely overcome by rest, because during the time of undisturbed rest the body is more capable of mastering such attacks. It is, therefore, wise to recommend absolute rest for certain illnesses. Now, the degree of rest different people require varies greatly, and what will suffice for one may not do for another; we cannot measure the rest required by yards, but have to consider each individual. Many people have become sick only because they have to work beyond the limit of their strength and cannot take the needful rest.

EXERCISE

A certain amount of exercise is just as essential for the body as rest. Every part of the body which does not daily, or at least frequently, have the required amount of exercise will droop and pine away and never gain the elasticity and capacity intended by Nature. A thorough development of all parts of the body promotes the change of matter, circulation of the blood and digestion to a high degree, and naturally prevents diseases, as accumulation of diseased substances in the body can rarely take place if the change of matter is an active one. In many diseases a cure can only be effected by daily proper outdoor exercise. All kinds of athletic sports, out-door games, etc., can be highly recommended to both young and old, particularly to those of sedentary habits. Indoor exercise is also very useful.

WARMTH AND CLOTHING

Warmth is a necessity to us; we could not live without it. Warmth is our vital force and animates all the functions of life; we usually feel much better in health in summer than in winter. Lack of sufficient warmth makes us ill, while in many cases warmth alone suffices to cure our organism. We protect ourselves against the changes of temperature by clothing and by the coverings of our beds. We should, therefore, never be careless as to how we clothe ourselves, as too thin clothing can be just as harmful as too thick. It is best that we should be accustomed from childhood to as simple and light clothing as possible, and that we always allow ourselves to be guided by our individual requirements.

This space is too limited to go fully into all questions pertaining to proper clothing. I will only say that, in advanced age, ramie or a linen mesh are doubtless the best and healthiest materials to use for garments.

The same may be said in respect to beds and their coverings. We should never accustom ourselves to too warm beds and too many coverings, but should cover ourselves only as warmly as we feel to be necessary.

BATHING

The healthiest bath is the river or sea bath taken in the open air and on a sunny day. It does most good when great heat makes us desire to take it. The old Spartans owed their iron health and athletic strength in great measure to their daily open-air baths. The value of these baths cannot be fully afforded by any artificially prepared baths. Those, consequently, who find it possible should lose no opportunity for taking river or sea baths during the summer months. People who are of a weak constitution should never remain longer than five minutes in the water. Besides their use as to cleanliness these baths give great strength, and it is greatly to be regretted that the general desire for bathing in summer seems to be less than it used to be some years ago. It must be remembered that in taking a bath we have the opportunity of enjoying an air and light bath at the same time, so that we derive benefit simultaneously from the three curative elements—light, air and water.

If one is not accustomed to open-air bathing he should be careful not to go in when the water is too cool; it is better to wait until the temperature is at least from sixty-eight to seventy-two degrees, and to choose a very nice warm summer day for the first trial. It is also good not to remain longer than from two to five minutes in the water for the first four or five times. It is very beneficial for the body if we expose it to the sun after bathing, in order to dry and warm it through and through. If the day is not sunny some exercise after bathing is recommended for the purpose of getting warm. If must also be remembered that we should never go into the water when we are overheated, but should wait until we have cooled off sufficiently; on the other hand, we must avoid cooling off too rapidly and waiting until we are chilled.

Every part of the body which does not daily, or at least frequently, have the required amount of exercise will droop and pine away and never gain the elasticity and capacity intended by Nature.

Frequent ventilation by open windows is the best way to obtain a good circulation of air.

SAYINGS

by Ella Wheeler Wilcox
The Naturopath and Herald of Health, (1904), V(1), 3. (1904)

How many of us throw away every day our real capital, squandering it in all sorts of folly?

Clear your mind of every gloomy, selfish, angry or revengeful thought; allow no resentment or grudge toward man, or fate, to stay in your heart over night.

Wake in the morning with a blessing for every living thing on your lips and in your soul.

Say to yourself: "Health, luck, usefulness, success are mine, I claim them." Keep thinking that thought, no matter what happens, just as you would keep putting one foot before another if you had a mountain to climb, no matter what mud or brambles you encountered.

Keep on—keep on—and suddenly you will find you are on the heights—"luck" beside you.

Ella Wheeler Wilcox Undertakes New Work

Favorite Author Becomes Associate Editor of The New Thought Magazine.

Best Writing She Has Ever Done Now Appearing in That Bright Publication.

The many friends and admirers of Ella Wheeler Wilcox will be interested to learn that this gifted author and thinker has connected herself in the capacity of associate editor with the NEW THOUGHT magazine and that hereafter her writings will appear regularly in that bright publication of which the aim is to aid its readers in the cultivation of those powers of the mind which bring success in life. Mrs. Wilcox's writings have been the inspiration of many young men and women. Her hopeful, practical, masterful views of life give the reader new courage in the very reading and are a wholesome spur to flagging effort. She is in perfect sympathy

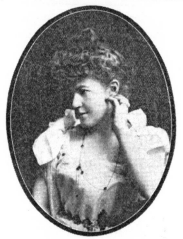

ELLA WHEELER WILCOX.

with the purpose of the NEW THOUGHT magazine. The magazine is having a wonderful success and the writings of Mrs. Wilcox for it, along the line of the new movement, are among her best. Words of truth so vital, that they live in the memory of every reader and cause him to think—to his own betterment and the lasting improvement of his own work in the world, in whatever line it lies—flow from this talented woman's pen.

The magazine is being sold on all news stands for five cents. It is the brightest, cleanest and best publication in its class and its editors have hit the keynote of all sound success. The spirit of every bit of print from cover to cover of the magazine is the spirit of progress and upbuilding—of courage, persistence and success. Virile strength and energy, self-confidence, the mastery of self and circumstances are its life and soul and even the casual reader feels the contagion of its vigor and its optimism.

FREE.—The publishers will be pleased to send a handsome portrait of Mrs. Wilcox, with extracts from her recent writings on the New Thought, free. Address

THE NEW THOUGHT
45 The Colonnades, Vincennes Ave., Chicago, Ill.

Announcement of Ella Wheeler Wilcox as Associate Editor of *The New Thought* Magazine.

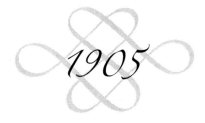

The Naturopathic System Of Therapeutics Or The Prevention Of Disease And Its Cure

Benedict Lust

Naturopathy

Dr. Carl Shultz

The Naturopathic Institute, Sanatorium and College of California advertisement.

THE NATUROPATHIC SYSTEM OF THERAPEUTICS OR THE PREVENTION OF DISEASE AND ITS CURE

by Benedict Lust

The Naturopath and Herald of Health, VI(7), 175-177. (1905)

The close of the 19th Century was characterised by two important advances made in the medical world, the discovery and use of anaesthetics by Lister and the universal acceptance of the germ theory of the origin of disease: the former discovery proving itself one of the greatest boons to suffering humanity, taking away the very sting and reproach from surgical operations, for up to this time many people preferred death rather than enter the operating room. It is in connection with Surgery that medical science has chiefly advanced and obtained victories of deathless fame and distinction. Of no less value are the revelations made by the Microscope of the infinitely small germs, good, bad and destructive; some are health promoters; some disease generators. Among the diseases due to bacteria are tuberculosis (consumption) causing 25% of the total Number of deaths; other diseases due to the tubercle bacilli are scrofula, abscesses, ulcer, tumours and diseases of the joints and bones, peritonitis (inflammation of the lining membrane of the abdomen) bronchitis, pleurisy, meningitis (inflammation of the covering of the brain) enteritis and catarrh; other bacilli produce cholera, leprosy, influenza, pneumonia, diphtheria and anthrax (splenic fever). The atmosphere is laden with micro-organisms and so is the surface layer of the earth. Much remains to be determined with regard to their disease producing possibilities; identity of form does not simply identify nature. Each species produces life that they are not destroyed by extremes of heat or cold, they will even live in acids; their greatest destroyer is Sunlight. Dr. Dallinger fixed the limit of vision for the microscope at the five-hundred-thousandth of an inch which gives 250,000 millions of germs on one inch of surface: in the light of this fact it would seem that finality in connection with micro-organisms were perhaps an unattainable realization: the results which up-to-date have been obtained are of the most marvelous nature and all tend for the good of humanity. Such studies have invested Chemistry with a halo of fairy romance.

The opening of the 20th Century has been distinguished by the general awakening of the people of all nations to take means to improve their health and physique and beget a more vigorous race, hence the attention now given to physical culture for building up powerful bodies, the grand basic condition for the development of powerful minds, a *sine qua non* in these days of International competition for the Mastery in Trade and Commerce, when every muscle must be strained and every thought concentrated so as to maintain our hold in the ever forward March of Commerce. Just as a chain is as strong as its weakest link, so it may be said of Nations that they are as powerful as the unit determines. Let us look after the units and the hundreds will look after themselves. The establishment of physical developments schools augurs well for the future. Physical regeneration is in the air as evidenced by our gymnasia, by our schools of natation and by our walking contests of both sexes. All this new activity proves that people are now realizing that health is the best wealth: that wealth does not determine happiness, but that happiness and wealth depend on health, and good health, and more than anything else promotes contentment.

A marked sign of our times is the disposition to take the advice of our immortal Shakespeare and "throw physic to the dogs". Notwithstanding the great increase of new chemical remedies, so great, that it is impossible for the ordinary medical man to give them a fair trial. A fact to be carefully considered is many doctors themselves have no faith in the drugs that they administer and these are proofs that even in cases where cures have been effected by drugs they have caused mischief in other direction as great as the one got rid of. Medicaments are now being renounced and men are reverting to first principles, maintaining health and combating disease by Natural healing factors as Water, Light, Air, Massage, Diet, Exercise, Electricity, Hypnotism and Rest. The ridicule and opposition of the medical faculty to these methods were to be expected and in this connection we may quote the pregnant words of Archbishop Whiteley: "In proportion as any branch of study leads to important and useful results and in proportion as it tends to overthrow prevailing errors, in the same degree, it may be expected to call forth angry declamations from those wedded to prejudices which they cannot defend."

Hydropathy as a healer is now an accredited fact and evidences are to be met everywhere of ailments apparently intractable which have given in under its kindly benign influence. Prof. Kussmaul has written: "It is not only among the educated but amongst all ranks of the people that a justifiable suspicion of drugs has now penetrated." This Nestor of the German faculty believed that every young physician ought to thoroughly schooled in the priceless therapeutic value of water and had withheld his signature from the new programme drawn up by the commissioners for medical examinations, because Hydropathy, as a subject, is excluded.

Bilz in his *Natural Method of Healing*: demonstrates how hydropathic modes need not a palatial establishment on some favored hillside for its remedial wonders, but can be practiced by every intelligent person in his own home, however, humble.

In Bilz all the different hydropathic appliances discovered by the great Priessnitz and adopted by Kneipp, as head bath, cold full-bath, tepid, shallow-sitz, eye, foot, leg and arm baths; sun and alternating baths, douches, and compresses find fullest and simplest explanation, a system of treatment says Dr. Gulley, father of the speaker of the House of Commons, which, when contemplated by the physiological eye is beautiful in its power, efficacy, and simplicity, but whose value can only be appreciated by comparing it with the results of medicinal treatment by having practised both.

Water for internal purposes is as important as air. Organic substances are often suspended in it. Bilz gives the most interesting particulars of the uses of water, as well as of the soils it runs through: of the removal of sewer and coal gas and the carrying away of all refuse from houses and streets: the purification of water is explained. Where to build a house and how to build it and to secure for it perfect Sanitations are fully treated of.

The value of air as a Natural healer is preventive of disease is now without dispute, though even now far too many only partially ventilate their rooms perfectly, close their windows at night, when the air is the purest. The most serious substance found in air is dust which partly consists of living beings. Pure fresh air is the sole grand cure for Tuberculosis and Consumption. Consumptives should spend all available time in the open air, and sleep all available time in the open air, and sleep in it, if possible, as at our best Sanatoria.

Most men and women are walking monuments of their ancestor's errors and to dare to go alone often brings upon one contumely. The time was, not very long ago, when we built our houses with the smallest of windows and our housewives pulled down the blinds to keep the sunlight out. Now we begin to see that Light and Heat are among our effective healers and in Bilz the value and use of Sun-baths, X rays and other rays are expounded in the most lucid manner.

Massage and Curative gymnastics have made progress by leaps and bounds and even the allopath practitioner, today, has his staff of Masseuses on daily attendance. The latest triumph of Massage, and most wonderful to say, has been in the inducing rhythmical movements of a heart which had come to a dead stop.

Electricity as a life giving power and stimulator is daily becoming more and more harnessed in the service of the Natural Healer and Hypnotism is becoming in the hands of the wise, pure and honorable men a power in creating and stimulating the moral sense so that there has, already, been established in Paris a Hypnotic dispensary for vicious children whose Natural tendencies beget anxiety in the minds of their parents for the future, so that the role of the neurologist and psychologist ought to be added to that of the teacher. By wise suggestion, control, self-control, the copestone of a well-balanced mind, can be developed and not taught. Without self-control life would be a regiment without a Colonel, a class without a Master, a family without a Father.

Changes for good come very slowly and we are long in learning the simple lesson that most of our bodily ailments are the result of our own follies and ignorance.

Food and Dietetics is a world and a subject fully treated of, in every aspect, in the *Natural Method of Healing*. Man acts contrary to his own best interests, as well as contrary to nature, when following the accepted customs of feeding. As a people we seem to live for the object of creating disease to support doctors. Often one, two or three days total abstinence from food would effect wonders.

Bilz pleads for a simpler mode of living, for the banishment of putrescent and fermented foods. Adopt a simple diet; give the stomach a rest and periodically, the body a good rest too. Cease from worrying and escape from all excitements and the best results will follow. Physical regeneration is the prelude to purity of conduct: the training of the body must reflect upon the mind. Hereditary taints are the causes of most miseries, the desolations of our homes and the filling of our prisons with lapsed men and women and our asylums with idiots. Jean de Bonnefon of Paris has said that three-fourths of the men who enter into the married state are impure and transmit the germs of infectious diseases: thus the dream of love is soon over for Many Noble Good women who retire to live the rest of their lives—a living death.

On all these subjects and many more every man and woman will find Bilz: *The Natural Method of Healing* a veritable treasure-house, a friend-in-need upon any emergency, as sudden illness or accident. There are two handsome vols. of 1000 pages each, 700 illustrations, 19 adjustable colored plates. It has gained gold and silver medals. It is in the hands of many crowned heads. It is a household word on the Continent. Thousands have made life worth living by adopting and practising its principles. It can be bought for $7.50 cash or $8.00 on installment system from the Naturopath, 124 E. 59th St., New York.

Medicaments are now being renounced and men are reverting to first principles, maintaining health and combating disease by Natural healing factors as Water, Light, Air, Massage, Diet, Exercise, Electricity, Hypnotism and Rest. . . . Water for internal purposes is as important as air.

NATUROPATHY
What it is, What it does, and Why it's Opposed by the Medical Trust

by Dr. Carl Schultz
The Naturopathic Institute, Los Angeles, CA.

The Naturopath and Herald of Health, VI(8), 216-219. (1905)

Naturopathy as a Science commenced nearly a hundred years ago. The first breach in the old-time honored method—the poisoning of the sick by THE physicians—came when Dr. Hahnemann (1755-1843) established the Homeopathic method. That he did not succeed in overthrowing the Idol "Drug-Poison" was because he did not go far enough and abandon the poisoning altogether, but continued to treat his patients with diluted proportions of drugs. But one thing he did, he forbid his patients all stimulants, such as beer, wine, coffee, tea, etc., and I am sure that this was to an extent his success in healing diseases. I am sorry that the majority of the Homeopaths of to-day have discarded Hahnemann's Rule.

At the same time that Hahnemann established his method, a common peasant in Germany of the name of Priessnitz, electrified the world and dumbfounded the medical fraternity by his numerous cures with water alone. Priessnitz the lay man, the common peasant, accomplished cures by the thousands—patients given up by the best medical doctors. No medical Trust forbid or stopped him, or had him arrested and put in jail; at that time permission from a medical Trust was not necessary. Priessnitz could cure the German people without being molested; but of course this was nearly a hundred years ago, and it was in the old Country, where people had no written Constitution, but they had love for liberty and a Constitution in their heart. We have a written Constitution granting every man the same rights and privileges, but the medical Trust tells you: "You must die if a member of our Trust cannot cure you—we command and you must obey; you, the free born American citizens—if you don't we send the men who are saving your lives after we nearly killed you, to prison!" And you the free citizens stand by and let the Trust do as it pleases, and the free press of the country keeps quiet, because they are afraid of the Trust. I say "the press" with exception of a few, as for example, the Editor of the "Care of the Body Department" of the *Times Magazine*, Los Angeles, Cal.

At the time when Hahnemann and Priessnitz were living and working for the welfare of the Public, there were other men at work for the same purpose. Jahn, commonly known in Germany as Father Jahn, and Henry Ling in Sweden, both taught the people how to live a simple life and to practice Physical Culture, known in Germany under the name, "Turnen", in order to get health and strength. Besides these men named, there were Schroth with his dry diet and water cure, also a German peasant; then came Hahn and Baltzer introducing vegetarianism. Then came others with pure water treatments, such men as Rausse, Munde, etc., etc. All these men laid the foundation of the present "Naturopathic School".

Then came Thure Brandt, a Swedish officer—but a layman, with Massage. I will say here that Massage as it is commonly understood is rubbing, is not what the Naturopaths and scientific Masseur understands. Massage as Thure Brandt taught it and men like Metzger, Reibritz and others developed it, is a complicated system of movements and manipulations, by which even the most sensitive organs, especially the female organs, can be put back in their places, so that an operation with the knife has become not only useless, but criminal in the majority of cases. Massage is the foundation of Osteopathy and is surely more thorough than the latter. Then came the sun, light, and air baths by Prof. Rickli in Germany, then Father Kneipp with his walking barefoot in the grass, his packs, gushes, and other water applications, his Herbal-Remedies, his linen underwear, his teachings of living a simple life. Another brought the old time Magnetism into credit. Electricity came, not invented by an M.D., but claimed now as their only right and privilege to practice it, notwithstanding the fact that the majority of the medical doctors do not know more of electricity than a child. Then came Adolf Just with his out-door life, etc. Then others with Suggestive Therapeutics; finally Chiropractic by D.D. Palmer, a method of knifeless surgery ahead of all other methods.

You will have noticed that all these men were laymen, not hampered by a lot of theories and unnecessary rules laid down by a Medical Trust; as a laymen they had not learned a lot of nonsensical theories, and used only common sense.

Nearly all the founders of Naturopathy were men of the common people. This is not strange; whatever is really good and near perfection or divinity has most always been accomplished by plain men—"Christ the Carpenter's son", Abe Lincoln, for example. These various systems have been combined by us and are practiced under the name, "Naturopathy".

Now as to what Naturopathy does: First: Naturopathy teaches the people how to keep well and how to raise healthy children and by that a healthy Nation. We also claim and prove by facts, that Naturopathy cures all diseases if the patient has vitality enough left, even if nearly killed with drugs. (Here the speaker stated nearly sixty cases; all these had been given up by the best medical doctors.) I have not given the names of the medical doctors, but will do so if the gentlemen in question or the medical Trust want them.

I will state here that we have no hard feelings against the members of the medical fraternity or any other school, if the Physician is at least honest and does the best for his patient. But we have no use for a Physician, who for the sake of making money, keeps his patient in ignorance or even tells him that Naturopathy or any other method will kill him.

A man who becomes a Physician must be a man of high moral character, a man with sympathy for suffering humanity—he must feel for his patient. A man who enters the profession of healing for the sake of making money will never become a good Physician. A Physician is like an Artist, he is born, not trained, especially not in a medical college. What a Physician needs is common sense, the gift of observance, love for his fellow men, love for Nature, the gift to understand Nature, and the ability to teach others how to live and to understand the laws of Nature. A Physician should be a teacher as well as a healer.

We Naturopaths do not heal but teach how to live and keep well. Naturopathy has worked its way into all countries and is acknowledged even in Russia, and the books of Kneipp, Just, Brandt, Bilz and other writers of Natural-Healing are translated and read in all living languages. Still the Naturopathic Physicians in this country instead of getting honors and laurels, are arrested by spies of a medical Trust—for what? For keeping your wives and sisters from the operating tables, for keeping your brothers and husbands from becoming cripples and Opium, Morphine, and Whiskey fiends, for saving the lives of your loved one. Arrested by the Police as common criminals at the instigation of spies, who do this dirty work because they could not get an honest job for years and who take up this work for a Trust larger and meaner than any other Trust on the Earth. Arrested at the command of a medical Trust—a Trust whose members kill, maim, cut and unsex your wives, sisters, and children and foster the Whiskey, Opium, Morphine, and Cocaine habits upon the Public, protected by law. A Trust whose members poison the baby in the mother's womb and create the desire for alcoholics by telling the mothers to take wine, whiskey, and other stimulants and poisons, making them believe they are helpful and good for themselves and their coming Babies, and then say, "Behold, we only are competent; all other healers are quacks and frauds; we command and you must obey." And you, the free American people bow low to the command of this Trust. Shame! But I believe you will break of help to break this Trust if you understand the question right.

Some of you may say, "What is all this fuss about? Why don't you Naturopaths get your license?" Yes, take out your license, get examined by a medical board whose members have not studied our Materia Medica? Have not studied Electricity, Massage, Hydropathy, Chromopathy, Suggestive Therapeutics, Orthopedic Surgery, and Chiropractic? I say a board whose members never studied these sciences but under the present Medical law alone entitled to use them? But suppose we did ask for examination, do you think they would examine us? No, they simply would say, "You do not come from a school we recognize," and if some of our members come from such a school being also Naturopaths, they would fare like many old-school Physicians who come here from other states, and who are not wanted here because the medical Trust do not want competition. Well, I hear some of you say, "That is strong." It is, but it is true; I will give you a few instances. Dr. S—, medical practitioner for 26 years, Professor of the University of Michigan, Professor of a Medical College in Los Angeles, a licensed Physician in two other states, failed in two points because he did not get his license. Dr. D—, graduate of a regular medical college, a Physician of good standing in another state, was allowed to practice prior to his examination. Failed in theoretical questions. No License, practiced without license, was arrested at the instigation of the Board of Examiners and fined $100.00

I ask you this question, who is more competent, a man who has practiced for years or a young man who just comes from college without any practical experience? These two cases are not the only ones; we could bring a number of similar cases. Will the Board of Examiners deny this? Do, if you can, gentlemen! If this is done with men of long experience, men of their own school, how do you think we should fare?

Now as to why the Medical Trust opposes Naturopathy, The Medical Trust opposed Naturopathy because it teaches people how to keep well; it teaches how to raise healthy children, and by this is a strong healthy Nation; by doing so it takes the from the Trust the power to fleece the public—it is easy to tell the patient, he suffers from some disease and inject a dose of morphine or fill him up with opium or quinine or whiskey, or write up a prescription, the ingredients generally not known to the Physician himself, coin in the money and let the patient die, or operate for the sake of having the name of a Surgeon (Butcher would be better). Yes, all this is easier than to cure your patient with natural means.

Now ladies and gentlemen, it is for you to say if the men who protect your health, save your mothers, wives and children from the knife and from death, shall have equal rights with the medical practitioner or not.

Whatever you do, the time will come when Naturopathy will rule in the whole world, not by force of Police or penal laws, but by virtue of its incomparable results in leading humanity to wisdom, health and longevity and to the pinnacle of happiness. Naturopathy will be the only future healing method of the world.

First: Naturopathy teaches the people how to keep well and how to raise healthy children and by that a healthy Nation.

A Physician should be a teacher as well as a healer.

1906

TEN COMMANDMENTS
BENEDICT LUST

VITAL FORCE IN MAN
SAMUEL A. BLOCH

DR. BURKE'S SANITARIUM.
Burke (nee Altruria), Sonoma Co., California.

THIS INSTITUTION is situated 54 miles North of San Francisco, California, near **Fulton Depot** on the California & Northwestern Railway.

It is situated on Mark West Creek, as it enters the great Sonoma valley, in a small valley to itself. Nature has here supplied an ideal location, which of itself is a sanitarium. The hills encircle it except on the Southwest giving shelter from winter storms, yet allowing the Southwest ocean breezes to temper the summer heat.

Nothing could more fitly harmonize with the work of the institution itself, for here, to aid in curing disease, Nature's remedies have been most thoroughly exploited. Fresh air, balmy sunshine, heat and cold, internal and external applications of hot and cold, mechanical therapeutics (Osteopathy), baths of every kind, electricity in its various forms, phototherapy, X-ray, are used scientifically. Foods nourishing the different systems of the human body, are given in proper combinations and proportions; these with other kindred remedies are employed with satisfactory results to patrons of the institution.

Rheumatism, neuralgia, nervous exhaustion, all skin affections including lupus and tuberculosis of the skin, dyspepsia, constipation, catarrh in all parts of the body, Diseases of the Liver, Hemorrhoids, Fistula, Diabetes, Obesity, Insomnia, Bronchitis, Paralysis, Dislocations of Vertebra or elsewhere, Tumors, etc., etc., are successfully treated at the Sanitarium.

Charges are according to room, including board at the public table, treatment and ordinary medical care. Prices are $17.50 and upward. Extra charge for surgical work, obstetrical cases and special nurses.

Persons confined to their rooms by chronic ailments, or afflicted with hysteria, melancholia or epilepsy, and persons to be treated for drug habits, cannot be received into the Sanitarium except by special arrangement. Address for particulars:

Dr. Burke's Sanitarium, Burke, Sonoma Co., California.

Paterson Naturopathic Institute.
841 Main St., Paterson, N. J.

Every branch of the Natural Healing Method skillfully applied Kneipp's System a Specialty. Best results in all acute and chronic diseases. Terms moderate. Depot for the genuine Kneipp Articles, Lust's Hygienic Foods, Agency for 'The Naturopath" and "Return to Nature"

JACOB LANG, N. D.   Mrs. J. A. LANG, N. D.

Members of the Naturopathic Society of America. Graduates of the American School of Naturopathy.

American Headquarters
FOR
Health Literature and Vegetarian nutritive food articles.

F. H. BENOLD, Prop.

413 E. North Ave.,   Chicago, Ill

On receipt of $2.00 I will send express prepaid to all places east of Omaha, Neb. and north of Louisville, Ky. one sample box of my Reform Health Foods and descriptive literature. Price list free. Write for catalogue.

ST. PAUL
Naturopathic Institute,
366 Hope Street.

EDW. LINDENAN, N. D.

Naturopathic Physician gratuated in Germany.
Member of the Naturopathic Society
of America.

Office Hours from 5 P. M.

Advertisements for institutes, headquarters, and sanitariums.

Ten Commandments

by Benedict Lust

The Naturopath and Herald of Health, VII(1), 7. (1906)

About 180,000 people die annually in America of pulmonary consumption. In view of this fact it will be found well worth while to observe the following ten commandments:

1. Love pure fresh air, and be careful to avoid breathing impure air.

2. Walk a great deal especially in the forests or at the seahore, and climb mountains.

3. Take breathing gymnastic exercises in forests or in any fresh, pure air; try to inhale deeply and to exhale perfectly, so that the lungs may become thoroughly cleansed, even to their utmost parts.

4. Drink a great deal of milk and of pure water.

5. Avoid beer, wine and spirits – in a word, all alcoholic drinks, and do not smoke tobacco in any form.

6. [In original documents item six is absent.]

7. Avoid dust and smoke.

8. Do not breathe through the mouth, but through the nose.

9. Avoid the company of people suffering of pulmonary diseases.

10. Never give way to bad temper, but always be cheerful and trust in the Lord.

Vital Force In Man

by Samuel A. Bloch

The Naturopath and Herald of Health, VII(7), 255-258. (1906)

I n order to most readily recognize any abnormal condition of the body, we must primarily comprehend what constitutes a normal body; we must observe what laws govern health, so that we can easily discern any deviation from these laws. Only after carefully studying the normal functions of our organs shall we be enabled to comprehend the causes which lead to the derangements of these organs and occasion dis-ease.

The body is a perfect unit, formed of millions of infinitesimal atoms, blended together in such an excellent manner, that a slight disturbance of any part will cause disorder in the whole system. Normal health pertains to the mental and physical conditions; the former is so intermingled with the latter that the mental condition influences the physical and vice versa. We have normal health when all our organs perform their functions naturally and unconsciously. It is our imperative duty to thoroughly comprehend these organs and the normal manner in which they should perform.

It is our purpose to show how we may know when our organs are performing normally, so we will examine the anatomical construction of man. Our body consists of many parts, bones, muscles, nerves, etc. The bones form the framework of the body; the muscles are attached to this bony structure; the nerves, although devoid of the power to contract, cause the muscles to do so. All the motions of the body are results of muscular contractions. The nerves control the muscles by a peculiar power called *vital force*. This power is constantly developed by the process of digestion and assimilation, and is stored in the brain, spinal cord and ganglionic system, to which one set of nerves run and from which another set starts. The nerves act as conductors of this force.

All of our organs are enveloped in what is called the skin. The skin is not merely a covering, it serves many purposes; for instance, the skin contains numerous perforations called pores through which oxygen is absorbed from the air, and the toxic carbon dioxide is eliminated, this process being a true respiration similar to that performed by the lungs. The skin is also full of nerves which inform the brain of the presence of foreign objects with which it comes in contact.

The body is composed partly of liquids and of more or less solid matter; all the parts are continuously changing in such a manner that the oldest are being constantly eliminated from the system. This work is performed by the depurating organs: the lungs, skin, bowels and kidneys. But so that the healthy body should maintain its normal weight we must replenish this loss by adding new material. The material thus absorbed is called food, and embraces solids, liquids and inhaled air. The solids and liquids are acted upon by the organs of digestion and assimilation which render it fit to take the place of the dead of effete matter. The soft part of our bodies is changed every year, while the bony formation requires seven years; thus we have possessed during seven years seven bodies of muscle and one of bone.

The various organs of our body are composed of myriads of very small parts called "cells" that can only be discerned through a microscope. The cells, on their part, are built up of atoms. The food we absorb, becomes vitalized, attains life as it were during the process of building into cells, but it remains there for a very short time only and in turn makes room for new substances. The old material is evacuated as soon as it has spent its vitality by contributing some manifestation of life—the conception of a thought or movement of a muscle. Vital force is the *breath of life*, so to speak, with which each individual is endowed at its birth. It is a fund supposed to last until our body has run its appointed length of duration. It is in our power to so economize this vital force, and to recuperate it (to an extent) that we live at least to 150 years of age; but it is impossible for us to add to our vital force in any manner whatsoever after it is once spent.

Our vital force is expended in the different activities of man's life, for instance upon all physical and mental actions, every sensation, painful or pleasant, involves an expenditure of our vital force. Life stands as an expression of all these actions, whether conscious or unconscious. Thus we see that *vital force is life*, they are both identical; in fact, the word "vital" is taken from the Latin word *vita*, meaning "life." Now we all concentrate our energies towards the continuation of our vital force for the present or the future, either in ourselves or offspring, or in the impression made by us on other people's mentality. This end is most thoroughly reached by longevity. A long life always depends upon this vital force which is stored in our systems and which we are forever expending. The wish to perpetuate pleasant sensations or to banish painful ones, demands the use of our intelligence to decide how best to accomplish these ends, and thereupon our will power impels the muscles in the chosen direction. There are two sets of muscles for expansion and contraction to correspond with our double sensations of pain and pleasure—one set to repel disagreeable sensations, the other to draw desirable objects towards us.

Now all of these exertions use up considerable of our vital force and the fund would soon be exhausted, were it not for our replenishing it within certain limits with the food absorbed. Is it not then wisdom for us to learn how to economize this vital force, and how to avoid wasting it? If the instincts of man were not so perverted they would unconsciously lead him in such a manner as to secure the greatest amount of good with the smallest expenditure of vital force. But, in man's present state, his will wavers and his unnatural cravings make him follow a course that is most ruinous to his health and opposes his best interests.

Those peculiar sensations which inform us of the need of fresh nutritive supplies are called hunger and thirst. It is described by Dr. Trall thus:

"Hunger and thirst, the sensations of which are referred to the stomach and throat, are indications of the wants of the general system. The rather ancient doctrines that hunger was produced by gastric juices in the stomach, and thirst by a dry condition of the mucous surface of the fauces (throat) are clearly erroneous. Both are sensations of organic instincts which communicate the need of the body for solid or liquid aliment to the common sensorium."

The intensity of the sensations of hunger and thirst depends mainly upon the amount of solids and liquids used up by the system, which in turn depends upon the amount of mental and physical activities, the quality of air inhaled and other expenditures of nerve force. Food enters the system in solid and liquid form via the mouth and in a gaseous form via the lungs and skin. Now, since the purpose of food is to restore vital force, naturally the quality of the food should be a matter of considerable importance.

To receive the greatest amount of vital force from foods we must eat it as Nature intended, and not as manufactured by man. We all know that the process of adding chemicals to the food destroys the life germ; that is, it destroys that which contains the vital force. In the destruction of the life germ we then have foods that build up dead tissue. Cells constructed out of the proper foods will not disintegrate and become dead matter, to be replaced by new cells in the fraction of the time it takes the cells formed by adulterated foods to disintegrate; hence there is considerable less vital force expended in the perpetuation of life and normal bodily conditions. It is a practical impossibility to rebuild and reconstruct healthy cells out of dead material. The dead cells must be replenished with nitrogenous material, if we wish to rebuild on a perpetuating plane.

The vibrations of the sun's rays fill everything with which they come in contact with vital life-giving energy; and all foods that grow in the sun contain the greatest amount of vital force. There is no doubt that "Mother Nature" intended her children to live on natural foods, already seasoned with all flavors to suit every individual taste; but man in his supreme wisdom endeavored to improve (?) on her handiwork by adding preservatives to the foods, and as in everything else proved a colossal failure. But when he enters into a copartnership with "Mother Nature" there is such an harmonious intermingling of all interests, that normal intoxicating health appears on the scene, hence, a greater amount of vital force is the consequence.

Health is maintained—as long as the food is of proper quality (that is foods that contain and yield the greatest amount of nutriment); as long as the production from the food is sufficient to counterbalance the expenditure; as long as all the organs perform their functions normally and unconsciously (that is, as long as the foods are properly digested and assimilated and the dead effete material eliminated); and as long as the vital force is not recklessly and criminally squandered by excesses (promiscuous sexual intercourse, alcoholism, late hours, etc.)

The carbon (C) of the food is burned up, as it were, while passing through the system, and thus by a transmutation of energy, mental and physical phenomena arise. This change is affected similar to the light and heat of the sun, stored up in all plants, reappear in the animals that feed upon them; they are evident in the muscular and other manifestations of the life forces. The action of the sun's vibration upon the bare skin has the similar beneficial effects as in plants, and is a valuable aid in recuperating expended vital force. The blood and nerves are the vehicles of this vital power, therefore the vitality of any organ is due to the amount and quality of blood supplied to that organ, and the condition of the nerves leading to that organ. The amount of blood in any organ is due to the principle of reaction—for instance, as in the case of bathing:—A cold bath taken by a normal, healthy person, brings the blood to the surface; while a warm bath leaves the skin bloodless (anaemic); the operation is thus explained. The impression made on the surface of the skin by cold water is communicated to the central station of vital force, and this power directs an extra quantity of blood to the cooled spot to make up the deficiency. In the case of the warm bath the central station relinquishes its efforts, as the temperature of the skin is already too high. The resulting consequence of continued warm baths is a gradual and permanent lowering of the vital force.

The natural tendency of the vital force is to equalize the temperature of the system. If any organ is especially active, an extra amount of blood is sent to that place. For instance, while in deep thought the blood is drawn to the brain and when eating the stomach is surcharged. Only one action should take place at one time, otherwise the blood cannot decide where to go—and then some positive injury will result to some spot. The harm resulting from bathing after a meal is an instance of the hesitation on the part of the blood where to go to, whether the skin or the stomach should have the necessary extra supply. That part of the vital force which is supposed to propel the blood acts by stimulating the heart. This in its turn propels the blood to the lungs. The intensity of a person's appetite for nourishment is in direct proportion to the energy with which the blood is propelled through the lungs. Thus we see a complete circle of expenditure and recuperations of the vital force, for in properly satisfying the craving for food by eating pure, unadulterated foods—we again build up our vital force. In reality there is no loss of life-force in any normal action of our system; even in the act of procreation, all of the vital force sacrificed by sexual intercourse reappears in the offspring.

The energies of the sun are changed into muscular energy of all animals, into the power of the steam-engine, into the heat of a stove, into the brilliancy and force of electricity. Force cannot be destroyed; it is as indestructible and eternal as matter. But force can be transformed; it can reappear in various forms. This condition exists also in the human engine; all fuel foods are converted into a corresponding amount of energy—such as muscular and mental force and power or sexual activity. When you economize one form of energy the others will be benefited thereby and gain in power.

Vital force is expended by the following actions: Supplying all the organs with energy, blood and new material, eliminating dead material from the system, by mental and physical overwork, and by the sex-act. If this act is performed as nature intended it to be, i.e., where love exists in the participants, there is no loss, as it gives pleasure to the actors, and as the vital force reappears in the offspring. Vital force is supported by proper vitality-building foods, it is economized by rest and leading a continent and chaste existence, and is recuperated by sleep and procreation. Our sexual organs have been given to us for the sole purpose of securing offspring; and their abuse through prostitution is a certain and permanent injury to the vital force. If promiscuous sexual intercourse is natural would nature punish us with the most loathsome diseases? It has been proven that one sexual act may effect fecundation; in order to enjoy normal and perfect health for themselves and offspring they should refrain from further approach. This idea will meet with ridicule and jest from many people who seem to think that such continence is impossible. Of course when the people's diet and mode of existence is unnatural and has a tendency to stimulate sexual inclinations, they think it is natural. If they would only change to a natural mode of life, eating natural vital foods, bathing regularly, exercising properly, etc., they would be enabled to know the difference.

The partaking of food serves a double purpose—to produce both heat and energy. This can be seen in the steam engine, where the power drawn from the coal, reappears as heat and force. Then again this force is utilized in various forms--to drive an engine, produce electricity, etc. Thus human energy reappears under different aspects—in the offspring, physical and mental activities, etc. When the vital force is once expended in a certain direction, it cannot again be used in a different way. Thus, mentality and promiscuous sexual actions act reciprocally. The more we indulge in the latter the greater is the power drawn from the physical and mental energies. If people acted in accordance with this knowledge the result to this race—physically and mentally—would be so ennobling and uplifting that it would be far beyond the realm of human conception.

THE PURPOSE AND METHOD OF NATURE CURE

BENEDICT LUST

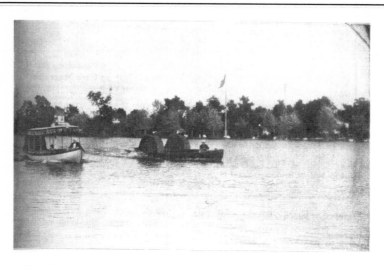

Orchard Beach Sanatorium NATURHEILANSTALT

(DURING THE WINTER IN CHICAGO) McHENRY, ILL,
DR. CARL STRUEH, Prop. 100 State Street (Room 1409), Chicago, Ill.

The sanatorium is located in the beautiful Fox River Valley, only 1 hour's ride from Chicago. Absolutely private location. Conducted on the "simple life" plan. Rural surroundings and home life. Twenty acres of ground, with large river front. Ideal home for the cure of chronic diseases and for convalescents. Special Department for delicate and sick children. Facilities for vacation guests.

Kneipp Water Cure, Diet Cures: Vegetarian, milk, grape, raw food diet. **Schroth's Regenerating Cure. Fasting. Open Air Gymnasium. Sun and Air Baths.** Sleeping Outdoors. All kinds of outdoor exercises, lawntennis, swimming, boating, fishing, gardening, etc. Extensive meadow for walking barefooted. Strictly **Individual treatment.** Terms moderate. Long distance telephone. Write for our illustrated booklet, or any desired information.

Advertisement for Dr. Carl Strueh's sanatorium in Chicago
and Dr. Lust's sanitarium, Yungborn, in New Jersey.

The Purpose And Method Of Nature Cure

by Benedict Lust

The Naturopath and Herald of Health, VIII(3), 68-70. (1907)

> *Serve humanity with every breath of your life.*
> *Make every day immortal by your acts.*
> —Lavater

Great changes take place on all planes of life. Progress is noticed everywhere. Whatever is old and whatever has become useless has to give way to new forms, to new conditions. These changes are of no greater beneficial results than in the treatment of diseases, or still better, in the prevention and total conquest of disease. In this conquest culminates the acme of medical science.

This medical treatment is directly based on Nature's laws; it takes man as a child of Nature which has to be educated according to its mother's laws and has to learn to follow them, though hard this may ever be for the highly civilized man and the fastidious lady of fashion. The reward for doing so is great, immensely great; this will only be fully realized by the next generation which will then appear as a tangible and undeniable proof of this great change in medical treatment. This treatment, as said before, will consist in strictly living up to Nature.

Humanity is still very far from this goal; the education to a natural life is still in a state of embryo; the ideal health is only a dream as most people suffer of this or that disease they have to be made acquainted with the fact that Nature alone is the true and lasting healer.

There is no country in Europe where this method has not yet been introduced and where it has not become the favorite cure of all well balanced people. And everywhere nature cure associations sprang to life.

This method is certainly not an enemy to science, though medical science treats the man who has transgressed the laws of Nature in harmony with those transgressions, instead of helping him adjust himself to those laws which are thoroughly contradictory to the life of refined society; to this scientific treatment the poor patient, deprived of all strong will power, gives in, until his body thoroughly decays and—dies.

The natural method of healing has not such results. She is like a severe parent; she demands exact adaptation and strict obedience to her laws; she wants man to know and to study these laws, until he has become familiar with them, that he cannot help but love them, and, consequently, submit to them. The consequence of these studies, of this submission, is strong, unimpaired health, accompanied by a healthy mind; and these are the chief or rather, the only factors for a successful life.

The study of Nature's laws, that is, of God's laws, challenges any criticism. Nature's method is pure and simple, is quiet and inoffensive in her progressive march and never condescends to criticize or belittle medical scientists. These methods belong to the past and will soon be swallowed up in the abyss of time, while the Natural Method helps to inaugurate the Millennium, the Golden Age, the time when we shall have done away with sickness, physical weakness and deformities. Nor does Nature Cure attack vaccination, vivisection or whatever name medical resources may have; these evils will die out as everything has to pass away that is detrimental to human progress.

The natural methods quietly resists or tries to resist the general degeneration as is revealed in the lower degree of popular health and the premature death of millions of people in their very bloom of life.

Millions of people, either out of ignorance or because of the hard social conditions under which most human being live, transgress Nature's laws. The natural method is taught by lectures and by literature. Everywhere true and genuine reformers raise their voices and preach the real regeneration of the body which has to precede that of the spirit; and in untold pamphlets and books this gospel of the body is proclaimed in all languages, in all countries.

Whoever belongs to this movement, goes boldly forward, attracting congenial minds and rousing the searching, inquiring spirit in the opponents. Nature Cure is beyond all religious and political parties; it appeals to rich and poor, to educated and uneducated, to scholars and workingmen alike, for its aim is health, pure and simple, the first requirement of each and all.

NATURE ALONE HEALS

Nature alone heals is the motto of Nature Cure. The power that after the winter awakens the earth to new beauty; the power that develops the chicken out of the egg; the infant out of the mother's womb, this power lives in each human being and whoever knows how to use it, may regenerate after sickness or when his system has run down, or his years declined. How often do we not meet with people who declare they have been cured by themselves; that means Nature helped them.

There is scarcely one person, who, when sick, has not been restored to health with the assistance of a regular physician. Wounds in plants, animals and human beings heal by themselves. Splinters and musket balls have entered the flesh have become encapsulated in the flesh and saliva without injuring in the least the human body. In thousands of autopsies these wounds were found to be thoroughly healed and cicatrised.

Vomiting and diarrhoea after the consumption of rotten or poisonous food, eczema, boils, inflammation, fevers are nothing else but self regenerating processes. That therapeutic medical treatment which is based on Nature or on self power; a treatment that supports, vitalizes and leads to regeneration and health is the method of nature cure.

The Limit Of Individual Power And The Factors Of The Healing Method Of Nature

The individual healing power has its limits; in specially hard cases it needs to be supported. This support is found in the remedies that are necessities in the days of health. These remedies are: Air, light, exercise (gymnastics, massage), the right nourishment, dry and humid warmth in the way of water, steam and hot air baths, packs, compresses, douches in the manifold variety. The natural healing method does not work miracles, nor is it able to cure any disease, the less so, as there are cases which have already been touched by the hand of death. Besides, this method is usually applied when all vitality has left the human body, when all human help is too late. The impossible can never be expected, and conditions of sickness which have taken many years for their development, cannot be cured in a trice. As long as there is one spark of life left, and the nature physician masters his art, the patient may be restored to health, even then, when all other methods have failed.

Why Does Nature Cure Reject All Drugs?

1. Because there is no sickness which might not be cured without drugs.
2. Because no healthy man needs drugs in order to remain in good health, and no sick man needs them in order to be cured.
3. Because drugs are no remedy at all. Many of the famous medical authorities of all countries reject drugs as powerless in any disease whatever. Prof. Dr. Natnagel says: "Drugs can never cure a disease; but may cause a new one."
4. Most drugs, extracted from poisonous plants, would injure healthy bodies and are therefore not fit to cure sick people.

Prof. Dr. Kobert says in his text book on *Intoxication*: "We physicians are bound to confess that thousands of people are killed by improperly or wrongly dosed medicines."

Expert nature doctors apply only such remedies that sooth and alleviate pain only in intense suffering and indispensable operations.

The nature cure method recognizes the necessity of surgical processes and recurs to operation only in virulent tumors, acute deep suppurations, accidents and so forth, but demonstrates continually through facts that countless other operations (especially in female troubles) about 90% might be avoided.

WHAT ARE THE EFFECTS OF THE NATURAL HEALING METHOD?

The hundred and one applications of water, air, light, exercise and so forth have the following results:

1. They clean the body inside and outside; as the disgusting mixture of dirt, dust, sweat, tallow, scales can be removed from the skin, thus all morbid matter, the retrogressive metamorphosis of the blood and all poisonous matter may be evacuated out of the organism by absorption and evacuation.

2. Water appliances will cool the feverish, hot body, as well as any burning wound.

3. They will calm the feverish breast, the over-excited nerves and the highly palpitating heart.

4. They will soothe the high and life-endangering fever.

5. In any congestion or inflammation they will draw the blood from the brain and heart.

6. They will soothe burns, or any goutic, rheumatic or convulsive pains.

7. By means of compresses and vapor baths they will dissolve and evacuate any morbid matter.

8. They stimulate, strengthen and vitalize all secretory organs, the circulation of the blood, the nervous system, the digestion, and the formation of blood and humors.

WHAT ADVANTAGES DOES THE NATURE CURE OFFER?

1. The cure is effected in a very short time.

2. The cure is sure, thorough and without any secondary disease.

3. The treatment by the natural method is cheaper than any other.

4. The natural cure may be applied everywhere in any family, at any home, without any loss of time and long before the sickness has fully developed, even then, when the evil is of long and old standing, when all human help seems to be exhausted.

5. By avoiding the countless causes of disease and by correct energetic and timely acting; the partisans of the Nature Cure movement have created a bulwark of health; from whence they will protect themselves against any attacks of the enemy called sickness, with all its horrid accompaniments.

In fact, Nature is the very first factor in our many and varied reform movements; for whoever has health, has the sesame, the wonderful key that unlocks every other treasure.

1908

DOCTORS AND THEIR EXORBITANT FEES
S. T. ERIEG

NATURE AS A DOCTOR
C. S. CARR, M.D.

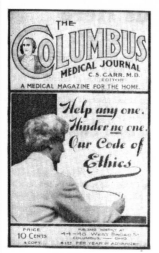
Dr. C. S. Carr was the editor of *The Columbus Medical Journal*,
a magazine to increase public health awareness..

Doctors And Their Exorbitant Fees

by S. T. Erieg

The Naturopath and Herald of Health, IX(1), 14-15. (1908)

It is rapidly becoming a conspicuous reality that the affairs of life are getting extremely stringent, and the tension is becoming greater day by day. The trusts are two great millstones grinding with relentless activity, and the grist is human beings. Their seal is set on all commodities of life, and the humblest home cannot escape the levy. Their slimy tentacles enter the poorest homes and fasten on everything, even the spool of thread which the poor mother finds necessary in making clothes for her shivering children, and she must pay twice the price for a spool of thread as formerly.

Among the various experiences the city of Williamsport, Pa., has encountered, that had made a heavy levy on the family purse, is the recent combined move of the city doctors in compelling the people to pay enormous fees for their services. It is expensive to be born now, and still more so to die; but to get well, most expensive of all. While the doctors' move might not be classed with the trusts, it means the same thing when it comes to dollars and cents.

The Williamsport doctors have unceremoniously and without any feeling for the people, announced a new schedule for fees, and all the city doctors have signed their names to the new schedule with perhaps two exceptions. They have raised their charges for office and home calls all the way from fifty to one hundred per cent, over the old rates. For office calls they charge $1, for house calls, $1.50, and for night calls they charge the small sum of $3; for surgical and other services the doctors charge proportional high rates.

However rosy the doctors pictured the acceptance of the new schedule by the people, they have now had reason to change their minds, for the people have received increased rates with indignation and protests. There is now on foot a move to boycott the city doctors. The beginning of this move had its growth in railroad men, but has since had many other adherents. There was a meeting held in the west end of the cozy with the object in view of getting out of town doctors. And if there were any hazy ideas entertained by some as to the possibility of this move materializing effective for results, the mist has entirely cleared away. The meeting was successful in every way. Not only the west end, but the east end citizens and representatives of every part of the city were present. A committee was appointed with the necessary officers and the committee is now ready to consider the procuring of out of town doctors, or, if any of the city doctors wish to offer their services at old rates, they will be considered the same as doctors from other cities.

A reason given by physicians for the increased rates is that living and other expenses have increased. This is true; but they have not increased so much as fifty or one hundred per cent. And it must be remembered that expenses have increased for all, and for those especially who will be most burdened by the increased rates. The doctors for a five minute call, and or even less time, take what most men work a while day for, so it is seen that the poor man has burdens enough without doctors placing additional ones on his back. The doctors are well cared for; they build fine houses, have automobiles and horses, and their families look prosperous. While those upon whom doctors' bills lay most heavily are satisfied to use their legs as a means of conveyance.

Another reason given is that some do not pay their doctors' bills. Now it would be just as much common sense for a tailor to charge fifty or seventy-five dollars for a suit of clothes which formerly could be purchased for twenty-five dollars because some do not pay for their clothes, as it is for doctors to raise prices for the same reason. It is certainly the portion of common sense to assert that if some can not pay their doctor bills at lower rates, raising them will not assist in their paying them.

Of course people should pay their doctor bills as well as their other bills. The laborer is worthy of his hire. But there are some life vocations in which men dare not conscientiously enter with the simple object of making money. Among the two foremost of these are the ministry and healing of bodily ills. When a man goes into the ministry or medicine simply for his living, it is a sign that he should stay out.

The most precious thing in this world is the soul of man, and the work of the minister is to save souls. But if the ministers were to get together and demand a certain fixed salary it would be considered an awful thing; yet increased cost of living and everything is shared by ministers, and they must go through years of hard study before they can enter their life work, but the ministers are poorly paid. The doctor should not enter his profession with the object of getting rich; if this is the object, business is the place for him. He should enter the profession for the love of humanity, to save life and alleviate suffering, just as the conscientious preacher enters his work to save souls. Of course all should be well paid for their work; but as we all know, the doctors are well paid.

It is hoped that the doctors have seen their mistake and will rectify it. Ruminating on this recent turn of affairs, we are reminded of the biblical dictum concerning the burdens thrust upon the people by doctors and lawyers.

There are some life vocations in which men dare not con-scientiously enter with the simple object of making money. Among the two foremost of these are the ministry and healing of bodily ills. When a man goes into the ministry or medicine simply for his living, it is a sign that he should stay out.

The doctors for a five minute call, and or even less time, take what most men work a while day for, so it is seen that the poor man has burdens enough without doctors placing addi-tional ones on his back.

The doctor should not enter his profession with the object of getting rich; if this is the object, business is the place for him. He should enter the profession for the love of humanity, to save life and alleviate suffering, just as the conscientious preacher enters his work to save souls. Of course all should be well paid for their work; but as we all know, the doctors are well paid.

NATURE AS A DOCTOR

by C. S. Carr, M.D.

The Naturopath and Herald of Health, IX(6), 180-181. (1908)

Nature's tendency is toward the normal. Every force that nature is capable of is directed toward producing symmetrical, normal and well balanced organisms. This is especially true of the laws that govern the human body. If disease attacks the body nature brings to bear all her forces to resist this disease. If a poisonous medicine is taken at once the powers of nature are summoned to resist the intruder. What we call the operation of a drug is simply nature's method of getting rid of a foreign substance. What we call symptoms of disease are simply nature's efforts to restore the body to a normal condition. A quick pulse, a high temperature, rapid breathing, a dry skin, or a moist skin; all these are the tactics which nature adopts to readjust the body to its environment.

What, then, should a doctor do when he witnesses nature's desperate attempts? He notes the efforts which nature is making. Should he help or hinder nature? It would certainly seem he should help. If he cannot help nature in her time of trouble he had better go away and leave the patient to himself.

In what way can he help? Manifestly the only help he can bring is to increase the power of nature to resist. If the physician notes that the patient's temperature is too high he will render no help by forcing the temperature down with drugs. If he notices that the pulse is too quick he will not help nature by making the pulse go slower with some drug. Indeed, he is fighting against nature when he does these things. The high temperature and quick pulse are nature's struggles to rid herself of disease. To weaken these struggles is to join the disease in over-coming nature.

All that a doctor can do in acute, diseases to which human flesh is heir to is to take all hindrances away so that nature and disease can have a fair fight, putting no obstructions in the way of nature, and, if possible, prevent disease from continually adding reinforcements to its powers. If the disease is due to some unsanitary or unwholesome environment, of course, such environment ought to be removed at once else the disease will be constantly reinforced.

The physician should do exactly as men do in the army, at the mines or in a logging camp. Two men have a quarrel and they start to fight. The crowd immediately forms a ring about them so as to shut out all interference. "Fair play," everybody cries, "give each man a fair chance." If either of the men have friends in the crowd they are carefully watched and kept from rendering assistance. "Let them fight it out," the cry goes from all sides.

This is what the physicians ought to do in all cases of acute ailments. Draw a ring of protection around the patient and let nature and disease have a fair fight. Don't allow any sort of deleterious thing to come in and assist the disease. Shut out everything that will harm the patient. Noise and confusion, bad odors and solemn talk, nasty medicine, sloppy foods—all these should be kept away from the patient in order to let nature have a fair show. On the other hand, plenty of light and good air giving the patient a small quantity of whatever he calls for, cheerful attendants, assuaging pain or nervousness, itching or aching, throbbing of burning, by such harmless and local applications as are within reach.

All this can be done so that the disease can take no unfair advantage of the patient. Now if there is anything else that can be done it is simply this: The patient's power of resistance, the patient's strength to fight the enemy may be increased by something that stimulates and strengthens his natural powers. What the physician could call *vis medicatrix naturae* should be strengthened. Exactly as the pugilist retires to the corner for the rest and refreshment at the end of each round, so at the proper intervals should the victim of disease be strengthened and nourished by the physician. The patient's own wishes should be largely consulted in these matters.

If he wants water, give him water; if he wants milk, give him milk; if he wants something sour, give it to him; give him whatever he wants within reasonable limits. Do not force him to take something he does not want. His own feelings are a better guide than all the physicians in the world.

Is there no medicine that would help? We believe so. Any medicine that would make the patient temporarily feel stronger and better during health will also have the same effect if he were sick. What would a well person do if called upon to endure some physical strain almost beyond his powers to bear? A gentle, non-irritating stimulus has saved many a life by rallying the forces of nature to make one more effort after nature had practically given up the fight. Stimuli are not good things for habitual use, but to meet some crisis where all the powers of nature are required quickly, else the battle be lost, a stimulus becomes an invaluable agent for good. What is still better than a stimulus is that combination of stimuli and invigorants known as a tonic. A small and oft-repeated dose of some well-devised tonic during the ordeal of acute disease will often turn the scale in favor of the patient, but this should not be carried to excess.

At first the powers of nature should be left to cope with the disease without the assistance of any drug, but when, in spite of all auxiliary assistance, nature seems to be getting the worst of the fight, a little medicinal assistance at the right time is very valuable. Quinine at such a crisis is often very useful, but the use of quinine at the onset of the disease is quite baneful, as it is altogether too early in the struggle for artificial assistance to be of use. A wise athlete will accept no stimulus at the beginning of a contest. It is only after his natural powers begin to flag when some last ordeal is required that seems too much for his natural strength that he will accept a little assistance from artificial sources.

This is exactly as acute diseases ought to be treated. The physician should be watchful and careful, never allowing himself to give any medicine until the actual moment that it is required. Some physicians begin to give quinine at the beginning of every acute ailment. They continue the quinine day after day during the whole course of the disease. All this is very harmful. The quinine becomes the ally of the disease, making it much harder for the system to cope with it. Thus it is that the fight which nature makes against acute diseases can be assisted slightly now and then, but as a rule no medicine is required. As between the usual treatment for acute diseases and no medicine at all, every odds is in favor of no medicine rather than the ordeal of medicinal treatment that is usually given.

In cases of typhoid fever, measles, diphtheria, small pox or any other acute disease, it would be far better of the patient lived in a country where there were no doctors at all. The practice of hydrotherapy and the rigid application of sanitary science has done very much toward lessening the mortality of acute diseases, but with this blessing has always been associated the curse of drug-giving, which in some instances well night dissipates all their benefits.

What we call symptoms of disease are simply nature's efforts to restore the body to a normal condition.

Draw a ring of protection around the patient and let nature and disease have a fair fight.

The Effect Of The Mind On The Body
E. G. White Et All

A Suggestion
C. M. Corbin, M.D.

Medical tourism before its time.

The Effect Of The Mind On The Body

The Naturopath and Herald of Health, XVI(11), 697. (1909)

Mind is the master-power that moulds and makes.
And man is Mind, and evermore he takes
The tool of thought, and shaping what he wills,
Bring forth a thousand joys, a thousand ills
He thinks in secret, and it comes to pass
Environment is but his looking-glass.

The condition of the mind affects the health to a far greater degree than many realize. Many of the diseases from which men suffer are the result of mental depression. Grief, anxiety, discontent, remorse, guilt, distrust, all tend to break down the life forces, and invite decay and death. Disease is sometimes produced, and is often greatly aggravated by the imagination. Many are life-long invalids who might be well if they only thought so. Many imagine that every slight exposure will cause illness, and the evil effect is produced because it is expected. Many die from disease the cause of which is wholly imaginary. Courage, hope, faith, sympathy, love, promote health and prolong life. A contented mind, a cheerful spirit, is health to the body and strength to the soul.

—Mrs. E.G. White in *Ministry of Healing.*

We are just beginning to understand the part that good thinking holds in good health. Our thoughts are just as real a part of us as are our bodies. A man who persists in thinking unhealthy thoughts can no more keep sound and healthy in body than a man who violates all the physical laws of his nature.

—Dr. Gulick in *The Efficient Life.*

Do not go about repeating the statement that nothing affects the temper like diseases of the stomach; it would be better to say that nothing troubles the functions of the stomach like moody tempers.

—Dr. Paul Dubois.

The more we study the processes of recovery, the more we are convinced that they depend, not upon the introduction of drugs from without, but upon the activity of forces within the body. . . . This power depends upon the ability of various organs in the body to produce protective and antidotal substances which destroy the poisons produced by microbes, or even kill the microbes outright. Such a substance may be produced in the liver or in the pancreas or in the bone-marrow or in the thyroid gland or elsewhere. But these tissues, like all others, are subject to the control of the nervous system. . . . We can readily understand that the trophic (nutritive) influence of the nervous system is diminished by worry and multiplied by hope.

—Dr. C.W. Saleeby in *Worry*.

I suspect that neither the nature nor the amount of work is accountable for the frequency and severity of our breakdowns, but that their cause lies rather in those absurd feelings of hurry and having no time, in that breathlessness and tension, that anxiety of feature and that solitude for results, that lack of inner harmony and ease, in short, by which, with us, the work is so apt to be accomplished.

—Prof. W. James in *Talks to Teachers*.

There is not a natural action of the body, whether voluntary or involuntary, that may not be influenced by the peculiar state of the mind at the time.

—Dr. John Hunter.

A Suggestion

by C. M. Corbin, N.D.

The Naturopath and Herald of Health, XVI(12), 769. (1909)

Imagination rules the world.

The above was given to us by Napoleon, the greatest fighter the world has ever known or ever will know; for the people that live today are of a different type, believing that the great world, by a greater God is ruled and that God is Love, therefore that Love is King and Love is the arbiter of all things of lasting natural law will fulfill all requirements needful to mortal man; therefore, if we but pause to think, we will know that the law of love will compensate for all, in all, over all.

The student of healing, teaching, preaching and true living is known today as a Naturopath, and to be all things that are good, he must truly live the life in all its fullness, which he will do in spite of environment, inclination or previous methods or habits of life, if his **intention** is good.

Dear reader, I have never had any reason for not feeling more thankful every morning and each succeeding day, that I have kept up the struggle in my endeavor to find the true light which is the guiding star of Drugless Healing, viz. naturopathy.

It might not be amiss at this time for me to tell you who it was that finally helped me to get the broader view, the higher idea. His name you all know and to know Him and His struggles is to love Him; to follow Him step by step as He has labored to establish a standard that is at once broad, yet easy of comprehending, is to reverse Him and His work, for it is and has been, truly a great work of love, for His fellowmen, giving as He has, the best His heart and soul possessed, at a price which in no wise compensate Him, from a financial viewpoint. And yet in His goodness he is steadily growing a bigger, better man, recognizing the truly great God consciousness that "lies within" as a force that will carry Him and His students, patients and followers to heights and realms undreamed of by many of us, that might be led away from the divine plan of Unity.

"In union there is strength" and this old quotation can never be used to better purpose than right now in the naturopathic movement of America. There is room for ten thousand Jungborns, right here in the United States, where there is a constant cry for relief from the great mass of people, who have leaned on the old schools of medicine only to find that their faith had been outraged and the law of "Ethics" (medical of course) placed in its stead and at a cost that cannot in its magnitude, be encompassed by the finite mind, yet the man who is devoting his very life, with all his vital and spiritual force, to the teaching of the great truths of Naturopathy (which is to my mind the grandest work under the sun) should have greater encouragement than he has heretofore received.

I, for one, am going to push a little harder. Are you? I, for one, am going to live a little closer to nature's divine laws. Will you? I, for one, am willing to make greater sacrifices to my pride of personal individuality, that the great whole may stand with an unbroken front which shall be as solid as "The Rock of Gibraltar". Are you?

Dear reader, if you and I will do this, Dr. Benedict Lust's life will have been lived and worked out in a way that will not only stand as a monument for all time to come, but countless hearts will be made happy, light and free, because of his work as a standard bearer and to this end I am willing to lighten his burden, by assuming my share of it with **others** that have so royally stood by him through the thick of the fight, but some of us are dozing, feeling or rather thinking that "all things will come to those that wait." But I have found out it is much better to "hustle".

If this does not land in the basket, I will give the readers of *The Naturopath* the results of some of the experiences I have had with a few so-called incurable cases.

There is room for ten thousand Jungborns, right here in the United States.

I, for one, am going to push a little harder. Are you? I, for one, am going to live a little closer to nature's divine laws.

1910

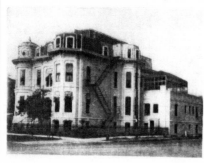
Advertisements for Dr. Lindlahr's sanitarium and Nature Cure.

Nature Cure In A Nutshell

by H. Lindlahr, M.D.
The Naturopath and Herald of Health, XV(1), 30-31. (1910)

Primary Cause Of Disease

Barring trauma (injury), advancing age and surroundings uncongenial to human life, all causes of disease may be classified as follow:

I. **Violation of Nature's laws** in thinking, breathing, eating, clothing, working, resting and in moral, sexual and social life.

II. **Lowered vitality** due to Cause I, overwork, nightwork, excesses, stimulation, poisonous drugs and ill-advised surgical operations.

III. **Accumulation of waste matter, morbid matter and poisons due to** Causes I and II, and to faulty food selection, overeating, the use of alcohol, tobacco, coffee, tea (and last, but not least, to **the suppression of acute diseases** Nature's healing and cleansing efforts) by poisonous drugs and surgical operations.

Resulting In The Following Secondary Causes Of Disease

I. **Hereditary and constitutional diseases** of sycosis, psora, syphilis, scrofula, mercurialism, cinchonism, iodism and many other forms of chronic drug poisoning.

II. Fevers, inflammations, skin eruptions, ulcers, abscesses, germs, bacteria and parasites.

III. Weakening and loss of reason, will and self-control resulting in negative, sensitive and subjective conditions which in turn open the way to nervous prostration, insanity and to control by other personalities. (Hypnotism insanity, double personality, etc., etc.)

In correspondence with the primary causes of disease, Naturopathy recognizes the following

Three Great Methods Of Cure

I. **Return to Nature,** or the establishment of normal surroundings, which necessitates:
> **a.** Extension of Consciousness by popular and individual education.
>
> **b.** The constant exercise of reason, will and self-control.

c. A return to natural habits of life in thinking, breathing, eating, clothing, working, resting, and in moral, sexual and social life.

d. Correction of mechanical defects and injuries by osteopathy, surgery, etc.

II. **Economy of Vital Force,** which necessitates

a. Stoppage of all leaks and waste of vital force.

b. Scientific relaxation, rest and sleep.

c. Proper food selection, magnetic treatment, etc.

III. **Elimination,** which necessitates

Pure food, judicious fasting, hydrotherapy (water cure), osteopathy, massage, exercise, physical culture, light and air bath, homeopathy and simple herb remedies.

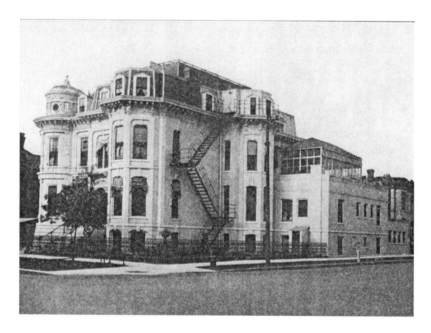

The Lindlahr Sanitarium, 525-529 Ashland Blvd., Chicago, IL.

CATECHISM OF NATURE CURE

by H. Lindlahr, M.D.

The Naturopath and Herald of Health, XV(1), 32-35. (1910)

Dalendo est Carthago!

For many years in the Roman Senate, Cato concluded every speech with these words. Again and again he repeated them in order to impress upon the consciousness of his fellow citizens the necessity of destroying their dangerous rival across the Mediterranean. The persistent SUGGESTION did its work. Carthage was destroyed and for many centuries Rome remained the undisputed mistress of the world.

The great and beneficial truths of Naturopathy must in like manner be reiterated over and over again before they can uproot and destroy the errors and sophistries of pseudoscience. In order to accomplish this we shall follow the method of the old Roman and repeat again and again by means of charts and diagrams the facts, laws and principle underlying the Science and Philosophy of Naturopathy until they become ingrained into popular consciousness. In all our future articles we shall have occasion to refer constantly to these definitions and diagrams. It is therefore not for the purpose of filling space that we shall republish these and similar tables in succeeding issues of this magazine, but in order to build the new consciousness of right living, natural healing and constructive morality.

Basing our deductions on the laws and principles enunciated and demonstrated in Volume I of the Nature Cure series, and in the full-page diagram, "Nature Cure in a Nutshell", we can now proceed to sum up the evidence therein presented and formulate it into a Catechism of Nature Cure.

As we proceed on our journey into the domain of rational science we shall make additions to this catechism by defining as precisely as possible certain words and phrases which convey meaning and ideas peculiar to our philosophy.

This becomes necessary, because every science embodying new modes of thought requires exact modes of expression and some new definitions of already well-known words and phrases.

Nature Cure and Diagnosis from the Eye are new sciences, dealing with newly discovered (or re-discovered) natural laws and principles, and with the application of these to the phenomena of life, disease and cure.

The student of Nature Cure and kindred subjects will do well to study closely these definitions and formulated principles, since they contain the pith and marrow of our philosophy and greatly facilitate its understanding.

1. **What is normal or natural?**
   That which is in harmonic relation with life purposes of the individual.

2. **What is Nature Cure?**
   Nature Cure is a system of man building in harmony with the constructive principle in Nature on the physical, mental and moral planes of being.

3. **What is the constructive principle in life or Nature?**
   It is that principle in life or nature which builds up, improves and repairs, which always makes for the perfect type, and whose activity in nature we designate as evolutionary and constructive.

4. **What is the destructive principle in life or Nature?**
   It is that principle in life or nature which disintegrates and destroys existing forms and types and whose activity in nature we designate as revolutionary or destructive.

5. **What is health?**
   Health is normal and harmonious vibration of all the elements and forces comprising the human entity on the physical, mental and moral planes of being, in conformity with the constructive principles in individual life.

6. **What is disease?**
   Disease is abnormal on inharmonious vibration of the elements and forces composing the human entity on one or more planes of being, in conformity with the destructive principles of individual life.

7. **What is the primary cause of disease?**
   Barring accidental and surgical injury to the human organism and barring surroundings hostile to human life, **the primary cause of disease is violation of Nature's laws.**

8. **What is the effect of violation of Nature's laws on the physical organism?**
   The effect of violation of natural laws on the physical human organism is:
   1. Lowered vitality, and,
   2. Accumulation of waste matter, morbid matter and poisons.

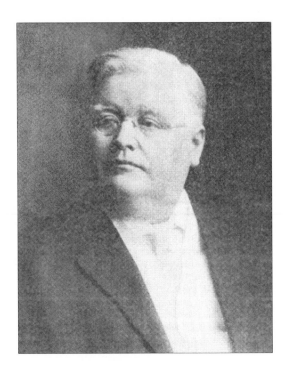

Dr. H. Lindhahr.

These conditions are synonymous with disease, because they tend to lower, hinder or inhibit free and harmonious vibration and because they promote destruction of living tissues.

9. *What is acute disease?*

What is commonly called acute disease is in reality the result of Nature's efforts to eliminate from the organism waste matter, foreign matter and poisons, and to repair injury to living tissues. In other words, every so-called acute disease is the result of a healing and cleansing effort of Nature. The real disease is lowered vibration and accumulation of waste matter and poison.

10. *What is chronic disease?*

Chronic disease is a condition of the organism in which lowered vibration (lowered vitality), due to the accumulation of waste matter and poisons, with the consequent destruction of vital parts and organs, has progressed to such an extent that Nature's constructive forces are no longer able to re-act against the disease conditions by acute corrective efforts, or healing crises.

A SECOND DEFINITION OF CHRONIC DISEASE

Chronic disease is a condition in which the healing or constructive forces of Nature have been forced to the defensive by the ascendency of disease conditions, thus preventing acute reaction or healing crises.

A THIRD DEFINITION OF CHRONIC DISEASE

Chronic disease is the inability of the organism to re-act by acute efforts or healing crises against constitutional disease conditions.

11. Are all acute reactions healing crises?
No, there are healing crises, and disease crises.

12. What is a healing crisis?
A healing crisis is an acute reaction, resulting in the ascendency of Nature's healing forces over disease condition. Its tendency is towards recovery, and it is, therefore, in conformity with Nature's constructive principle.

13. What is a disease crisis?
A disease crisis is an acute reaction resulting in the ascendency of disease conditions over the healing forces of the organism. Its tendency is toward fatal termination, and it is, therefore, in conformity with Nature's destructive principle.

14. What is cure?
Cure is the readjustment of the human organism from abnormal to normal conditions and functions.

15. What methods of cure are in conformity with the constructive principles in Nature?
Those methods of cure are in conformity with the constructive principle of Nature which:
(1) re-establish normal surroundings and natural habits of life in accord with Nature's laws.
(2) Which economize vital force.
(3) Which promote the elimination of waste matter and poisons without in any way injuring the human body.
(4) Which, in the highest possible degree, arouse the individual to the consciousness of personal accountability, intelligent personal effort and self-help.

16. Are poisonous drugs and promiscuous surgical operations in conformity with the constructive principles in Nature?
Poisonous Drugs and Promiscuous Surgical Operations are **not** in conformity with the constructive principles in Nature.

(1) Because they deal with acute diseases or crises as in themselves harmful and suppress them.

(2) Because poisonous drugs and promiscuous operations are in themselves harmful and destructive to human life.

(3) Because such treatment fosters the belief that poisonous drugs and surgical operations can be substituted for obedience to Nature's laws and for personal effort and self help.

17. Is metaphysical healing in conformity with the constructive principles In Nature?

Metaphysical Systems of Healing are in conformity with the constructive principle of Nature, in so far as they do not interfere with or suppress Nature's healing efforts, and in so far as they awaken therapeutic faith. They are in conformity with the destructive principles in Nature:

(1) In so far as they fail to assist Nature's healing efforts.

(2) In so far as they ignore, obscure and deny the laws of Nature and defy the dictates of reason and common sense.

(3) In so far as they substitute, in the cure of disease, a dogmatic belief in the wonder-working power of prayer and metaphysical formula, for intelligent co-operation with Nature's laws, personal effort and self-help, and in so far as they thereby weaken the consciousness of personal accountability.

18. Is Nature Cure in conformity with the constructive principles In Nature?

Nature Cure is in conformity with the constructive principles in Nature:

1) Because it teaches the absolute necessity of conforming our lives to the laws of Nature.

(2) Because it teaches that disobedience to the laws of Nature is the primary cause of weakness and disease, and that we are therefore, personally responsible for our own status of health and for the hereditary traits and tendencies of our offspring.

(3) Because it arouses the individual to the study of natural laws and to the necessity of strict compliance therewith, strengthening the sense of personal accountability and encouraging personal effort and self help.

(4) Because it adapts surroundings and habits of life to strict conformity with natural law.

(5) Because it promotes elimination of waste matter, foreign matter and poisons from the system by simple, natural means, which are

within the reach of every one and in no wise poisonous or destructive to human life.

19. *What are the natural methods of cures?*
We classify natural Methods of Cure into five groups and call them the Great Five of Natural Cure.

20. *What are the great five Of Nature Cure?*

(1) **Return to Nature:** IN thinking, breathing, eating, drinking, clothing, working, resting, moral, sexual and social life, etc.

(2) **Elementary Medicines:** Water, air, light and earth cures, magnetism, electricity, etc.

(3) **Mechanical Medicine:** Massage, physical culture, healing gymnastics, surgery and osteopathy for the repair of mechanical injuries and lesions.

(4) **Suggestive Medicine:** Normal Suggestion, sincere prayer, rational faith.

(5) **Chemical Medicine:** Scientific Food Selection, Homeopathic Medicine, Simple Herb Remedies.

Barring accidental and surgical injury to the human organism and barring surroundings hostile to human life, the primary cause of disease is violation of Nature's laws.

. . . every so-called acute disease is the result of a healing and cleansing effort of Nature.

Chronic disease is a condition in which the healing or constructive forces of Nature have been forced to the defensive by the ascendency of disease conditions, thus preventing acute reaction or healing crises.

How To Live Long

by Prof. Irving Fisher, Yale College

The Naturopath and the Herald of Health, XV(1), 4. (1910)

Avoid poisons—poisoned air, poisoned water, poisoned food, poisonous thoughts, poisonous emotions, and just plain poisons, like alcohol, tobacco and drugs.

Breathe deeply of pure air, eat abstemiously of foods demanded by appetite.

Exercise for the delight of physical expression, not to win a game or because you think you ought to, and exercise the intellect and emotions as well as the muscles.

Wear as few clothes as possible, and these of porous materials, so disposed as not to weigh heavily upon, constrict or destroy the balance of the body.

Bathe frequently enough to keep the skin in condition for performing its eliminative function.

Keep cheerful.

Don't worry.

SOCIAL HEALTH AND PERSONAL HEALTH

by C. J. Buell
President of the Minnesota Health League
The Naturopath and Herald of Health, XV(8), 454-457. (1910)

ARTICLE II.

SUPPRESSING SYMPTOMS

There is really but one cause of physical disease, and that is "violation of the natural laws of our being." This fundamental cause produces multitudinous forms of disease symptoms. Each separate manifestation of this one disease cause has been given by the doctors a specific name, just as if it were a disease by itself, entirely independent of all others.

The principal work of the doctors has been the naming of these symptoms and trying to find ways of suppressing them. Very little attention has been paid to finding the underlying cause; very feeble have been the attempts to teach people the *Return to Nature*, thus enabling them to avoid both the internal disease and the external symptom. Figuratively speaking, the doctors have stood by with a club to knock the symptoms in the head as soon as they show themselves, thus driving the real disease back into the system and making it many times more dangerous to the health and life of the patient.

Just so, in the social and industrial world there is really but one disease. That disease is the failure of society to learn and to obey the natural laws that govern social evolution.

This one social disease manifests itself in many forms—it has many symptoms: lack of employment for willing workers, and voluntary idleness for rich nabobs; tramps who ride brake beams and besiege our back doors for cold victuals and old clothes, and the far more dangerous tramps who tour the earth in automobiles, private cars and million dollar yachts; sky-scraping tenements surrounded by vacant lots; the low saloon at one extreme, the gilded club house at the other. Labor unions and strikes for the workers, trusts and lockouts for the privileged monopolists; bread riots and free soup houses for the poor, and banquets beyond the dreams of Epicureans for the rich; petty graft among the lower classes, and the wholesale purchase of city councils, state legislatures and national congresses by our foremost business men. For the petty thief, the policeman's club, the workhouse, jail and prison; for those who make laws for others but themselves evade and misuse them, the high places in church and the state, the judicial bench and the senate; prostitutes who huddle in city brothels and women who for the sake of a home or to gain the bauble of a glittering title sell themselves in loveless unions.

All these are the surface symptoms of the one deep-seated social disease. They correspond to the boils, tumors, fevers and catarrhs in the man or woman who has violated Nature's fundamental law of physical health.

As medical men have spent most of their time and energy in treating and suppressing symptoms of physical disease, so the political quacks and social reformers have devoted their efforts to covering up the symptoms of social disease.

We deplore the unhealthy condition of our cheap tenements and vainly pass laws to compel their owners to give a few more feet of air space or a little more light to the miserable dwellers therein; while at the same time we place a heavy tax on buildings and a low tax on vacant lots, thus doubly discouraging the erection of more and better tenements. We seldom or never ask why so many people are forced to live in such unwholesome dens. The stench of the sweatshop offends our nostrils and we pass laws in a fruitless attempt to make them a little more tolerable; but every time a man erects a new shop or factory we lay upon him an additional burden of taxation.

Thousands of workers are maimed or killed by unguarded machinery, therefore we besiege the legislature to appoint factory inspectors; we spend vast sums for labor bureaus, compel the adoption of safety devices, and then, in our stupidity, tax every one of these improvements. It never occurs to us that there must be something radically wrong, or laborers would refuse to work in dangerous and unsanitary surroundings.

We establish compulsory education, and at the same time levy a burdensome tax on every bit of material that enters into the construction of schoolhouses.

We club and imprison hobos, petty thieves and paupers, but use up very little gray matter in any attempt to find out why society is infested with such human vermin. We curse the trusts and monopolists, but refuse to repeal the laws that create them and which make their plundering possible. We despise the vulgar rich and the vulgar poor, little dreaming that they are both the legitimate offspring of the same unwise statutes.

Drunkenness is a terrible curse to society; but how many of us realize that our special and enormous taxes on liquors and our unholy practice of selling the privilege of saloon keeping are the sole bases of the blighting and corrupting influence in our politics of the united liquor interests?

Over and against all these social evils we ought to paint in letters large enough to be read miles away, the word *WHY?* and then rid society of the bungling and stupid statutes that are the primary cause of social disease.

"Behind every social evil you will find a social wrong." Thus wrote one of the wisest statesman of any age or nation; and the evils will never disappear until the wrongs are righted. Unjust laws lie at the bottom of all social disorder; in fact, unjust laws creating and maintaining unequal opportunities among men constitute the only real social disease, and all these evils that we deplore and try to suppress are only the natural effects of underlying social injustice. You might as well try to cure the small-pox with a club, or annihilate consumption by arresting and fining its victims, as to attempt to remedy the evils that curse society by filling the workhouses and jails with petty offenders and by building poorhouses and asylums for those who are too weak to stand the strain of an unjust artificial environment, created by *violation* of the *natural laws* that *govern* social and industrial life.

There are such natural laws—good, kind, beneficent laws—that will work without police or prisons, without force or compulsion, if only we will repeal and abolish our bungling statutes that prevent society from obeying the social laws of Nature.

Until society is freed from this incubus of *Ours* that we find confusion of thought. And yet the law of *Ours* is just as simple as the law of *Mine* and *Thine* when once we grasp it.

It is only when we come to the law of legislation and given a chance to Return to Nature, it will be impossible for men and women to enjoy the kind of social environment necessary to a strong, healthy, pure and noble life.

Where, then, is the path by which society may Return to Nature?

THE WAY OUT

The individual who really wants to return to Nature and live a free, pure, healthy, natural life, must, first of all, cease to do wrong. He must first find out in what ways he has been violating the laws of his personal body, and then he must stop transgressing those laws. Nature, the only real healer, will then restore him to health as fast as possible.

Just so, when we would cure Social disease, we must first learn wherein society has been violating a social law of Nature. To him who thinks, it must be plain that the laws of Nature that govern social development must work perfectly, if only they are not interfered with; and it must also be plain that the only way the natural social laws can be interfered with is by some man-made statutes that set up artificial barriers to the working of the natural social laws.

Man, by his legislation, cannot overrule or repeal the laws of Nature; but he may set up statutes that will cause the natural laws to work great harm to certain classes of people; and this is the way social disease is always brought about.

Here, then, is the social problem—to find out the man-made statutes and customs that produce the disease in the social body—get rid of those statutes and customs as soon as possible, and then let things alone. Nature will then cure the social disease very quickly.

Again, the person who thinks, must see that each man, woman and child has just as much right to be in the world as any other man, woman or child; and that the bounties of Nature—the air, the sunshine, the water, the soil—all the boundless resources of mine, and forest and fertile plain—of river, lake and ocean—that all these gifts of Nature are as much for one as for another.

So, also, it must be plain that all the benefits of social growth and development must be regarded as the common property of all the people of any social unit—of any community.

In every community there are certain places that are more desirable for homes, or stores, or factories than others. For these specially desirable places people will be glad to pay more than for less desirable sites.

Now as the gift of Nature belongs to all equally, and as the benefits of social progress also belong to all equally, it follows that whatever may be the value of these specially desirable places, must, in all fairness and justice, be considered the common property of the people of the village or city whose growth and progress have produced these values. Here we shall find the natural fund to meet the common public needs of each social unit.

If these values are taken to meet the necessary public expenses for making and maintaining streets—for city water, gas, electricity—for police protection and public schools—in short, for all the various public expenses that are incident to every town or village or city—then there is no need for taxing people's houses, clothing, furniture, stocks of goods or other personal belongings.

Here we see a great natural law—the law of MINE, THINE and OURS—the law of giving and receiving.

Every individual is the owner of himself—all his strength of body—all his power of mind—all his qualities of soul and spirit are his to use for his own benefit, so long as he does not encroach upon the equal right of each and every other person to do the same. This is the law of *Mine* and *Thine*—a law that has been recognized and insisted upon by all social philosophers in all ages.

Give me an equal chance—what I produce by my labor of hand or brain is *Mine*. No one else has any right to it nor any part of it. If I choose to give it to another that is my own affair, but no other has any right to compel me to do so. If John D. Rockefeller has honestly earned, under a "square deal," with no favor or privileges, all the many millions he calls his own, then he has a right to all those millions, and no one else has any right to deprive him of a dollar of them. But the trouble is he hasn't earned his millions in a "square deal." He and all the rest of the great millionaires have enjoyed the special favor that others did not possess. They have been able to get *something* for *nothing*, and just to that extent, others have been obliged to take *nothing* for *something*.

And here we can get an idea of the source of swollen fortunes. They are derived largely from what is *Ours*. A man has a title deed to a valuable mine, or forest or oil well—a water power, a wharf site or a city lot. These places become enormously valuable, not because of anything the owner has done especially, but because of the demands and needs of all the people. These values are *Ours*—all the people have produced them, and all the people naturally and properly own them. They are the values that Nature has provided to meet the common expenses of the community. But we let those who own the title deeds also own the values which attach to the lots or lands covered by those title deeds. Here we, the people, violate a law of Nature. We let our natural public revenue go into private pockets to create swollen fortunes, and then to get funds for streets and schools and other necessary public needs we pass man-made statutes by which we rob the people each year of a part of the value of their food, their clothing, their houses, their stock and farm implements, their merchandise, and all sorts of other things by which the people earn a living.

In this way we make the poor and the common run of workers and business men yield up each year in taxes a part of their own earnings for public purposes while we let natural public funds—the values that are *Ours*—go to swell the fortunes of those who already possess the best parts of Nature's gifts to all. This is one of the ways by which we make millionaires and paupers with all the train of social diseases that follow. We have violated the natural law of *Mine* and *Thine* and *Ours*. This is not the only cause of social disease, but it is the biggest one. Other causes will come to light as we proceed.

> *. . .the person who thinks, must see that each man, woman and child has just as much right to be in the world as any other man, woman or child; and that the bounties of Nature— the air, the sunshine, the water, the soil—all the boundless resources of mine, and forest and fertile plain—of river, lake and ocean—that all these gifts of Nature are as much for one as for another.*

THE NEW PARADISE OF HEALTH, THE ONLY TRUE NATURAL METHOD

By Adolf Just (Copyrighted)
The Naturopath and Herald of Health, XV(12), 711-717. (1910)

The Jungborn—The True Return to Nature and Its Importance for the Body, Mind and Soul

We wish now to show by the institutions of the Jungborn in the Harz Mountains how men must return to nature in a right way, so they will experience true joys and delights of life by a natural conduct of life, and sickness will be cured much quicker and better than we to-day may believe.

THE BATH

The higher developed land-animals and birds take a bath from time to time. We must guess therefore that a special bath has been destined also for men from the beginning by nature besides the frequent involuntary showers of rain. But what kind of bath, is the question. Which form in the use of water is the right one? The full bath by which the body is for the most part in the water, is not at all in accordance with nature for the men. Man also took originally the bath following his instinct. But this having been lost by the long unnatural life of man, we must learn again from the happy creatures who have this safe guide of life, how to recognize the right bath. At the bathing puddles of the animals, at the so-called sloughs of the wild boar, the stags in the woods we can learn to know the bath which nature prescribes. In the Jungborn the arrangement is made now for the natural bath (not a full bath).

A demand of nature is being obeyed again by taking the bath in the open air. In cold weather only the bath is taken in the house. The rain shower in nature is replaced by this bath while a massage is added by a natural way. As all that is bountiful in the sense of nature, overwhelms us in a certain manner with a feeling of comfort, streaming from a horn of plenty, such is also the case with the bath which I established according to nature. Every trial will confirm this fact. My book: *Return to Nature!* contains a complete instruction in taking the natural bath.

Water will do, to be sure.
—Rausse

More sublime yet is air,
Most glorious is the light.
—Rickli

LIGHT AND AIR

Man is the highest light- and air-creature, no aquatic animal. He cannot live in water like the fish. Man can use the water for his benefit only only at times in a certain form, while he cannot dispense with light and air for one moment without the greatest injury. The water bath, though excellent results can be had from the natural bath, is, nevertheless, only a secondary expedient. But light and air are in contrary the proper elements of man within which nature has originally placed him without any garments.

The good health of man rises and falls in the same ratio as he is provided with light and pure air. Light and air are just in days of sickness of the highest necessity for man. Man must in all disease, acute and chronic, breathe always as much fresh air as possible, especially the air of the forest. He also must to-day at times expose again his whole body (not only the head) to the light and air without being dressed and draw in again through the pores of the whole body fresh air, which has not been contaminated by the vapors of the body. This is called the light- and air-bathing.

The most beautiful air of the Harz Mountains, being very aromatic and full of ozone, blows in the Jungborn.

The air in the houses, however, though they stand in the woods, is always much corrupted by the joint living of many men, by the vapors of the kitchen and the cellar, by closets, piles of rubbish, by stonewalls, etc. In the light- and air-huts and houses, however, which stand in the open air under trees, there can always be perfectly fresh and unspoiled air.

The guests in the Jungborn live and sleep in charming and friendly little air- and light-houses, which are no huts and show various decorations. Every house stands fully in the open air, surrounded by shrubs and trees. It contains only two rooms, one for each person, so that each room is fully free at three sides. The two rooms can be connected by a door. The little houses are entirely constructed of wood (at present with two walls, made of boards), sufficiently elevated above the ground, and protect as every room in any other house against any unfairness of the weather and are even pretty warm in cooler temperature. They are provided at all sides with blinds, windows, air-valves, etc., which can at every time be kept open or closed.

The Jungborn has two great light- and air-parks with high, dense and protected planks. In one the light- and air-houses for ladies are situated, in the other those for gentlemen. The ladies and gentlemen can therefore live and sleep here, just as they please, in fully open light and air-houses, fully undisturbed by changes of weather. They can sleep also under the open sky if they please and if the weather is fair. Besides everybody can at any time, especially in the early morning, immediately when coming from his bed (which is of the greatest importance), take the whole day, if convenient, light- and air-baths and sun-baths, lightly or half-dressed, with a bathing suit or with the light- and air-bathing mantel of the Jungborn, which is made of a light fully porous linen, or he can go fully naked, which is the best. There is also an opportunity given in each park to take a natural bath in open air. Everybody can in the rain step out of his house and take a showerbath—i.e., he can go naked in the open air when it rains. This is again a full regular use of the water which also is productive of perfect well-feeling and good health.

No feeling of constraint oppresses us in the light- and air-parks in spite of the high planks, as the parks are very large and the valley of the Ecker, the high mountains and the romantic rocks present everywhere to the eye their natural beauties by the favorable situation of the Jungborn.

There are also little light- and air-houses in another more open, great and beautiful park in the Jungborn, which are open to everybody, especially families whose members do not wish to be separated. The circulation of the air during the night can in these houses be produced by valves, lids, etc., which are constructed all around above the windows and others. It is self-evident that the guests in these houses can also use the light- and air-parks for bathing in light, air and sunshine.

Good care is being taken for the order and safety of the guests when living and sleeping in the light- and air-houses and while taking the light- and air-baths.

The light- and air-houses are elegantly furnished with very fine furniture. I set a great value especially upon comfortable and warm beds (woolen quilts, similar to the Steinert reform beds). These are very necessary for sick people.

In the Jungborn, therefore, the closest adaptation to air and light is combined with the greatest comfort and all commodities. The patient who has been carried away from all the wrongs of the world and rests now in a light- and air-house, entirely in the lap of nature where balmy airs blow and the trees of the forest rustle, or who pitches his bed entirely under the open sky where his eyes are turned to the stars in fair weather and gently zephyr breezes fan his sick breast, they all enjoy the beneficent and refreshing impressions which are the most salubrious balm to them. They first of all render him conscious of all those eternal and mysterious powers of the grand nature which are so eager to cure the unhappy man and return to him happiness if only he accosts them again.

> Then softly in his gentle moods
> Godfather wanders through the woods.

Plants and animals decease and die in the dark, but when exposed to the light they at once show life again and freshness. The same change is caused in the body of man when it comes out of the darkness of the garments into the light. The digestion is also in the body greatly promoted, while all the organs begin at the same time to exert a very lively activity to cure all the frailties and sufferings of the body. The body is being pervaded in the light- and air-bath as by a new life and an unknown freshness.

The dining-room in the Jungborn stands also in the open air, as to render the sojourn here most salubrious and agreeable.

There are, during the cooler season, easily heated rooms in the Jungborn besides the light- and air-houses. Friendly winter-houses have lately been built in the Jungborn for the guests, which can be heated and are practical in every way and much liked.

Man to-day misunderstands very often the wise, kind nature and its healing workmanship. This easily explains why men, especially beginners, make often mistakes when adapting themselves to the light and air and taking the light- and air- and sun-baths. As great injuries can evolve from them, it is necessary to give a right instruction in the light- and air-cult and the bathing in light, air and sun.

THE EARTHEN POWER

Animals and men are but moving plants; they have dissolved themselves from the earth after a higher development. But they also draw even yet strength and freshness out of the earth.

When Hercules, as the Greek legend relates, was engaged in combat with Antaeus, the son of goddess of the earth, about the golden apples of the Hesperides, he observed that Antaeus became weak and frail as soon as he had lifted him from the earth, but regained his strength, health and freshness as soon as he stepped on the earth again.

The animals in the woods (rabbits, roe, stags, etc.), who follow their instinct, the general officer of health, remove all the leaves and branches when lying down to be in immediate connection with the earth in their repose.

There is offered now in the Jungborn the most favorable opportunity to use the earthen power, the strongest remedy of nature, by going barefoot, by taking in light, air and sun, and at night when sleeping, which is of the greatest importance.

But almost incredible cures can also be made by earth when healing wounds, ulcers and other diseases of the skin, when dissolving strange matter (in the breast, the abdomen), when appeasing pain (also toothache and headache), when soaking out poisons (after poisoning, etc.).

It is often surprising what great results can be had by the forceful remedies of nature, water, air, light and natural nutrition, but nothing can so much cause our admiration than the earth in its healing power (adhibited as earth force or earthly mass). The animals also (like the elephant) and the barbarous tribes use earth for their wounds.

In all sicknesses a so-called universal treatment of the body with water, light, air and natural foods is of great importance, but not less a local treatment a direct interfering with the sick spot and for this purpose earth is the only true, natural and efficacious remedy. Earth is the proper element of man.

For dust thou art and into dust shalt thou return.
—1. Moses, 3, 19

Earth in combination with water is the only natural remedy which has the greatest future yet, in daily occurring cases of vulneration, inflammation, pain, etc.

The Diet

In the undisturbed tranquility of nature which art did not invade yet, man in our climate would only find berries and nuts as a nutriment and these nuts by far in greatest quantity during the longest part of the year.

In the freedom of nature every creature selects its foods, following its instinct and taste, i. e. it eats the food, the taste of which it likes best, in the unchanged, uncultivated state of nature.

The curse: "A fugitive and a vagabond shalt thou be in the earth" must fulfill itself or no cause can be seen why man gives up the simple means which nature gives him to recognize his true nutriments and tries to find out his nourishment by laborious and obscure researches, by chemical, anatomical and physiological studies, by examining the teeth, the bowels. The last method which is averse to nature, must always turn out erroneous. Let us shun it therefore by all means.

There was no danger imminent in the original pure nature that the creatures selected any other foods than nature had destined for them. First when man had discovered the fire, he could neglect the natural laws in his nutrition and could produce all possible things (meat, vegetables, cereals, potatoes, bread, alcoholic drinks, medicals) and could render them eatable and tasteful.

And Prometheus, who stole the fire from heaven, as the Greek legend relates us, was for punishment enchained to the Caucasus, the vultures came and devoured his liver which was ever growing again, so that the vultures ever returning found their food again. The anger of the gods has never been expressed in a more fascinating way then by this legend about the purveyance of the fire.

Strange materials (a diseased matter) originate now by the unnatural nutrition of man which the fire made possible. They produce after a while ulcers, eruption, fever and other forms of disease. These external symptoms are now removed by cutting, burning, by salves and medicines but the disease always breaks out again from the internal hearth of the malady, and the cruel operation is always taken up again with the man who is enchained to-day to the rock by his ignorance.

For man nature has destined the most beautiful and excellent that was produced in the vegetable kingdom, the precious fruits, berries, grapes, and especially nuts. Nature has covered the table very abundantly for man. If we add to our fruits the many tropical fruits, dates, figs, oranges, almonds, etc., there is given him for his nutrition the greatest and most beautiful variety.

The young mammalia in nature, before adopting the food of the grown animals, retain for some time yet the natural breast.

Milk is also for men with their diet of fruits the best transitory expedient which they can retain at first. Their spoiled stomachs must be also treated at times like a baby.

There are offered in the Jungborn besides the multi various precious kinds of fruits and nuts especially many berries of the forest, bilberries, raspberries, and especially whortleberries, the healthiest food imaginable. Swollen fruits which had been made to rise by manure of the stable, or the artificially prepared, are excluded as much as possible. The nuts and the other fruits are sometimes prepared as naturally as possible if bad teeth or other special conditions require it, and also for the purpose to give to spoiled men some more delicacies of their choice (fruit salads, etc.). To the nuts and fruit diet is besides some good bread, also the milk of goats and cows, added who pasture the whole day in the woods and on the meadows; also sour milk, good butter, soft cheese with cream, etc.

No art, not even the most perfect culinary science, can give foods the relish by which nature has endowed the beautiful raw fruits for man. The unnatural foods and delicacies of to-day, especially alcohol, tobacco give only vicious pleasures. The unspoiled taste struggles at first always against these, but finally becomes accustomed to them like all poisons and is firmly attached to them, though he perceives almost every time that they really are nauseous (like tobacco-juice, when smoking) and are undermining his health always more and more. If we have avoided such unnatural things only a short time, then the fruit diet will offer again true pleasures and joys.

The nutriment which nature has destined for a creature is only for this one really easily digestible and gives alone real strength, health, pure blood and freshness of life. By the fruit- and nut-diet alone the further development of all strange materials in men's body is arrested at once, and the right juices and stuffs, which are necessary for the development and strengthening of the body, are introduced to it again. Man, therefore, delivered now of heavy fetters, breathes again in new strength and delights and young again he rises like the phoenix out of his ashes.

The danger of overeating is excluded by the raw fruit diet.

The fruit-, nut- and milk-diet in the above described composition is appreciated with the greatest enthusiasm in the Jungborn since the first year of its existence, first on account of the beautiful pleasures of the table given by them, and then for the great successes gained.

The vegetarian diet of to-day, vegetables, cereals, potatoes and the bread, lack principally sufficient fat, which nature has provided for men in the nuts, and this especially constitutes a danger to health and explains fully why so many men abandon it again.

It is self-evident that the right composition and in certain cases the necessary preparation must, regarding the quantity and quality, be done without mistake and that the symptoms which appear in the body are well understood to avoid the mistakes and not to lose the greatest profits or even engender injuries. The prescripts of nature must also be obeyed in regard to the hours of eating.

Nobody must attack the liberty of man. Everybody in the Jungborn, therefore, retains the liberty regarding the diet. The most tasteful vegetarian foods (vegetables, potatoes, etc.) and even meats are willingly presented at any time as requisite and to one's wish. It is also allowed to take only partly the natural foods. If it is too difficult to adopt the natural nutrition at once, it will be recommended to keep up part of the foods to which one is accustomed. Nature offers, it is known, many more strong foods which, if used in the right way, as in the Jungborn, have great effects even without a full natural nutrition. That only is really salubrious to man what he does with a full conviction, voluntarily and with pleasure in his natural mode of life.

No opportunity is further given in the Jungborn to indulge in debauchery and ebriety, the swamp in which the maladies spring up like marshflowers.

IMPRESSIONS OF THE SOUL

We can influence the soul immediately by the body and also vice versa we can subject our body to the influence of the soul. The outward impressions and relations of the patient, therefore, his surroundings and treatment, are of the greatest importance.

The original paradise was a forest and the forest is therefore the proper home for man. When man after his fall from nature became restless, he was always more driven into his ruin. He refused the foods which so bountifully the woods presented him from the beginning voluntarily and without his efforts and always cut down the woods more and more to engage in agriculture. The curse was fulfilled:

> Cursed is the ground for thy sake, in sorrow shalt thou eat of it all the days of thy life. Thou shalt eat the herb of the field. In the sweat of thy face shalt thou eat bread till thou retunst into the ground; for out of it wast thou taken.
> —1. Moses, 3, 17-19.

Man has attacked nature the most by destroying and cutting down the woods; he has caused by it conditions, and especially dangerous climatic and aerial changes, which are to-day very detrimental to man and to beast. Many a country has by it become entirely unhospitable for man.

The sick who has arrived at the end of all human perversities and errors must go again back to the woods. For in the woods alone he can regain his health, in the magic enchantment of the woods, in the rustling music of the forest, under the green shady canopy of the trees, through which the sun is lurking, to the frolicsome chirping of the birds his feeble pulses beat with greater vigor and the grave fetters of his sickness are more easily dissolved. The Jungborn has for this reason been established in the middle of a great wood.

These woods are the Harz Mountains, the crown of the German forests. Who knows these mountains with all their grand and romantic beauties of nature, he is aware of the fact that man only here can forget the quickest his misery and the rest of the world. The Jungborn is situated in the mild and protected valley of the Ecker, the most beautiful part of the mountains.

The sick feels lonely in the world. Nobody understands him and therefore he often experiences a false treatment and bitter rancours. One sees only the weakness of the sick, his faults, his peculiarities and bad manners, his sins and vices, his laziness or restlessness, his disorders and want of energy, and condemns him, reproaches him and embitters the more and more his trist life, instead of looking deeper into his sick interior, to find here an explanation and an excuse for his demeanor, his acts and his mischief.

This especially is the case to-day with many patients whom nervous troubles ail. We often are here inclined to warn, calling:

Judge not and ye shall not be judged.

—Luke, 6, 37

There is another sun for man besides the one which daily circulates on the sky. Where that sun does not shine, all is dark and cold, desolate and trist. There the blood becomes obdurate and will not finish its circulation. The sun is love which refreshes the sick mind as the morning dew the tender little flowers. There is every care taken in the Jungborn for the sick by a right loving treatment of them and great indulgence. The writer of this paper, who has sufferings of the sick, all the misunderstandings and condemnations of the world, knows well the patients and their right treatment.

Man has been destined by God for a social life and happiness.

This also is not being neglected in the Jungborn. Though the pilgrim, being exhausted to-day in the atrocious struggle of life amidst unnatural surroundings, finds the most and best joys and delights in the tranquility and peace of the beautiful romantic nature around the Jungborn, there are besides social intercourses and entertainments provided for the guest, entirely as they please and need it, also by art and music. These pleasures must elevate the soul and strengthen the health. But the pleasures of to-day are nothing but a wild intoxication with alcoholic drinks and tobacco fumes, which soon cause pain and disgust.

> Man is free! By his chart of creation is free,
> Though born amid fetters still free-born the same.
>   —Schiller

Liberty, especially the liberty to which in his ways of life he is entitled by his reason and his higher faculties, gives him foremost the higher rank among the creatures on earth, even if he uses this liberty to his ruin and misfortune. Every hard constraint which the sick puts on himself so often by a false judgment of his condition, or is being put on him by others, is harmful.

The quicker and the more complete the sick returns to nature, the more favorable it is under all circumstances. But when beginning a new phase of life according to nature, one must not suffer from great uneasiness, strong depressions and torments, as he might be greatly displeased by it. This depends on the measure, how much his organs, especially the digestive one, are spoiled already. Everybody can feel and judge the best by himself how far and how quick he can lead again a truly natural mode of life, so that his maladies can be cured and in every way his pleasures and delights of life increased.

Nature had certainly certain intentions when giving to man a special liberty which only brought ruin to him so far. Man probably will some-time, after much misery and unhappiness, contracted by his voluntary departure from nature, seek eagerly nature's friendship and thus arrive at the highest state of happiness on earth. Providence can have the same intentions with single men if led by some impetus or all by themselves they quickly and with enthusiasm return to nature, while others prefer to perish by themselves. The desire and interest in the return to nature depends also on the load of strange materials which they bear. Old and deep-rooted ideas and prejudices cannot be conquered at once. Man, therefore, must retain his liberty.

Every guest in the Jungborn is during the whole cure in possession of his liberty. Every one may use the cure by water, light and air, earth, diet, etc. as long and as much as he wishes. But I always assist him by advice and explaining everything. I always refer the guests to nature, our great mistress, that they learn from her again clearly and distinctly how they will become again healthy and happy.

The Jungborn is no infirmary in the sense of to-day, but a kind of pension with an opportunity of a true natural method of living and winning health with an opportunity of a true natural way of life and health restoring is taught.

Everybody in the Jungborn shall learn to become his own physician or to make rather his mistress, the wise and benign nature, his adviser and physician again. Just this must be our principal aim, that man does not confide any more his health to other men, thoughtless and without a will, as is done to-day.

> Man errs as long as lasts his strife.
> —Goethe, Faust

Nature only is true and does not err. Man must directly learn again from nature alone, every one for himself, what is necessary for his well-being and happiness.

> *The nutriment which nature has destined for a creature is only for this one really easily digestible and gives alone real strength, health, pure blood and freshness of life. By the fruit- and nut-diet alone the further development of all strange materials in men's body is arrested at once, and the right juices and stuffs, which are necessary for the development and strengthening of the body, are introduced to it again. Man, therefore, delivered now of heavy fetters, breathes again in new strength and delights and young again he rises like the phoenix out of his ashes.*

1911

J. Austen Shaw Explains Yungborn Nature Cure
J. Austen Shaw

Preventive Medicine
J. W. Hodge

How To Avoid Pain And Sickness
Louisa Lust, N.D.

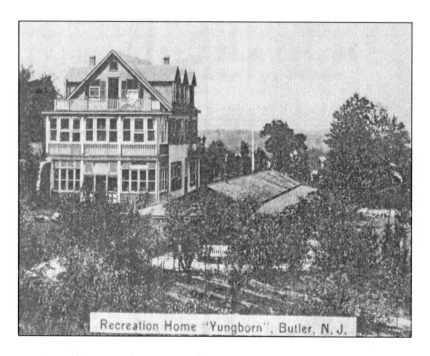

Recreation Home "Yungborn", Butler, N. J.

Just an hour away from New York City, the Butler Yungborn offered an
oasis for those in search of health.

J. Austen Shaw Explains Yungborn Nature Cure

by J. Austen Shaw

The Naturopath and Herald of Health, XVI(3), 145-56. (1911)

A Unique Institution In The Ramapo Mountains—
Sun, Air And Plunge Baths, Many Kinds Of Rhythmic Exercises And The Best Of Natural Foods

J. Austin Shaw, of Brooklyn, lectured before the Franklin Literary Society, at the rooms of the society in the Johnston Building, his subject being, "The Return to Nature at Yungborn in the Ramapo Mountains." He spoke as follows:

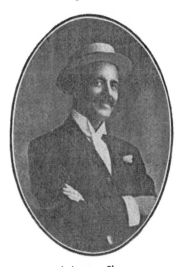

J. Austen Shaw

You shall hear how Hiawatha
Prayed and fasted in the forest,
Teaching men the use of simples,
And the cure of all diseases:
All the sacred art of healing!

And the Master of life, who sees us,
He will give to you the triumph,
In the last days of your fasting,
Make a bed for you to lie in
Where the rain may fall upon you,
Where the sun may come and warm you,
Lay you in the earth and make it
Soft and loose and light above you.

Let no hand disturb your slumber,
Let no weed nor worm molest you,
'Till you wake and start and listen,
'Till you lean into the sunshine.

So sang one of your favorite poets—a man illustrating in his own life, a closeness to nature, a knowledge of the laws of health, and the glory of a ripe old age.

Every one of you has visited, or read about the natural health resorts of Europe. I question if one of you has ever visited any of the American 'health homes;' not even the best one of them all, which is right at your very door.

Few of you have even heard of 'Yungborn.' But you have read about, and perhaps seen, the beautiful Ramapo Hills and Mountains; and perchance you have been at Butler, some thirty-nine miles away on the winding Susquehanna Railroad, and as the crow flies, little over twenty miles from this great city, with teeming millions.

But to see Butler resting at the foot of the hills, is to see only an ordinary village of 2,500 people. Less than a mile away, on the edge of the mountains, climbing the gentle activity gradually, you come to these sixty acres of forest and fruit, of hill and dale, of glorious vistas, now the centre of an amphitheatre of rainbow foliage, the very sight of which is a perpetual inspiration.

THE SURROUNDINGS OF YUNGBORN IN THE RAMAPAO MOUNTAINS

On this acreage rises a miniature mountain, called 'The Cat's Back,' from which on every side for twenty miles spreads out the gold and bronze and crimson of the Indian summer, as the great trees of all the hills, in the sweet sunlight, turn their foliage from emerald to every fascinating hue. Only a mile away rises 'Kickout Mountain' from whose summit may be seen seven scintillating lakes, flashing their silver radiances, while afar rise the towers and spires and giant buildings of our own great city. The view at night is a 'fairy land,' with none of its noise and turmoil and strenuosity to weary us.

Now you have seen the lovely circle of which 'Yungborn' is the center. 'Yungborn,' with its springs and purest water, its trout streams dashing over rocks, and spreading out their arms to give you welcome on their bosoms; its great trees of chestnut, butternut and oak, that have spread their protective arms around and above this Eden spot for centuries.

Now that we are here, let us see what there is of practical account to interest you and me and make it worth while to give this nature-recreation and home our serious consideration. For if it is not worth while, we waste our time to give it thought at all.

I judge you wish to know what has been my personal experience; and so I presume upon your patience and consideration by telling you what I have learned and seen and enjoyed while resting a few happy days in the waning summer season amid its interesting developments.

As you perhaps know, Benedict Lust and his charming wife—both naturopaths—are the joint owners of this paradise, and from small beginnings in 1896 they have built up an enterprise which, through great discouragement and local opposition, has risen to so fascinating a repute that its charms and benefits are known all over the civilized world; and all the year round enthusiasts may be found there, enjoying its restful quiet, its closeness to nature, and the healthful ozone that, laden with the aroma of its pines and cedars, bring 'healing on its wings.' As many as one hundred at a time, during the past summer, have evidenced to growing popularity.

How To Add Many Years To One's Life

You must come up with me for a month next summer and add a quarter century to your life.

You shall have sun baths and air baths; you shall sink into healthful sleep at 9 o'clock, soothed to sweetest slumber by the music of the crickets and the katydids. You shall rise with chanticleer at dawn, refreshed as you have never been before, and as the sun is peeping o'er the mountain tops, you shall plunge into the pure cold streams, as it dashes from the hill top sources, and so your inspiration of the day begins. Shall I described to you a day, from dawn to dewy eve, just as I found it and just as you shall know it, if you will?

Just banish from your consciousness any of your fake-modesty ideas, for you will be garbed in nature's apparel only, before I send you to pleasant dreams!

I must not forget to assure you of many wonderful cures that old Dame Nature has made in this delightful home—not the least, the recovery of Dr. Lust himself, long given up by doctors as 'incurable.'

Mrs. Lust, too, is a practical demonstration of her own theories, having completed the other day a fast of twenty days, the only sensible and sure method, as I know, and some of you, for the eradication of disease.

'Yungborn' is equipped with the best of facilities for natural healing. In summer, the sun and air baths are given in the open; in winter, under the sheltering roof of the sanitarium, with sun parlors and all modern improvements. In summer the light and air cottages are utilized, and their windows, screen protected, are open on every side. There is purity of air and water and food, the aids and incentives to purity of life.

Perfect Drainage, Sanitary Heating And Electric Light

There is perfect drainage, sanitary heating and electric light.

'Yungborn' is not for men only. Ladies seem to gather the keenest enjoyment and greatest benefit from this nature life. Separate sections of the sixty acres are set apart for the sexes, where the greatest freedom from dress restrictions may be enjoyed. Men and women meet at meal time and in the evenings, but at other times each one goes his or her own sweet way, unmolested and unafraid.

Clothing is only a concession to modesty, and far from a necessity. The only serious diseases are nervous disorders that yield rapidly to the better life. No cases of contagious diseases are admitted. There is, therefore, perfect safety for all who go. Many spend their vacations, and some their summers there, because of its quiet, rest and change from the conventional city life. Its novelty appeals to you. Your food is fruit and nuts and milk and vegetables. Some try the raw food diet. You are free to use your own judgment as to this. If you desire advice, expert medical intelligence is at your service.

You wear sandals. You walk barefoot in the dewy grass. You can go hatless and collarless, if you choose. You will find neither meat, nor drugs, nor tobacco in this elysium. You do not need any of them. You never would if you lived rightly, and if you are ill and worn out and poisoned by wrong eating and drinking, here is a delightful spot in which to let old Dame Nature make you new again.

You can have a fruit breakfast, if you want it. The majority have found the no-breakfast theory best, as I have found it for more than eight healthful years. You can fast if you need to, and you will have excellent company.

MANY PROMINENT PEOPLE MEET AT THIS HEALTH RESORT

You will meet some most interesting people there. Last summer Wu Ting Fang, the Chinese ambassador, put in nearly a week of experience there, that included everything from cue to toe, and he seemed to find everything a delight. You ask me what kind of people do we meet? I met there a Spanish consul, a wealthy New England shoe merchant, a German artist, a count, a genius and a poet, a mental scientist, a number of seasoned athletes, a Canadian philosopher, a charming octogenarian from San Francisco, and a wonderful old man of seventy-eight from Boston, renewing his youth and busy with the buoyancy of a man of forty—every moment he is awake.

Then—in a 'higher class, by themselves'—there was a score of ladies, whose very presence overshadowed all the place with an atmosphere of purity and placidity, and to mention them separately would be nothing less than sacrilege. Suffice it to say, their nearness was a benediction.

But I promised to tell you in detail just how a day sped on, from cock crow until the evening shadows fell, and I will now complete my obligation. Then you must realize by personal experience whether or not I have been dreaming.

You know the lights are out at nine. From then, your only glimmer is a candle or the phosphorescent gleam from the glow-worm or the lightening bug. And such a restful sleep, for you are weary—and you're off to 'the beautiful land of dreams' the moment your devoted head is laid down upon the downy pillow, close to the open window, with sweet mountain air pouring in upon you.

You breathe health with every inhalation, and the voice of chanticleer at five announces rising time, you spring refreshed, from sweetest sleep into the light and sunshine, alert and ready for your long and strenuous

day. Now, follow me, and when the lights go out again at nine, tell me
if you are not the tiredest, happiest, healthiest thing you ever knew, and
then begin to think, with me, that health is, after all, the best thing in the
world.

Make An Early Start And Climb The Mountain

Don't rise at 5 unless it pleases you so to do. Rest for an hour in the
land of sweet content and happy memories. Your mind will be alert, your
senses quickened, your muse, perchance, inspired. Don your negligee cos-
tume and your sandals and walk with me a mile or so through these fra-
grant woods and up these hills to the summit of the Cat's Back Mountain,
the top of Yungborn's sixty acres. Drink half way up as you are climbing,
a glass of pure spring water from a never-failing source; and now, as the
mists are rising and the glory of the early sunlight floods, the enchanting
landscape, breathe deeply the first zephyrs of the new day, laden with
health, as they are, right to the very brim.

Now you are ready for the easy journey down the declivity to the
plateau where men's park spreads out before you amid the great trees,
but open long enough to gather up the sunshine and spread its warmth
and comfort over and through you, as disrobed and perspiring from your
early exercise you plunge into the running brook and feel the thrill of the
delightful reaction that follows it.

Drying yourself in the air and sun and with your hands, in a few minutes your whole body is aglow with healthful color, and again you dress
and journey to the central section of the grounds where, for half an hour,
you, barefoot, walk on dewy verdure.

Now, for those who care to eat, the big bell sounds welcome; exactly
as the clock rings out the hour of 7, and a bountiful breakfast of fruit and
whole wheat bread and cocoa or barley coffee awaits you. Better come
with me and read your morning papers or one of the interesting books
from the home's big library, or walk, if you prefer, through more of these
'lovers lanes.' Cross the rustic bridge and see how well your lady friends
have been cared for in *their* 'secluded park,' for they will not close the
doors of their hearts' delights before the hour of ten. Here they have, you
see, seclusion, sunlight, pure, fine sand for parks and baths, and their *own*
rippling stream of water, where they bathe and rest and absorb health
and weight so rapidly you declare 'the age of miracles has not yet passed.'

An Hour Of Rhythmic Exercise In The Morning Air

But this must not concern us longer, lest there should be ambitious
and early bathers among the fair sex, and so, at 8.30 promptly the bell is
calling us to 'morning exercises.' Here, on the plateau overlooking Butler,

and our eyes entranced by glorious views on every side, while under the shade of overhanging branches, we have a strenuous program of every kind of rhythmic motion which the expert and gentlemanly teacher has devised, and for half an hour we pose and turn and swing our comfortably-clad bodies, breathing deeply, filling the lungs to their limit with the sweet mountain air, and, by our strenuous muscular exertions, exciting the capillaries to healthful effort, until, perspiring freely and delightfully tired, we end the formal energies of the morning.

I suppose you think you are through for the day, and now should come sleep and rest again. You haven't *yet begun*. Now, while the ladies wander to their secluded park for delightful air and sun baths that so rapidly bring health, we will 'follow our leader' to the bathrooms, where for an hour warm or cold or sitz or spray or stream or lightening ablutions are our portion, according to our need.

Careful judgment is exercised in each individual case, but you and I will just try them all, and perhaps you will decide as most delightful of the surprises that here come to you, there isn't anything so inspiring as the *lightening spray*. Let Felix play that hose on you from head to foot awhile and a 'boiled lobster' has not half as ruddy a glow, and never before did your blood so wildly dash through all your arteries and veins.

Don't dry yourself. Put on your clothes while covered with the spray. They all do. You won't feel chilly. You won't 'catch cold.' Do as I tell you. Isn't that glow delicious? You feel so comfortable, you want to shout in your ecstasy and you can if you wish, for it is 'the land of liberty.' Now it's only 9.30, or maybe nearly 10; and hungry as you are, having had no breakfast, there will be no dinner bell till 12. Everything is methodical here. You'll soon get used to it and like it, too.

Sun And Air Baths In The Garb Of Nature

Now we have two glorious hours ahead of us. We will go up, over the sandy road, in the woodland paths, to our own park, where no intrusion ever need be feared or expected and laying aside the modern garb, we will awhile return to nature and let the sun and air do their good offices in our behalf.

Isn't the sun warm and the air delightfully caressing? We will lie on the grass awhile. We will try the mud baths and cover our bodies with their healing magnetism. For an hour we will lie in the embrace of nature and, covering our eyes from the sun's rays, we'll sleep a dreamless sleep, unless the flies and bees grow inquisitive and awaken us all too soon.

Now it is after 11, and the time has not dragged a moment, and we have almost lived a lifetime of surprise and benefit since we arose.

Let's step in the brook and cleanse our bodies from the clay. Then in the clear, cold waters lie, or swim, or plunge, cold as it is, from living springs, and always flowing on and on. Now rub yourself briskly in the sun and let its rays and the warm air dry you.

There is time for throwing the ball—and you used to play, you know— why should the years destroy your interest in any legitimate sport? They have not mine, and here is a splendid game for the forenoon's last hour, a game of quoits.

DELICIOUS FOOD FOR DINNER AND A HEARTY APPETITE

And now I hear the dinner bell. It is time to dress and eat. I know you're hungry and I promise you a dinner your memory will hunger for many a year. Eat slowly and enjoy it. If eating gives pleasure, why limit it by rapidity? The *longer* you chew your food, therefore, the *greater* must necessarily be your satisfaction. Just remember that when you return to the busy city and become a 'chew-chew' man. Note the abundance of flowers on the table from Yungborn's gardens, the big dishes of assorted nuts, brazils, pecans, almonds, etc., the plates of nut butter, and the liberal supply of fruit of many kinds, according to the season, not a little of it from the orchards which help to cover these practical sixty acres.

You need not put on any anxious meat-eating expression, for there is none of it to satisfy your excited and unnatural stomach, and before many days have flown by you will wonder why you ever thought it was a *necessity* at all. Try this delicious soup, uncontaminated by the flavor of any dead animal, made palatable, as you remember, by spices and con- coctions that lead you to forget when you absorbed these excitants to abnormal desires and passions. This soup depends upon nature's sources for its healthfulness and nourishment. I thought you would enjoy it. Yes, you can have another plate of it. Certainly. There is no stinting here of generosity.

But I will not reveal the secrets of the Yungborn larder, nor tell you how the meatless dinners satisfy, upbuild and delight you. Every variety or vegetables, puddings of unpolished rice, better even than 'mother used to make,' everything in abundance and so delicious that the only danger is that you will eat too much. One little lady from Arden gained in weight a pound a day.

But your slow and thorough mastication will *prevent* your over feed- ing, and the novelty of so much that is tempting on the laden table will not affect you, as your consciousness of the wisdom of 'temperance in all things,' grows upon you. You surely have eaten about *twice* what you needed by this time, and no wonder. 'They all do it,' but 'do not let it happen again.'

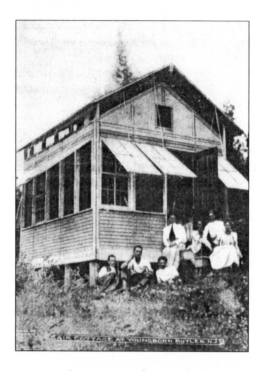

Air Cottage at Yungborn, Butler, N.J.

AN HOUR'S NAP AND THEN MORE SUN AND AIR BATHS

Now, for an hour you can read, sitting where the sun can fill you with its genial influence, or, if you wish, you may sleep an hour, just to realize the comfort of a nap at midday, a luxury you can't 'afford,' you think, in the hurry and rush and worry of the city.

See that you are ready for the park at two, where you repeat the sun and air baths of the morning. Take your choice of recreative games, ball or quoits or bowling in the big gymnasium. Next year you will have a big swimming pool there, and lawn tennis courts adjoining it, and billiards and a running course of a mile through the woods, already almost completed.

You can have a mud bath again, if you desire. You can sit in the sun and read or doze. The afternoon hours fly. The bath again in the running stream is irresistible. Some take a plunge at hourly intervals. It is never warm. The reaction is quick and certain. The sun and horizontal bars, and games or exercise of many kinds will soon banish the moisture from the brook! How you wish the days were longer. It is nearly six, and at the very moment the village bell rings out the hour, you hear your own call to the evening meal.

I forgot to tell you, however, of the call to breathing exercises on which all engage on the plateau from half past five until the call to supper. This is one of the most beneficial half-hours of the happy day. Deep breathing, difficult perhaps at first, becomes so natural that soon you go around with head erect and chest expanded *all the time.*

Supper Is Abundant In Surprises And Variety

This supper, too, is most abundant in surprises and variety. Don't forget the lights are out at 9, and eat lightly. 'That's all.' Why make you hungry now by elaborating on all the dishes and making your mouths water in anticipation?

Now you can walk again through these charming lovers' lanes, or, perhaps, a lecture or entertainment at the village may draw you for a mile's walk down the hill, but don't forget it is up-hill coming back and you should be in bed at 9. I don't think you will care to leave 'Yungborn' anyway, no matter how long you stay here.

In the well-lit parlors you can indulge in music or whist or euchre or any recreative games, and the library is close at hand. Dr. Lust or one of his visitors may lecture to you on 'health' and kindred subjects. Your new-found friends have much of interest in common to talk about; there isn't an instant when the time drags heavily. At 8 the ladies take their nightcap of herb tea, and you can have a cup too if you want it.

It is 9 o'clock before you know it. The lights are out; here is your candle and yonder is your cottage, screened, but open, on every side, with air, air, air all around and over and beneath you. Such comfortable beds! Such entrancing music by the tree toads and the 'katys'; such a dear, sweet song by the cricket on the hearth! 'So tired.' Deliciously, deliciously tired you are! Unconsciously, you drift out on the great wide ocean of dreamless sleep!—and so I'll say:

"Good night, good night, till we meet in the morning!"

As you perhaps know, Benedict Lust and his charming wife— both naturopaths—are the joint owners of this paradise, and from small beginnings in 1896 they have built up an enterprise which, through great discouragement and local opposition, has risen to so fascinating a repute that its charms and benefits are known all over the civilized world; and all the year round enthusiasts may be found there, enjoying its restful quiet, its closeness to nature, and the healthful ozone that, laden with the aroma of its pines and cedars, bring 'healing on its wings.'

PREVENTIVE MEDICINE

by J.W. Hodge, M.D.

The Naturopath and Herald of Health, XVI(11), 711-717. (1911)

[This paper by Dr. Hodge is one well worth reading. He treats of "The Past," with its mercury and calomel in this number. Other subjects treated are diet, clothing, exercise, habits, causes of disease, how to prevent sickness, increase the average length of life, etc., etc. You get in these articles the best thoughts of Dr. Hodge's life on the subject of "Keeping Well."—Benedict Lust, Ed.]

Preventive medicine, as sanitary science has been sometimes called, has of late years rapidly advanced in public interest as well as in the actual development of practical knowledge pertaining to the causes of disease, and the means of prevention, especially in communities, have been obvious, numerous and great. Not until the last few decades has the preventive art in medical practice received anything like the attention it deserved. The conception that the maladies which afflict mankind, and which have received the name of diseases, can be prevented is of modern times—I may say practically of the century that has just passed, the last few decades of which were marked by very great activity in the development of knowledge pertaining to hygiene, i.e., the science and art of conserving health and preventing disease.

The Past. The ancient and once worldwide belief, that disease is a visitation of special Providence, or that it is due to the vengeance of offended Deity, although now generally abandoned as regards individual cases or limited localities, still lingers in the minds of some illiterate and superstitious people with regard to great epidemics which are believed to be either inevitable, or, at least, to be averted only by prayer and fasting.

By the intelligent student of medicine, however, causes and effects are not regarded as belonging to totally different classes, for although he admits the close relationship existing between vice and disease, yet he considers their influence as reciprocal and that in many cases they are only different names for the same thing. The crude idea which descended almost to us who now live was that diseases of every kind were a portion of the necessary suffering which might by some art, conjuration, or divination be removed, but which could not be avoided or prevented. For this reason the so-called curative art, the art of palliating or removing diseases, took naturally a first place in the course of human progress. The curative art, useful in many of its applications, could not, however, be expected forever to remain the be-all and end-all of human endeavor against disease.

It was considered wonderful while it combatted the unknown and the invisible. But in the course of the natural development of knowledge the unknown and the invisible passed away, in so far as belief in them was concerned, and there was left in the mind, in place of that belief, the conviction that not one of the diseases long thought to be supernatural, and out of the range of inquiry as to causation, was supernatural at all. Each one was traceable by the acquirement of correct knowledge, and when traced was found to be largely and effectively preventable by a further extension of the same acquirement. In this manner have originated and developed the science and art of preventive medicine.

In early times doctors knew so little about hygiene and paid so little attention to natural laws that for hundreds and hundreds of years they did not allow a patient suffering from fever to partake of a drop of cold water. Doctors in those days declared: "Cold water in fever is certain death." "Do not give the patient a drop." "Give a dose of calomel and a teaspoonful of warm water." Fever patients were denied not only pure cold water—nature's remedy—but sunlight and fresh air were also withheld from the sufferers and they were salivated with mercury, physicked with jalap, depleted of their life-blood by the lancet, and starved until they gave up the ghost.

The doctor with his mercury and his lancet made the weary hours of sickness a crucifixion, and left hundreds of thousands of human wrecks by the wayside. In those days it required a very robust constitution to withstand the combined assault of the disease and of the doctor with his heroic remedies. Even as late as fifty years ago it was a very serious matter to "fall sick with a fever" and have a doctor. I mean the doctor was the serious part of the business, for in those days the doctor still declared "Cold water is death," and fathers and mothers were warned not to give a drop to the child tossing with a raging fever and vainly pleading like Dives for "just a drop" to cool the parched and burning tongue.

Owing largely to the advances made in hygiene and in sanitary science, and to the discovery and application of the homoeopathic law of cure with its mild medicines, single remedy, small dose, and brilliant results, the harsh and drastic, modes of treatment which were common half a century ago, have been dropped one after another by the profession until now the instinctive calls of nature are being more and more heeded by the medical practitioner, and the profession as a whole is daily approximating nearer and nearer to the constructive art of healing which takes more cognizance of sanitation and hygienic living and far less account of poisonous drugs.

Calomel and bloodletting have had their day and the good will of some doctors, and during that terrible day the sick-room was a veritable torture chamber, a gloomy and dreadful place, and the doctor's visit the most dreadful part of the composite calamity.

Bloodletting had been erected as a horrible fetish and at its altars were sacrificed for centuries hecatombs of human victims.

But, thanks to the advancing forces of science, among which was Hahnemann's great discovery, times have changed. The lancet is rusting away. The healing sunshine, and the pure fresh air which in those days were sedulously excluded from the sickroom are now freely admitted as the welcome harbingers of health.

The pure cold water which was once looked upon as a messenger of death is now plentifully supplied to the sick as one of nature's most beneficent remedies for the cure of disease and the restoration of health. The physician who studies from a hygienic standpoint the cases of those who entrust themselves to his care, and give judicious advice regarding the regulation of diet, clothing, exercise, condition of dwelling, and habits of life, performs his duty with far greater fidelity to the requirements of his profession, and with much more benefit to his patients than he who places his chief reliance on the exhibition of drugs and medicines for the restoration of health.

Prevention is far more logical than cure in the philosophy of medicine.

I believe that it is fair to presume that if physicians generally were to devote more time to the discovery and removal of the causes of diseases and less effort to seeking out indications for the use of drugs, much more good might be accomplished. I have reasons for believing that the time is not far distant in the future when the well equipped family physician will deem it his duty to apologize when he administers drugs to any members of a family whose physical welfare he supervises. He will feel that it was his fault that they became ill, for he should have guided them in such hygienic and sanitary paths, that illness should not overtake them. The truth must now be candidly admitted that the system of relieving mankind of his load of diseases can no longer rest alone on what is called curative skill. We have entered upon an era in which the preventive art must be put into service. We must make a steady effort not only to cure the disease, but to cure the cure.

The legitimate function of the modern physician, it seems to me, consists not so much in curing diseases as in curing their causes. He should strive to trace diseases back to their origin, and, so far as he is able to seek the conditions out of which they spring. He should endeavor, further to investigate the contributing conditions, and ascertain how far they are removable, and how far they are avoidable. The success of his efforts in combating disease will turn on the success with which he is able to carry out this analytical and practical design. Unless he is able to detect and remove their causes, he cannot logically hope to cure diseases quickly, safely, and pleasantly, by the administration of drugs, however skillfully prescribed.

When we look around us and contemplate the condition of the world, the abundance of life and its appalling waste, and when we note the condition of the human race and consider what it might be, as compared with what it is, its wonderful endowment of mind, its capacity for happiness and its cups of sorrow, its boon of glowing health, and its thousands of diseases and myriads of painful deaths, we exclaim, he must indeed be gifted with sublime endurance and undying faith who can still believe that out of this chaos, order can come, or out of this suffering universal happiness and health can be achieved. But as ages roll on, hope in some measure grows. With all our errors we are certainly gaining knowledge, and that knowledge tells us in no uncertain terms that the fate of mankind is largely in his own hands.

To what extent the prevention of disease, the prolongation of life, and the improvement of the physical, mental, and moral powers of mankind may be carried in the future, it is impossible at the present time to state. No doubt the tendency of those who write and speak on this subject is to be unduly optimistic. It does not seem probable that the conditions of perfect personal and public health are obtainable except in rare and isolated cases and for comparatively short periods of time. Yet it appears highly probable that the average length of human life may be much extended, and its physical powers greatly augmented.

It is apparent to the scientific hygienist that preventive medicine is destined to become the medicine of the enlightened future. At present, however, we have to deal with the facts before us, viz., that there are a great many diseases actually existing which must form the subject of investigation. While the business of the physician is, therefore, necessarily to a large extent the cure of disease, or where that is beyond his power, as is frequently the case, to relieve suffering and secure temporary ease for his patient, he is, nevertheless, especially called upon to ascertain so far as lies within his power and to discover, the means of obviating or destroying these causes.

Hundreds of deaths from typhoid fever have occurred in Niagara Falls and the Tonowandas during the past few years. Niagara River is used jointly as a carrier of Buffalo sewage and as a source of domestic water supply for this city. It is a sad commentary on our modern civilization that man is his own worst enemy, that human interests, instead of being mutually helpful, morally uplifting, and productive of real brotherhood, are largely destructive and antagonistic to health and happiness. The cornerstone of modern society is self-interest, and in its service we do not identify our neighbor's with our own, but rather sacrifice our neighbor's life that our own selfish interests may the better thrive.

Buffalonians exercise especial care in safe-guarding their own water-supply from sewage-pollution. The great trunk-sewer of the city of Buffalo is so constructed as to belch its Niagara of infective filth from man and beast, both sick and well, into the waters of Niagara River at a distance of two miles below the city of Buffalo. Thus while guarding their own water-supply from pollution the people of Buffalo deliberately poison and pollute the drinking water of three neighboring cities and two villages by discharging their raw sewage into the Niagara River. What could be more atrociously criminal than such procedure on the part of Buffalonians?

It is obvious that the science of preventive medicine is necessarily and intimately related to the art of so-called curative medicine. Conceding that the study of prevention and cure should proceed conjointly, it is obvious that he is the most perfect sanitarian, and he is the most accomplished and useful physician who knows most of the preventive art, as well as of the nature and correct remedial treatment of diseases. The foregoing assertions in reference to the great importance of prevention in medical practice may appear somewhat dogmatic; still I believe that they will receive the ready assent of every physician who has carefully studied the subjects of hygiene and sanitation, and made himself familiar with what has recently been accomplished along this line of work in certain limited localities. As one of the many notable examples of the great advances in this direction I may point to the glowing accounts with which medical literature has recently abounded in regard to the signal triumph over yellow fever, which has been accomplished in Cuba during the past few years by the chief sanitary officer of Havana, Surgeon W. C. Gorgas, U. S. Army.

I believe it is the consensus of opinion among sanitarians that by the adoption of proper modes of living on the part of both individuals and communities nearly one-half of all existing diseases are preventable or avoidable and might be abolished by the judicious exercise of appropriate sanitary measures. There are logical reasons for believing that the present mortality-rate might be very greatly reduced by a more rigid adherence to the general rules of hygiene, and less frequently recourse to the use of poisonous drugs and serums.

The saddest pages in the history of all nations are those that record the wholesale sacrifice of human life through ignorance or neglect of the simplest means of preserving health and averting disease. It is no disparagement to the art of healing to state that more human lives have been sacrificed to neglect of the simplest means of conserving health than could have been saved by the most skillful medical and surgical treatment.

In a large proportion of the cases that come under the care of the medical practitioner, it is desirable that he pay special attention to those circumstances which affect the general health of the patient, and to give directions for his client's guidance in matters that pertain rather to the province of hygiene than to the practice of physic. Indeed, it very frequently happens that the only remedial measure which the competent physician feels called upon to prescribe consists of a change from bad to good habits of life; from an unhealthy residence or locality to a healthy one; from intense application to study or business to repose of mind and complete change of scene and occupation. In a certain class of cases change of climate is the logical remedy, and is of more benefit to the patient than all the drugs mentioned in medical books. A locality suitable to the particular disease or state of health of the patient has to be chosen.

By such hygienic regulation of the habits, and residences of their patients, physicians are performing their duties by saving many valuable lives which could not be saved by the most skillful exhibition of drugs.

It is clearly obvious to the scientific sanitarian that every year within this commonwealth thousands of valuable lives are lost which might have been saved; that tens of thousands of cases of sickness occur that might have been prevented; that a vast amount of unnecessarily impaired health, physical debility and suffering exist which might have been avoided; that these preventable evils require an enormous expenditure of money, and impose upon the people innumerable and unmeasurable calamities, social, physical, mental and moral, which might have been averted; that means within our reach exist for their mitigation or removal, and that the timely application of appropriate measures for the prevention of disease is destined to accomplish far more in the future than all the drugs administered for the cure of disease.

One of the best illustrations of the extent to which ignorance and carelessness nullify the utility of the advances of the knowledge of methods for the prevention of disease is found in the fact that smallpox still continues to appear here and there as local endemics, and sometimes with great mortality. If anything is definitely known in preventive medicine it is that this loathsome malady is a filth-disease. Smallpox is a member of the group of diseases described as zymotic which thrive only in unwholesome conditions of life, and in common are diminished or prevented by the reduction or removal of these conditions. Long before the time of variolous inoculation and vaccination we find this disease to have been identical in every respect with that of to-day. Smallpox appeared at sundry periods, sometimes not returning during an entire century and was at certain times virulent and at other times mild. Into whatever country it penetrated, among whatever people it found a home, and wherever its ravages decimated the population, the conditions which favored its development and its diffusion were one and the same. It had its stronghold in filth and its victims where uncleanliness and untidiness dwelt under the same roof. Ignorance and superstition had caused man to view this pestilence as a thing of supernatural origin, and a punishment for national sins, whereas, it is too true that smallpox and cholera, like the plagues of centuries past, owe their existence to the uncleanly conditions by which we are surrounded, and to the unhealthful and unsanitary modes of living which characterize large numbers of people. Until scientific sanitation began to engage the attention of state and municipal authorities, the plague returned as punctually to the cities of Europe as smallpox did during the eighteenth century. At present the fatality, not only from smallpox but from all other zymotic diseases, is steadily declining as sanitation becomes more rigidly enforced in crowded districts, notwithstanding the pernicious effects of vaccination and other reactionary devices which the drug doctors from time to time, aided by tyrannical and unjust legislation, have inflicted upon mankind. Isolation and sanitation have robbed smallpox of all its terrors and vaccination has unjustly claimed the credit. While it is freely admitted by its promoters, that vaccination has destroyed the lives of tens of thousands of healthy children, I challenge the entire profession to produce any kind of proof whatever which is worthy of intelligent consideration, that vaccination ever saved a single life or ever benefitted in the slightest degree any member of the human family or that this operation ever prevented a case of smallpox except by killing the person vaccinated.

CLEANLINESS THE GREAT PROPHYLACTIC

Cleanliness is the great scientific protection against diseases, and especially against the contagion and infection of zymotic, or filth diseases. All other so-called prophylactics or protectives are viewed by the practical sanitarian as worthless subterfuges. Pure air, pure water, internally and externally, plain, wholesome food, temperate habits of life, and plenty of exercise in the open air, are nature's health-producing disease-repelling agents. Attention to diet, clothing, exercise, place of residence, and habits of living is a well-known safeguard against disease. It is obvious that hygiene is a subject of scientific interest, not only to the student and to the medical man, but also to the political economist, to the legislator and to the people generally.

Its discoveries ought, therefore, to be of great practical importance to all. But when we examine the extent of knowledge as to the causes of disease which is actually possessed by the majority of fairly well-informed and intelligent people, and note how much of it is mere vague conjecture, untested theory, and baseless assumption, and withal, how hopelessly unconscious these people are of their own ignorance of the subject, and how promptly and confidently they will undertake to advise what should or should not be done to prevent disease, we cannot wonder that the public at large is confused at the very contradictory assertions made to it, and consequently hesitates as to what should or what can be done to prevent disease. The truly scientific sanitarian will promptly admit that his knowledge is scant and defective that he cannot assert that the measures he proposes are the best possible measures, but only that they are the best he can at present devise, and that in the present rapid progress in sanitary science and its application for the benefit of mankind, it may be that within a few years, at farthest, some better means may be devised for the attainment of the results desired.

Imperfect as is the progressive physician's knowledge of the causation of disease and the prevention thereof, it is, nevertheless, far in advance of the popular practice.

The greatest obstacle the scientific physician encounters in the practice of preventive medicine is the fact that the mass of mankind is unwilling to sacrifice present comfort for possible future benefit. Sanitary measures, to be most effective, should be carried out at those times when lay men see no special cause for anxiety and often, therefore, appear to involve unnecessary worry and expense. When such measures are most successful their value may be least appreciated. If the expected disease does not appear, the physician's warnings are considered to have been a false alarm, and the precautions taken to have been excessive if not unnecessary.

The relatives and friends of the typhoid fever-patient, who will not fail to gratefully remember the care and assiduity with which the attendant physician may have treated the patient, would no doubt have thought the same physician obtrusive and troublesome had he taken one-half the trouble to see that the cause of the fever was avoided. That the labor required in the pursuit of personal sanitary measures often becomes in itself a source of pleasure, as for instance the preservation of personal cleanliness by ablution, and that the expense incurred in most cases is the best possible investment of capital, is not and cannot be appreciated by the masses. It is nevertheless an encouraging sign of the times that in the work of sanitarian the general public is growing more and more interested and more in sympathy with the movement to prevent disease and prolong life. The people are becoming more and more enlightened daily and more disposed to entrust matters of sanitation to those who have spent years of labor in perfecting themselves in these branches. On the other hand when we hear of the great fortunes accumulated by the venders of patent medicines vaccines and anti-toxins, we are reminded there are still opportunities for the higher education.

Prevention is far more logical than cure in the philosophy of medicine.

It is apparent to the scientific hygienist that preventive medicine is destined to become the medicine of the enlightened future.

How To Avoid Pain And Sickness

By Louisa Lust, N.D.

The Naturopath and Herald of Health, XVI(2), 99. (1911)

Nature cure teaches that pain may be avoided only by knowing and avoiding the causes. Pain warns us of the disorder that sets in with our organs.

Nature cure teaches and shows us that any method or remedy that paralyzes, poisons, overstimulates or depresses, produces sickness or pain with any healthy person and is very injurious to the sick person. Sunshine, pure air and right living are the elixirs of life and health that will stand the test of time and not be found wanting. Pure food furnishes all the mineral necessary to sustain our bodies.

If mothers would learn how to live, how to prepare simple healthy good and by example teach their children the all-important lessons of how and what to feed the body, sickness would be outgrown and forgotten in one generation. What a revolution and revelation this would be in every well-ordered house in one year's time. But in its stead the children are either overfed or underfed.

The necessities of good health are pure food, pure air, water, sun, heat, light and thinking in a right way. We all recognize the comfort and pleasure experienced from cleanliness even while we are healthy. A daily bath will do more to counteract disease than any remedy to method yet discovered; therefore, the daily cool natural bath should be as regularly taken as the meals. A hot bath, with a cold shower afterward, may be taken once or twice a week to advantage. If the circulation is sluggish and a chilly condition exists the body should be slapped and rubbed with the hand until a warm glow is produced. This can be well accomplished by brisk exercising as well.

Such a daily cool bath in the morning before dressing is very beneficial, and the children should be taught to take one every morning, thus saving them from pain and many a disease.

Never take a cold bath when you feel cold; first warm up with exercise, or walking, or a hot lemonade. The best time for a cold bath is in the morning when getting up, and never take a full bath soon after a meal, not before two hours have passed.

Air-baths can be taken freely. Cold air-baths of 5-10 minutes duration are very beneficial.

Water, air and sunshine are three curative agents; they are priceless if their proper application is understood. The sunrays increase vibration, strengthen and sweeten the temper and disposition.

Among the producing causes of rheumatism, neuralgia and nervous affections are sunless, ill-ventilated sleeping and living-rooms. DO not, under any circumstances, shut out the air and sunshine from your home.

Do not mind if the furniture, curtains, draperies, etc., will fade. It is better to let them fade than you should.

Overwork is destructive to life and health, and it is wiser to dispense with trifling luxuries of dress and of the table than to be compelled to get these at the price of hard work.

Do not bustle, worry or get excited; keep your nerves and muscles perfectly under control of your good common sense.

Do nothing in a careless manner. Order is law, and to be happy we must obey all of nature's laws.

To be free, happy, harmonious and contented, one needs to understand what life signifies. To see that means more than selfish gratification of pleasure seeking and of money making. If we are living in harmony with nature, we will sleep well, and while we are sleeping, resting, every part of the physical organism is being built up, healed and invigorated.

Rest you can, rest you must, or rest you will when you are in your grave.

The "Yungborn" is open all the year round. The nature cure is highly beneficial in the winter. Few things are as invigorating and enjoyable as the cool air bath, especially when alternated with vapor baths and other beneficial and pleasant water treatments.

"Yungborn," Butler, N.J.

Nature cure teaches that pain may be avoided only by knowing and avoiding the causes. Pain warns us of the disorder that sets in with our organs.

Nature cure teaches and shows us that any method or remedy that paralyzes, poisons, overstimulates or depresses, produces sickness or pain with any healthy person and is very injurious to the sick person. Sunshine, pure air and right living are the elixirs of life and health that will stand the test of time and not be found wanting. Pure food furnishes all the mineral necessary to sustain our bodies.

Everything needed to practice nature cure was found
in Benedict Lust's Supply Company.

1912

SICK PEOPLE
ARNOLD EHRET

—·—

HELP TO ABOLISH AN UN-HUMAN INDUSTRY
A. A. ERZ, D.C.

—·—

IN JUSTICE TO THOMAS AND TABBY
HELEN SAYR GRAY

Breathing exercises, dietetics, hygiene and water cure
were the treatments offered by early Naturopaths.

SICK PEOPLE

by Arnold Ehret

The Naturopath and Herald of Health, XVII(3), 166-170. (1912)

I. THE COMMON FUNDAMENTAL CAUSE IN THE NATURE OF ALL DISEASES

All the phases of the process of development of the medical science, including those of the earliest periods of civilization, have in their way of understanding the causal nature diseases that one thing in common that the diseases, owing to external causes, enter into the human body and thus, by force of a necessary or at least unavoidable law, disturb it in its existence, cause it pain and at last destroy it. Even modern medical science, no matter how scientifically enlightened it pretends to be, has not quite turned away from this basic note of demoniac interpretation. In fact, the most modern achievement, bacteriology, rejoices over every newly discovered bacillus as a further addition to the army of beings whose accepted task it is to endanger the life of man.

Looking at it from a philosophical standpoint, this interpretation differs from the mediaeval superstition and the period of fetishism only in the supplemental name. Formerly, it was an "evil spirit," which imagination went so far as to believe in "satanic personage," now this same dangerous monster is a microscopically visible being whose existence has been proven beyond any doubt.

The matter, it is true, has still a great drawback in the so-called "disposition"—a fine word!—but what we really are to understand by it, nobody has ever told us. All the tests on animals, with their symptom-reactions, do not prove anything sure, because these occur only by means of injection into the blood-circulation and never by introduction into the digestive channel through the mouth.

There is something true in the conception of "external invasion" of a disease, as well as in heredity, however not in the sense that the invader is a spirit (demon) hostile to life, or a microscopic being *bacillus*; but all diseases without exception, even the hereditary, are caused—disregarding a few other unhygienic causes—by biologically wrong, "unnatural" food and by each ounce of over-nourishment, only and exclusively.

First of all I maintain that in all diseases without exception there exists a tendency by the organism to secrete mucus, and in case of a more advanced stage—pus (decomposed blood). Of course every healthy organism must also contain a certain mucus—lymph, a fatty substance of the bowels, etc., of a mucus nature. Every expert will admit this in all catarrhalic cases, from a harmless cold in the nose to inflammation of the lungs and consumption, as well as in epilepsy (attacks showing froth at the mouth, mucus). Where this secretion of mucus does not show freely and openly, as in cases of ear, eye, skin or stomach trouble, heart diseases, rheumatism, gout, etc., even in all degrees of insanity, is mucus the main factor of the illness, the natural secretive-organs not being able to cope with it any longer, the mucus entering the blood and causing at the respective spot where the vessel-system is probably contracted owing to an over-cooling (cold), etc., heat, inflammation, pain, fever.

We need only to give a patient of any kind nothing but "mucusless" food, for instance fruit or even nothing but water or lemonade: we then find that the entire digestive energy, freed for the first time, throws itself upon the mucus-matters, accumulated since childhood and frequently hardened, as well as on the "pathologic beds" formed therefrom. And the result? With unconditional certainty this mucus which I mark as the common basic and main cause of all diseases will appear in the urine and in the excrements. If the disease is already somewhat advanced so that in some spot, even in the innermost interior, there have appeared pathologic beds, i.e., decomposed cellular tissues, then is also being excreted. As soon as the introduction of mucus by means of "artificial food," fat meat, bread, potatoes, farinaceous products, rice, milk, etc., ceases, the blood-circulation attacks the mucus and the pus of the body themselves and secretes them through the urine, and in the case of heavily infected bodies, even through all the openings at their command as well as through the mucus membranes.

If potatoes, grain-meal, rice or the respective meat-materials are being boiled long enough, we receive a jelly-like slime (mucus) or paste used by bookbinders and carpenters. This mucus substance soon becomes sour, ferments, and forms a bed for fungi, molds and *bacilli*. In the digestion, which is nothing else but a boiling, a combustion, this slime or paste is being secreted in the same manner, for the blood can use only the ex-digested sugar transformed from starch. The secreted matter, the superfluous product, i.e., this paste or slime is a foreign matter to the body and is being completely excreted in the beginning. It is therefore, easy to understand that in the course of life the intestines and the stomach are gradually being pasted and slimed up to such an extent that this paste of floral and this slime of faunal origin turn into fermentation, clog up the blood-vessels and finally decompose the stagnating blood. If figs, dates or grapes are boiled down thick enough we also receive a pap, which, however, does not turn to fermentation and never secretes slime, but which is called syrup. Fruit-sugar, the most important thing for the blood, is also sticky, it is true, but is being completely used up by the body as the highest form of fuel, and leaves for excretion only traces of cellulose, which, not being sticky, is promptly excreted and does not ferment. Boiled-down sugar, owing to its resistance against fermentation, is even used for the preservation of food.

Each healthy or sick person deposits on the tongue a stinking mucus as soon as he reduces his food or fasts. This occurs also on the mucous membrane of the stomach, of which the tongue is an exact copy. In the first stool after the fasting this mucus makes its appearance.

I recommend to the physicians and searchers to test my claims by way of experiments which alone are entitled to real scientific recognition. The experiment, the question put to nature, is the basis of all natural science and reveals the infallible truth, no matter whether it is stated by me or somebody else. Furthermore, I recommend to those who are brave enough to test on their own bodies the following experiments which I undertook on mine. They will receive the same answer from nature, i.e., from their organism, provided that the latter be sound in my sense. "Exact" to a certain degree reacts only the clean sound, mucusless organism. After a two years' strict fruit-diet with intercalated fasting cures, I had attained a degree of health which is simply not imaginable nowadays and which allowed of my making the following experiments:

With a knife I made an incision in my lower arm; there was no flow of blood as it thickened instantaneously; closing up of the wound, no inflammation, no pain, no mucus and pus; healed up in three days, blood-crust thrown off. Later, with vegetaric, food including mucus-formants (starch food), but without eggs and milk: the wound bled a little, caused some pain and pussed slightly, a light inflammation, complete healing only after some time. After that the same wounding, with meat-food and some alcohol; longer bleeding, the blood of a light color, red and thin, inflammation, pain, pussing for several days, and healing only after a few days' of fasting.

I have offered myself, of course in vain, to the Prussian Ministry of War for a repetition of this experiment. Why is it that the wounds of the Japanese healed much quicker and better in the Russo-Japanese War as those of the "Meat and Brandy Russians"? Has nobody for 2,000 years ever thought it over why the opening of the artery and even the poison cup could not kill Seneca, after he had despised meat and fasted in the prison? It is said that even before that Seneca fed on nothing but fruit and water.

All disease is finally nothing else but a clogging up of the smallest blood vessels, the capillaries, by mucus. Nobody will want to clean the water-conduit of a city, a pipe-system, which is fed with soiled water by a pump, the filters of which are clogged up, without having the water-supply shut off during the cleaning process. If the conduit supplies the entire city or a portion of it with unclean water, or if even the smallest branch-pipes are clogged up, there is no man in the world who would repair or improve that respective spot; everybody thinks at once of the central, of the tank and the filters, and these together with the pumping machine can be cleaned only as long as the water supply is shut off.

"I am the Lord, thy physician"—English and modern; nature alone heals, cleans, "unmucuses" best and infallibly sure, but only if the supply or at least the mucus supply is stopped. Each "physiological machine," man like beast, cleanses itself immediately, dissolves the mucus in the clogged-up vessels, without stopping short, as soon as the supply, of compact food at least, is interrupted. Even in the case of the supposedly healthiest man this mucus, as already mentioned then appears in the urine where it can be seen after cooling off in the proper glass tubes! Whoever denies, ignores or fights this uniform fact, because, perhaps, it goes against him or is not scientific enough for him, is jointly guilty of the impossibility of the detection of the principal cause of all diseases, and this, in the first place, to his own detriment.

Therewith I also uncover the last secret of consumption. Or does anybody believe that this enormous quantity of mucus thrown off by a patient stricken with tuberculosis for years and years emanates only from the lung itself? Just because this patient is then almost forcibly fed on "mucus" (pap, milk, fat, meats) the mucus can never cease, until the lung itself decays and the *bacilli* make their appearance, when death becomes inevitable. The mystery of the *bacilli* is simply thus: The gradual clogging up by mucus of the blood vessels leads to decomposition, to fermentation of these mucus products and "boiled-dead" food-residues. These decay partially on the living body (pussy abscesses, cancer, tuberculosis, syphilis, lupus, etc.). Now, everybody knows that meat, cheese and all organic matter will again "germinate, put forth *bacilli*" during the process of decomposition. It is for this reason that these germs appear and are detectable only in the more advanced stage of the disease, and disease-furthering only in so far as the decomposition, for instance of the lung, is being hastened by them, because the excretions of the *bacilli*, their toxins, act poisoning. If it be correct that *bacilli* invade "infect" from the exterior, then it is nothing but the mucus which makes possible their activity, and furnishes the proper soil, the "disposition."

As already said, I have repeatedly (once for two years) lived mucusless, i.e., on fruit exclusively. I was no longer in need of a handkerchief which product of civilization I hardly need even up to this day. Has anyone ever seen a healthy animal, living in freedom, to expectorate or to blow its nose? A chronic inflammation of the kidneys, considered deadly, which I was stricken with, was not only healed, but I am enjoying a degree of health and efficiency which by far surpasses even that of my healthiest youth. I want to see the man who, being sick to death at 31, can run without a stop for two hours and a quarter, or make an endurance march of 56 hours' duration—eight years later.

With this "mucus-theory", well confirmed by my numerous experiments, there is for the first time put up a thorough, etiologic, i.e., a cause—defining uniform conception of all diseases. If naturopathy here and there mentions certain affections of the blood as being the fundamental cause of all disease, this theory has proved insufficient because the food had been prescribed to be meatless or its contents of meat greatly reduced, at the same time, however, introducing so much the more mucus by means of bread, pap, milk, butter, eggs, cheese and farinaceous stuffs, especially starch food. That is the reason why most of the vegetarians in spite of their lauded bill of fare, are not healthy just the same. I myself was such a much—and mucus-eater for several years. If a considerable number of the vegetarians does not soon advance towards the only natural food, the fruit diet, or at least returns to eating little, there will be great danger of the shallowing-down of vegetarianism; not because the principle of "no meat eating" is bad, but because the healthful effects of the existing vegetaric nourishment are so inferior. The representatives of the vegetarian movement are still trying to prove what man is in need of as regards boiled meals, because they themselves as well as all the amateurs in this field have a fundamentally wrong conception of the fruit diet as a healing remedy, and go at it in a wrong way. The hobby of the vegetaric propaganda is the argument that man is not a carnivore and that, therefore, the eating of meat is unnatural. With perfect right says the opponent that the eating of meat is just as "natural" as that of bread, cabbage, milk, cheese, etc. Professor V. Bunge has reproached the vegetarians for inconsequence more than a decade ago, and he is right.

It is surely theoretically correct that man was a mere fruit eater in times gone by, and biologically correct, that he can be it even to-day. Or can the horse-sense of man not conceive, without any proofs and directly, of the fact that man, before becoming a hunter, lived on fruits only? I even maintain that he did live in absolute health, beauty and strength, without pain and grief, just the way the Bible says. Fruit only, the sole "mucusless" food, is natural. Everything prepared by man or supposedly improved by him is evil. The arguments regarding fruit are scientifically exact; in an apple or a banana, for instance, is everything contained what man needs. Man is so perfect that he can live on one kind of fruit only, at least for quite some time. This, however, need not necessarily be coconut (Kabakon). But a self-evident truth preached by nature must not be discarded just because nobody has been able to apply it in practice on account of civilizational considerations. From fruit only one becomes first of all ill, i.e. cleansed; this cleansing process, however, is better to undergo at home and not in the tropics. No man would have ever believed me that it is possible to live without food for 126 days, in which 49 at a stretch, during 14 months. Now I have done it, and yet

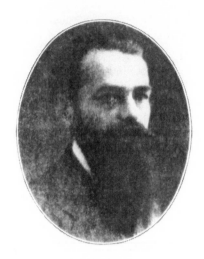

Arnold Ehret

this truth is not being understood. Hitherto I say and teach only that fruit is the most natural "healing remedy." Whether my calculation is correct will be proven by the next epidemic. I take, however, this opportunity to uncover the reasons why the self-evident is not believed in. When in the previous century somebody talked about telephoning from Berlin to Paris, everybody laughed, because there had never been such a thing. Natural food is not being believed in any more, because almost nobody practices it and, being a man of civilization, cannot easily practice it. It must also be considered that contra-interests fear that the prices of the other, artificial food-stuffs may drop, and others fear that the food-physiology may receive a shock and the physicians become unnecessary. But it is just this fasting and fruit cure which requires very strict observation and instruction—therefore: more doctors and less patients who, however, will gladly pay more if they get well. Thus the social question regarding doctors is solved—assertion already made by me publicly in Zurich several years ago.

First of all I maintain that in all diseases without exception there exists a tendency by the organism to secrete mucus, and in case of a more advanced stage—pus (decomposed blood).

If potatoes, grain-meal, rice or the respective meat-materials are being boiled long enough, we receive a jelly-like slime (mucus) or paste used by bookbinders and carpenters.

Hitherto I say and teach only that fruit is the most natural "healing remedy."

Help To Abolish An Un-Human Industry

by A. A. Erz, D.C.

The Naturopath and Herald of Health, XVII(7), 422-425. (1912)

You have heard of industrial or occupational diseases. Almost every modern industry or occupation has its own special form of disease. There is hardly a discovery made that will not develop some kind of a new form of disease, or aggravate an old one. And some of these afflictions are apparently inevitable. Such is life in these days of modern civilization, where not every accomplishment is really a proof of beneficial progression. For in these times of greedy commercialism and brutal industrialism, where private and public justice have hardly any place, things have to be done in our factories by those employed in the manufacture of the most common articles used in everyday life that often involve for the workers the most terrible diseases and sufferings, which, at the same time, are absolutely unnecessary. And I wish to call your attention to one of the most horrible industrial diseases known, which is not so new, but entirely needless to-day, and which ought to be stopped at last.

Everybody uses matches, but not everyone knows out of what material and how they are made, and at how great sufferings for those who work at the poisonous match-trade. For there are different kinds of matches, but there is one kind the manufacturing of which exacts the most awful penalty, not of those miscreants who are responsible for this outrage, though. As fate will have it, the poor victims are the scantily paid, ignorant tools of the greedy instigators of this unhuman industry, resulting in a most cruel affliction known as "phossy jaw," or phosphorous necrosis of the jaw-bone. It is the old style "lucifer" or "parlor" matches which readily strike anywhere, in the manufacture of which white or yellow phosphorous is used that causes all the trouble.

This peculiar malady of the lucifer match maker is a localized manifestation of highly poisonous infection resulting from continuous exposure to the fumes of white phosphorous, one of the most subtle and dangerous of all industrial poison. The insidious poison finally attacks the teeth and gums, gradually afflicting the cover of the jaw-bone, inevitably inducing a process of slow decay in the bone itself. Defective teeth and gums greatly aggravate the intensely painful condition, which, under the usual uncongenial medical treatment, soon reaches the hopeless stage.

The frightful condition of women and men afflicted with this awful industrial disease are beyond description. The physical and mental tortures of the poor sufferers mutilated in features and broken in health, stuns the imagination.

Their sufferings often last for many years, before a merciful death brings final relief. Toothless, with rotted gums, from which protrude fragments of decaying bone, with pus oozing from abscesses in jaw and mouth, the poor victims of phosphorous necrosis endeavor to tell of their awful experiences in a manner that is both appealing and appalling, some with the apathy of all hope lost, others by an inarticulate mumble, which is their only means of oral communication that is more convincing than the most eloquent speech.

Such is the tragic reality in outline of the life of the hopelessly suffering victims of phosphorous necrosis who seem to have passed beyond the recognized pale of human misery, and who are innocently paying the penalty of human greed of modern sordid industrialism and heartless commercialism. Yes, life often is but a tragedy.

The usual medical treatment involves either avoidable removal of the jawbone by destructive surgery, or a horrible, agonizing form of slow death, or both. Only under the most careful drugless congenial treatment can permanent relief and cure be obtained, provided the patient is taken in proper time. Those of you who have an idea about the marvelous advance in industrial ingenuity, or of the humanitarian tendency prevailing in our industries, can hardly believe that there should be so much danger attached to an industry like this, since all kinds of mechanical devices have been invented to do away with intervention of human agency.

Yet, in spite of the most ingenious devices to eliminate handwork, it is an undeniable fact that fully 95 percent of the women, 82 percent of the children, and 44 percent of the men employed in this damnable American industry, are directly exposed to the danger of contracting either "Phossy Jaw," with all the misery implied in this worst form of chronic phosphorous poisoning, or some other trouble characteristic of "phosphorus," such as dyspepsia, anemia, jaundice, yellow atrophy, aluminuria, etc.

For the danger of the subtle fumes of white phosphorous is still beyond any control and protection, in spite of all scientific efforts to find a certain escape from the menace of this most unstable and powerful poison. The laborers are constantly exposed to the treacherous vapor invariably produced by a combination of the poisonous fumes with the oxygen in the air. And the danger lies not alone in the air breathed; the deadly poison also becomes dissolved in the saliva by the unavoidable inhalation of fumes, and minute particles of phosphorous attach themselves to the skin of the employees. Thus every minute spent in the factory offers a menace to the matchmaker, and may mean untold suffering and untimely death to children, women and men employed in this barbarous industry.

And all on account of white phosphorous being three to five percent cheaper than either of the innocuous substitutes, our greedy and cruel manufacturers force poor children, women and men to run the needless risk of enduring what has been described as "all the torments of the orthodox hell!" For there are cheap and less harmful materials for the manufacture of matches that eliminate such disease dangers as well as fire dangers in a large measure.

Yes, all the terrible physical and mental suffering implied in the production of white phosphorous-tipped matches is a needless horror. And to our shame it must be admitted that the United States is the only important civilized country where this barbaric industry still prevails to the extent that some 4,000 match-workers must ever be exposed to all the dangers of phosphorous poisoning. Because the effort to stop the making of these dangerous matches meets constant objections at the hands of the interested manufacturer. And it was the fact that this American match still possesses especially tragic human interest which induced President Taft to make the following special appeal to Congress, concerning the protection of the poor match-workers, in his annual message: "I invite attention to the very serious injury caused to all those who are engaged in the manufacture of poisonous phosphorous matches. The diseases incident to this are frightful, and as matches can be made from other materials entirely innocuous, I believe that the injurious manufacture should be discouraged, and ought to be discouraged, by the imposition of a heavy Federal tax. I recommend the adoption of this method of stamping out a very serious abuse."

There is hardly a progressive country today which permits the use of poisonous phosphorous in any industry without the most severe restrictions. Finland stopped the manufacture of poisonous phosphorous matches altogether in 1872, and adopted the use of almost harmless red phosphorous. Denmark followed in 1874. Then the principal European countries found out that they could no longer withstand the pressure of outraged public sentiment. Even in countries where they still manufacture poisonous matches for export trade, and where they have apparently less regard for human life—such as Russia, Hungary, Sweden, Norway, and Japan—they enforce at least the strictest sanitary regulations, in an effort to protect the employees. Only the government of the United States has so far done nothing in the line of regulation and protection, in this matter. Our record of seventy years of indifference and criminal negligence is a disgrace to civilization.

And our State regulations amount to nothing. Our public Health Boards being merely political institutions for the benefit of certain medical interests have usually no time for matters of this kind. Most of our State inspectors are either neglecting their duties, or they are so ignorant of the risks offered to laborers in these factories, that a firm may be in operation for years before an "epidemic" of phosphorism among the poor ignorant employees would reveal to them the nature of the poison. It is only in the case of a few companies that the European sanitary regulations are voluntarily observed. The majority of our factories violate every sanitary principle of precaution known. While other countries have endeavored to eliminate the dangerous features of the industry by strict sanitary regulations, and, failing to banish phosphorous necrosis, have either prohibited the use of poisonous phosphorous altogether, or restricted and safeguarded its use by all known scientific precautions, the United States alone have remain indifferent.

Hence it is high time that pressure of legislative restraint be sought to compel the universal adoption of harmless material in the manufacture of matches. At the instance of the Association for Labor Legislation, a "bill to provide for a tax upon white phosphorous matches and for other purposes" has been introduced into the House of Representatives, in 1910, by the Honorable John J. Esch, of Wisconsin. This bill, which has since been awarded by its framers, is still before Congress, and ought to become a law. For the adoption of this bill would mean not only the prevention of "phosphorism," and "phossy jaw," with all their untold tortures, but also the saving of many lives which are annually lost through innocent children's sucking of poisonous matches. And it would eliminate the abominable use of readily available poison to produce criminal abortions, and commit suicides and murders. It would also lessen the enormous property losses by fire, and reduce the appalling waste of human life, incident to fires, which for years have called forth the protests of insurance companies against the use of the extremely inflammable phosphorous match.

As is usually the case in matters like these, the selfish "interests" are hard at work to defeat the passage of a Bill by our National Legislature. Even cries against the "match trust" are raised to befool the minds of the public and its representatives, and nothing is left undone to down the real question at issue—*the question of humanity*. It is high time that the public interest be awakened, and that we forward our protest against official inaction, and demand prompt action in this matter *now*, to stop so unnecessary a toll of suffering and loss of lives, at last.

Here is a chance for every reader to half win a good cause, to abolish a most unhuman industry, and to wipe out a blot that disgraces us in the eyes of the civilized world. All you have to do is to write a note to your own Congressman and United States Senator or the Honorable Oscar W. Underwood, M.C., chairman of the Ways and Means Committee, Washington, D. C., asking them to use their whole influence to secure a speedy and definite action on the Esch Bill, in order to stop the use of white phosphorous in the manufacture of matches, urging them that the honor of the United States and public justice demand that the stigma attaching to us should be wiped out, and an unhuman industry be abolished in the name of humanity.

This is a humanitarian work, demanding the support of all good citizens, regardless, of party, and politics. *In the meantime stop using any poisonous white phosphorous matches, known as "parlor" or "lucifer" matches, and get all your friends to join the protest and the boycott. Do it now.*

San Francisco, Cal.

I wish to call your attention to one of the most horrible industrial diseases known, which is not so new, but entirely needless to-day, and which ought to be stopped at last.

Yet, in spite of the most ingenious devices to eliminate handwork, it is an undeniable fact that fully 95 percent of the women, 82 percent of the children, and 44 percent of the men employed in this damnable American industry, are directly exposed to the danger of contracting either "Phossy Jaw," with all the misery implied in this worst form of chronic phosphorous poisoning, . . .

To our shame it must be admitted that the United States is the only important civilized country where this barbaric industry still prevails to the extent that some 4,000 match-workers must ever be exposed to all the dangers of phosphorous poisoning.

In Justice To Thomas And Tabby
(Medical Superstitions of the Twentieth Century)*

by Helen Sayr Gray, Portland, OR

The Naturopath and Herald of Health, XVII(8), 501-506. (1912)

[The following article is a number of paragraphs taken here and there from a pamphlet by Helen Sayr Gray entitled "In Justice to Thomas and Tabby". Its theme is medical superstitions of the twentieth century. She shows that medical superstitions were not sloughed off in the eighteenth century, but still survive and flourish in the guise of the germ theory of disease, serum therapy, vaccination, the use of drugs as medicines, and contagion and infection through germs. For the benefit of those who before they can shed one superstition demand something to take its place and ask, if germs do not cause disease, then what does, she quotes from writing of distinguished physicians who reject the germ theory and the other superstitions mentioned above and shows the function of germs in the body, the true cause of disease, and that drugs do not cure disease, but only relieve pain and suppress or mask symptoms.—Benedict Lust, Ed.]

Some weeks ago much was said in the Chicago papers about Dr. Charles B. Reed's invention of a cat-trap or gibbet to be baited with catnip and operated in back yards. I also read that he had found four dangerous kinds of germs on a cat's whiskers and is therefore urging the extermination of cats as a menace to health. Dr. William McClure, of Wesley Hospital, the same report stated, was examining miscroscopically hairs from cats' fur to ascertain how many different kinds of germs there are on it. From Topeka comes the report that six different kinds of deadly germs have been found on cat's fur and that the Board of Health has in consequence issued a mandate that Topeka cats must be sheared or killed! From time to time a health board official or other doctor gives out a statement for publication condemning handshaking as a dangerous and most reprehensible practice.

The hair of horses, cows, and dogs is full of germs, which they disseminate. Germs are everywhere. Why should cats' whiskers be an exception to the rule? If Thomas and Tabby could retaliate and examine doctors' whiskers, doubtless as many—or more—virulent varieties of germs would be found nestling there. In cities doctors usually wear a somewhat closely cropped beard, in villages, a frowsy, filthy lambrequin of the Jonah pattern that doubtless harbors not merely four deadly varieties, but forty-

---

seven. Doctors are a menace to public health, for they disseminate germs quite as much as do cats. Therefore, exterminate the doctors.

All the leading works on bacteriology admit that a person may have germs of diphtheria, typhoid fever, tuberculosis, pneumonia, or any other disease within his body without having any of those diseases. Since that is the case, it is obvious that germs of themselves cannot cause disease. They do no harm in a body that is in a healthy condition. But so daft is the medical profession on the subject of germs that the true causes of disease are overlooked and disregarded. The doctors are aboard a germ toboggan and cannot get off until they have run the course.

Among the four kinds of germs found on a cat's whiskers Dr. Reed mentions a germ "which causes a variety of infectious diseases, including kidney disease." As if anyone ever got kidney disease because he unwittingly swallowed some germs of the kind found in diseased kidneys, if he had not abused those organs by gross eating or gross drinking! But don't blame the booze.

It relieves the individual of all responsibility for the cat. There is no personal stigma attaching to such a cause; for it is commonly supposed that anybody is liable to be attacked by germs, that, like rain that falleth upon both the just and the unjust, germs attack both healthy persons as well as those whose bodies are saturated with autotoxemia.

An inspection of the family dietary usually reveals the cause of a man's untimely demise. But his death is piously attributed to an inscrutable visitation of Providence. His wife drapes herself in crape, observes all the conventions of grief, and overworks her lachrymose glands for a season. His friends pass resolutions of condolence, lamenting that their dear brother has been "called to his eternal rest," a flattering implication that he had so overworked himself during his brief span of life that he needed an eternity of rest in which to recuperate and was entitled to it as a reward. Whereas the only thing overworked was his digestive organs in disposing of his wife's cooking.

A few centuries ago witches were blamed for misfortunes. It was not known where else they could have originated. Therefore they must be due to witches. Now doctors lay the blame for disease on germs and sometimes on cats as accessory to the fact.

"Isolating children will not prevent the spread of diphtheria. Suppose in a thickly settled community there is a cesspool or a grease-trap that has not received attention for years; the pipes leading to it are broken, and the soil for yards around is saturated with decomposing matter which is sending out toxic gases that pollute the atmosphere in the locality for a block or more; what will happen? The children living in this particular environment will be prostrated by some form of so-called contagious or infectious disease. Every susceptible child or adult reached by this septic miasm will show its influence. Suppose the weather is favorable for the propagation and transmission of this miasm to the inmates of neighboring houses; what can quarantine do? Stopping the leak in the drain and using lime freely is the best quarantine. Can anyone set a limit to the distance that this emanation will be carried in the atmosphere? If the source of the infection remains unknown, which is often the case, it will be said that it was carried by teachers, children, parents, or the cat."

So, if deadly germs are found on cats' whiskers, what of it? It is as valuable a contribution to science to know how many and what kind of germs are to be found on cats' whiskers as to know how many devils can be balanced on the point of a needle. Verily, a fool and his time are soon parted.

That a cat has germs on her fur and whiskers does not prove that she is a menace to health; whereas, that doctors are a menace to health and to life itself can be readily proved. Most of the surgical operations performed are unnecessary and frequently result in death. Personally I am of the opinion that more operations are performed for $300 than ever were performed for appendicitis. Vaccination and the administering of antitoxins are frequently followed by death or impaired health. Nature holds a man accountable for his habits and makes him by an automatic arrangement pay the penalty for violation of law, but the doctors have taught him to think he can escape responsibility for his habits by taking medicine. One of the gravest charges against the prescribing of medicine is that they mask the symptoms and do not remove the cause of the disease but leave the patient to continue in the error of his ways until overtaken by the same trouble again or an equivalent that has cropped out in some other place; and by that time the malady has perhaps reached a fatal stage.

In some respects doctors are like cats; they caterwaul, and sometimes they purr. So here is a metaphorical bootjack thrown at the medical caterwaulers. Erstwhile they indulged in unmelodious caterwauling at the homeopaths and the Christian Scientists, and they still make more noise than a back yard full of cats, yowling in the press denouncing the irregulars. Now a director has charge of the Thomas concerts and has drilled the cats to join in the chorus and sing paeans in praise of the efficacy of their wonderful new serums, vaccines, and antitoxins, in order to foist their fallacious doctrines on the public by constant iteration.

When a woman patient calls at a doctor's office and he does not know just what is the matter with her nor what to do to cure her, if he belongs to a certain type in the profession, he holds her hand and purrs and is so sympathetic that she leaves his office in a transport, walks on air, and goes home convinced that no one understands her case as well as he does. Or else he tells her how beautiful she looked on the operating table. After such a subtle appeal to her vanity she pays without demur his bill of $300 or $400.

He takes great care not to offend his patients by telling them unpleasant truths but instead resorts to delicate flattery. If a woman comes to his office suffering from dyspepsia brought on chiefly by eating devitalized foods of unsuitable selection and eating too much, he purrs softly while he determines the latitude and longitude of her pain and gently inquires if she has had a shock recently. She thinks hard a moment and recalls that she has had, that the news of a death of a child of an intimate friend was broken to her abruptly. Yes, that must have been what caused her condition.

When patients have a cold or the grippe, instead of making plain to them what laws of health they have violated and that their illness is a direct result, the doctor, it not infrequently happens, tell them that it is "going around". Colds and grippe are consequently in the popular mind of mysterious origin, and the victims complacently regard themselves as blameless but unfortunate.

It is because the medical profession teaches people to look outside of themselves for the causes of their maladies that we see such spectacles as Caruso, obliged to break professional engagements that would have yielded him $100,000, ascribing his case of grippe to external influences. "I like everything in New York except its colds and grippe," he is quoted as saying in an interview. "I think I can boast that I have had the most expensive case of grippe on record. It has cost me $100,000. The public says I am a great singer. I should be a greater man if I were a scientist who could drive grippe out of the country. See if you can't drive it out of New York before I come back."

The germ theory delusion is in great vogue at present, but in time it inevitably must be discarded. The time is not very far distant when the contagiousness and infectiousness of disease through germs, vaccination, the injection of serums as preventives or cures, and the resorting to the use of medicines by deluded people as a substitute for correcting their habits of living will generally regarded as superstitions.

I know of a case of illness recently in Long Beach, California, in which a mother suspended a nutmeg on a string around her child's neck as a cure for throat affection. The child's father, being somewhat of wag, on seeing the device, suggested that, if the nutmeg did not work, she try a cocoanut!*

I recall another household remedy, one that I chanced upon among the health suggestions in an extensively used cook book: "Sufferers from asthma should get a muskrat skin and wear it over their lungs with the fur side next to the body. It will bring certain relief." O shade of Hippocrates! The remedy is worse than the disease.

---

* Cocoanut means coconut.

Note this: it was the medical profession that taught people to look to such means for cures and formerly prescribed just such grotesque remedies. In a leaflet reprint entitled *Bacteriophobia and Medical Fads*, Dr. J. W. Hodge quotes some of the prescriptions given in "the second edition of *The New English Pharmacopoeia and Dispensatory*, printed in London in 1752 and edited by R. James, M.D., an eminent old school physician of that period." Among the remedies to be taken internally were pulverized warts, dried earthworms, snails, and snakes, nanny tea made from sheep's droppings, live bedbugs, hog's lice (adult dose, nine swallowed alive), powdered toads, the dried blood of black cats, pulverized asses' hoofs and mules' hoofs, and "infallible powders," composed of the tails of lizards, snakes, white puppy-dogs, and dried toads. "This work was the official standard authority in the 'regular' school of medicine in those days and for many years thereafter. In it I find all the above mentioned substances highly recommended as specifies for the various diseases that afflict the human family."

If germs are not the cause of disease, then what is? To this Dr. J. H. Tilden makes answer as follows. I quote excerpts taken here and there from his writings in *A Stuffed Club* on the subject of the causes of disease, the germ theory, and contagion.

"Disease is brought about by obstructions and inhibitions of vital processes . . . . The basis—the first cause—is chronic auto-intoxication from food poisoning. This systemic derangement—chronic auto-toxemia—is brought about by abusing the body in many ways . . . by living wrong in whatever way . . . and is ready at all times to join with exciting causes to create anything from a pimple to a brain abscess and from a cold to consumption. Without this derangement injuries and such contingent influences as are named exciting causes would fail to create disease. This is the constitutional derangement that is necessary before we can have such local manifestations as tonsillitis, pneumonia, and appendicitis. . . . . Epidemics and endemics feed upon the autotoxemic and stop where there are none."

"I do not recognize germs as a primary or real cause of disease any more than drafts or any such so-called causes; at most germs can be only exciting causes. . . . Germs are victims and partakers of their environment. They act upon it and are reacted upon by it. They are in all bodies in health and in disease. As they must be amenable to environmental law, the same as everything else, they necessarily change when their environment changes. Because of a change in their habitat, the germs that are native change from a non-toxic state into one of toxicity . . . . They are not something extraneous to the human organism but are the products of lowered vitality in the individual, of lost resistance. My theory is that the toxicity of germs is due to being saturated with poisonous gases. The germs of typhoid fever, for example, are not poisonous until the patient is sufficiently broken down to cause the generation of toxic gases, after which all the fluids and solids of the body take on a septic state, poisoned by the absorbed gas . . . . Bacteria are not the cause of disease; wrong living, which puts the system into such condition that the bacteria can readily multiply, is the real cause; the bacteria are simply necessary results.

"The belief of the medical profession that contagion and infection pass from one human being to another—from a sick man to a healthy man—is an old superstition unworthy of this age. Disease will not go from person to person, unless they are in physical condition that renders them susceptible and unless environment states favor decomposition—those of the household and the general atmosphere where the proper amount of oxygen is deficient. So-called contagious and infectious diseases are self-limited. If it were not for this self-limitation, the world would be depopulated every time an epidemic of a severe character succeeds in getting a start. But the medical profession believes that vaccination and antitoxin do what nature has been doing since the world began, namely, set a limit to the spread of disease."

"Health is the only immunity against disease. If there is any state that man can be put into that will cause him to be less liable to come under disease-producing influences that full health, then law and order are not supreme and the world must be the victim of caprice, haphazard and chance."

"Tuberculosis is a seed disease. The seed must come from a previous case." Dr. J. N. McCormack, official itinerant lecturer of the American Medical Association and "mouthpiece of 80,000 doctors", as he very appropriately terms himself, is wont to declare in the plea that he is sent out to make all over the country for the establishment of a "national department of health and education to bring the benefactions of modern medical science to every household." But if one contracts tuberculosis from the germs of another case and he in turn from someone else, how did the first case that ever happened originate, as the leaders among those who reject the germ theory. Did the causes that produced the first case of tuberculosis, cholera, typhoid fever, measles, diphtheria, and other diseases commonly regarded as contagious or infectious quit the business after producing one case, disappear, and go out of existence, or do they still operate and cause all the cases that occur? That troublesome first case is the missing link in the chain of the theory; but it happened so long ago that it has been lost sight of, and doctors are seldom embarrassed by being asked to account for it.

I know a family in which all of the six children had adenoids. Adenoids are not regarded as contagious, so far as I have ever heard. So contagion cannot be made the scapegoat in this instance. The children had adenoids because the mode of living was the same for all. In like manner when several members of a family contract tuberculosis, diphtheria, or measles, do they not get the disease because they all lived in the same manner and were exposed to like influences, instead of through contagion or infection with germs? Disease is sometimes spread, however, through the contagion of fear and suggestion.

In Paris there is a museum—the Guimet Musee—in which are housed discarded deities—gods that once were feared and worshiped and prayed to and paid, until their congregations dwindled and the pews were empty, gods that have been put out of the deity business by the advance of civilization. This collection of monstrous theological superstitions is a most instructive exhibit.

Some day a philanthropist, instead of founding a library or a college, will establish a museum of medical superstitions, in which will be displayed the things that in the past were regarded as preventives or cures of disease, as well as those still in vogue at the present time; for it is not necessary to go back to the middle ages to find barbarous cures. There will be tablets and statues to commemorate the illustrious perpetrators of the serums, viruses, specifics, antitoxins, and elixirs that are so much extolled by the medical profession at the present time.

Among others there will be a monument to the eminent Frenchman, Dr. Brown-Sequard, who immortalized himself by discovering an elixir of life "and died five years after he found it;" to Jenner, who perpetrated vaccination on an ignorant and gullible public; to Dr. Flexner, because of his discovery of a serum for meningitis; to Prof. Ehrlich, who has recently set the medical world agog with his "epochal discovery" of 606.

This is a truly remarkable remedy. It is a sort of instantaneous cure, a medical miracle. One dose is all that is necessary. The attending physician injects some of it and says "sic'em". It does the rest. It runs around through the system and singles out certain germs and destroys them without disturbing any others. Wonderful! Selah. When it is discredited and discredited writers of "idiotorials" who heralded its discovery as a remarkable achievement of science and declared its efficacy "has been proved just as conclusively as that the earth is round," will then realize that their skimmers leak and will gracefully repudiate their former assertion by declaring that the scientific world never really accepted 606.

Such a museum would be most interesting and instructive and would greatly enlighten the community.

Germs are everywhere. Why should cats' whiskers be an exception to the rule?

1913

MEDICINE AND PSYCHOLOGY
A. A. ERZ, D.C.

—·—

REMOVE THE CAUSE
FRED KAESSMANN

—·—

SYMPTOMATIC TREATMENT, A WASTE OF EFFORT AND TIME
DR. CARL STRUEH

—·—

PRINCIPLES OF ETHICS
INTERNATIONAL ALLIANCE OF PHYSICIANS AND SURGEONS

THE MEDICAL QUESTION

The Truth About Official Medicine and Why We Must Have Medical Freedom

Medical Laws vs. Human Rights and Constitution. The Great Need of the Hour. What Constitutes the True Science and Art of Healing

By A. A. ERZ, N. D., D. C.

HERE is a book that cheers one like a draught of ozone after having breathed the mephitic vapors of the philosophy of official medicine, that exploits the immorality of vivisection, and swears by the unscientific and useless products of the torture trough.

It consists of 600 pages, written by the trenchant pen of one who is master of his subject. It embodies the revolt of the latest and most efficient school of medical healing against the tyranny and ignorance of the drug doctors, who, while attacking symptoms, fail to understand the need of the higher practice of treating the causes of disease instead. The charlatanry and inefficiency of official medicine has reason to be envious of the successes of the natural school whose philosophic practices are here fully manifested.

Dr. Erz makes very clear his position in the art of healing. He is an enthusiastic Naturopath. He believes that when a man becomes ill, he should employ the natural forces of hydropathy, diet, exercise, sunshine, electricity, mechano-therapy, massage, and all the healing agencies that have proven their worth as prophylactics, and their ability to arouse the inherent restorative power for health that resides in every organism. His information is illuminating in the highest degree.

He is the sworn enemy of the "scientific medicine" of the allopaths, that consists of poisonous drugs on the one hand, and the equally poisonous and wholly dangerous serums, inoculations and vaccines on the other, that form a body of medical superstition that is propagating disease rather than curing it. He discusses, one by one, the most loudly-praised products of medical research, and proves them either to be utterly useless, or of deadly danger to the duped and unsuspecting patient.

In support of his statements, he quotes the opinions of the greatest exponents of official medicine who confess that allopathic medicine has produced more misery and premature death than famine, pestilence and war combined. As Billroth says, "Our progress is over mountains of corpses."

He proves that the American Medical Association, and the various State and County Associations affiliated therewith, form one vast engine of oppression, armed with legal power to harass, crush, and if possible destroy, the true saviors of mankind, the exponents of natural healing, whose activities naturally discredit official medicine. By legally securing a monopoly of practising medicine, THEY ARE ABLE TO MAKE IT MORE OF A CRIME TO CURE A PERSON THAN TO KILL HIM.

He shows how easy it is to understand why the unthinking legislator favors official medicine to the exclusion of the natural school of therapy. The psychological pressure of an institution, no matter how despotic its use of power may be, or how false and deadly its products are, that has its roots deeply rooted in history, is vastly greater on the unenlightened mind, than a true and noble institution that was born but yesterday—where man does not know conservatism rules.

Dr. Erz fully proves that the so-called remedies of medical research are violations of every law of nature, of health, of life, and a disregard of every principle of physiology, biology and therapeutics.

The people were never consulted about these laws, and never asked for them

They are the product of medical feudalism, which means intolerance, injustice and brutality, instead of charity, justice and dignity. The people should rise in their might and stay the infamous activities of these medical malefactors.

It is a startling indictment of humanity that its saviors are never recognized until the advance guard, and many of the main army, are killed, or trodden underfoot, and official medicine in America, the glorious Land of Freedom, is busy at this moment, as it has been for many years past, in hunting down the drugless practitioner, whose only fault is the fact that he cures patients by natural methods, where the vendors of rotten pus have signally failed. He is arrested, and heavily fined, or thrown into jail for the offense of practising medicine without a pus-vendor's license.

Dr. Erz rightly advocates the urgent need of a great Academy of Natural Healing to convince the thinking masses of the superiority of the Natural Healing System, and to protect it against all misrepresentations and abuses, and assure its efficiency and permanent success. Medical Freedom is the great need of the hour to prove that Nature's constructive laws overshadow all ignorance, superstition and ambition. As the exponent of a standard of drugless healing, and as a monitor, mentor, and defence of humanity from rapacity and superstition, such an institution would be of enormous value to mankind.

Dr. Erz's work is a standard contribution to the great propaganda of Drugless Therapy that is sweeping over the land. No drugless practitioner can afford to be without its inspiring companionship. It marks an epoch in the history of the grand science and art of Natural Healing.

Price, in cloth, postpaid, $5.00; paper cover, $4.00.

THE NATURE CURE PUBLISHING CO., BUTLER, N. J.

Medical Laws vs. Human Rights and Constitution, a book written by A. A. Erz, N.D., D.C.

MEDICINE AND PSYCHOLOGY

by A. A. Erz., D.C., San Francisco, CAL.

The Naturopath and Herald of Health, XVIII(2), 81-85. (1913)

In these days of so-called Psychical Research and all sorts of New Thought cults and fads, so many works on Psychopathology, Psychotherapy, Psychopathy, Psychic Treatment are being offered the student that one might think psychology the science of the soul, belonged to those branches of science that have been mastered at last. And since there are so many prominent medical men openly professing their faith in "psychic treatment," it would appear as if medicine were ready to embrace this most important branch of higher science, and accord it the proper place in its course of study. As a matter of fact, real psychology has no worse adversary today than the regular medical school, and medical practitioners almost wholly ignore or neglect it. Although of all vital branches of medical knowledge, psychology ought more than any other subject to be studied by all physicians, since without its knowledge their practice degenerates into mere guess-work and chance-intuitions.

Our study of life brings us to face the facts of unity of existence underlying all life and form. Modern science speaks of one common hypothetical, undifferentiated substance, called protyle, or it speaks of self-existent motion. But there is a subtle something underlying the physical and co-ordinating with it: *Consciousness*, consisting the unity of existence, and manifesting life. Mind is only another differentiation of manifestation, more subtle, and intricate and expansive of life in tangible form. The objective world is not to be looked upon as essentially matter and force—as modern science considers it—but as Life and Consciousness. Life being divine in its essence, is involving and evolving, or manifesting itself for a definite purpose, in matter and form. There is Law, Intelligence and Purpose in and behind this evolution. There is One Existence whose consciousness is active at every point and in every particle in His cosmos. His life sustains all, His purpose guides all. All living beings love no other object than to carry out His Laws. The Law of Sacrifice is the law of the evolution of life and form. Man, the highest form of physical life, being a spark of Divine Essence, possesses the potentiality of unfolding into Divine Being.

Every living physical object has its origin in basic principles in the cosmos, by means of which principles the form comes into manifestation, all having a first cause and life functioning in every atom in the Universe which holds each form together. There are two basic principles, Life and Form, constituting the underlying foundation in all objects, and they must be studied before the object can be known. Modern science takes up the study of physical manifestations of forms and seeks to find the relations between them and the laws within which, and by means of which they act. True science takes the seed and observes the life principles at work and deduces from these principles the manifestations which appear as rootlet, trunk, branch and leaf. Modern science begins at the leaves, observes their shape, color and characteristics; it dissects them one by one, passes on to the branch, trunk and root. It is far more scientific to first study the forces and intelligences of nature that are building the things and producing manifestations.

Without the higher knowledge of the constitution of man in his

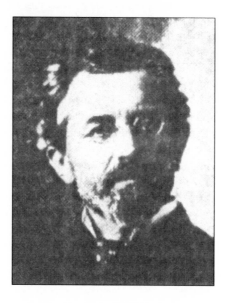

A. A. Erz, ND, DC.

triune nature, modern science is yet groping in the dark as regards many simple things. It tells as much about the diagnosis and the different stages of diseases, and loads of books have been written by different authors on pathological anatomy and kindred subjects; but even after a perusal of all these "learned" works, one still does not know what diseases really are and how they arise. Because medicine is lacking the knowledge of the true science of life which explains the nature and measure of life, and what is beneficial to it and what injurious. Life being the union of body, mind and soul, it is that which unites, the one thread that links all three together; it holds together the elements of which the body is composed; it constitutes the existence, and ever going and unbroken sequence. If this rope is broken, life no longer can flow from the higher to the lower body, and what is called death or disunion of body, mind and soul, follows.

The soul, the vital principle and divine breath of life, is eternal and immutable. Mind is the energy of the soul working within the physical brain. The soul links the divine spirit in man and his lower personality. The faculties are attributes of matter, and the senses are the instruments of consciousness. The soul is the divine eternal witness of our actions, without being itself affected by any of them; hence it is not affected by disease. Consequently we cannot have a psychopathology as a psychotherapy, in the exact scientific senses; although modern medicine uses these terms, which actually refer to the mind and not to the soul. Disease can affect body and mind only; thus we have physical and mental diseases. Body and mind are the subjects in which health and disease co-inhere, parity of correlation of the mental and physical forces being the causes or condition of health, or normal state of mind. The ultimate cause of all diseases is an adverse or excessive correlation, or a want of correlation, of the physical and mental forces. Disease is not merely the absence of health, it is not negative but it is something positive. Its prevention as well as its cure consists in the knowledge of the laws of nature and life, by means of which both the maintenance and the re-establishment of health are made possible. Hence all true healing systems must be based on the laws of nature and life, excluding everything injurious to health and life. Consequently, poisonous drugs and destructive treatments can have no place in any truly therapeutic system.

It has ever been the practice of the medicine wiseacres to resent as a heresy the least dissent from their antiquated doctrines, and though a popular, common sense curative method not as yet officially recognized, should be shown to save thousands of human lives, they will cling to the most fallacious theories, dangerous prescriptions and treatments, and decry both innovator and innovation until the official mintstamp of "regularity" has been obtained. Millions of poor sufferers may meanwhile perish under the old "regular" treatment; but so long as "professional honor" is vindicated and "medical authority and ethics" are upheld, the welfare of the people is a matter of secondary importance to the professional stickler of medicine

Theoretically the most benignant, at the same time no other school of science exhibits so many instances of petty prejudices, bigoted dogmatism, cross materialism, vulgar theism, and malignant stubbornness as official medicine. The predilections and patronage of the average leading medical practitioners, regarding certain average therapeutic methods, are scarcely ever measured by the usefulness of a practical treatment. One need only think of bleeding by leeching, cupping, and the lancet, each of which had its epidemic of popularity with medical men and has slain millions, but at last fell into merited disgrace when people refused to submit the wanton butchery. Water, now freely given to fevered patients, was once denied them, and the "regulars" would either let the suffering sick die before they permitted this "irregular" use of a cooling drink of plain, pure water to a patient burning with fever. Indeed, there never has been a lack of medical superstition and fetishism of the worst kind.

History repeats itself. We all recollect how the best medical authorities would decry "mental or physical treatments" as a mere humbug, and call any drugless healing system an outright fraud; while today, medicine tries to adopt the very same ideas and names of the once tabooed methods. However, it is well to remember the old truism, "When two are doing the same, it is by no means the same thing." Because, the average medical practitioner, owing to his previous one-sided education, is utterly unfit to comprehend any system of natural healing, and is hardly ever capable of practicing anything else in the line of healing methods, but medicine; and he will usually make a very poor drugless healer, as no matter how hard he may try to unlearn the ingrained habit of drugging people, and of looking at disease from the materialistic medical standpoint, which to him is quintessence of all science.

How many medical men are there who realize that there is an occult aspect of the known side of Nature? The study of true science in its entirety offers tremendous difficulties to those who have been trained in the familiar methods of modern medicine. The more they have of the one the less capable they are of instinctively comprehending the other, for a man can only think in his worn grooves, and unless he has the courage to fill up these and make new ones for himself, he must perforce travel on the old lines. And what does medicine really amount to? Any observant student of modern medicine becomes impressed by the vast extent of ignorance of medical men on every subject of their study. What is called medical science represents but a few palpable facts collected and roughly generalized, and an extended unintelligible technical jargon invented to hide our "learned" medico's ignorance of all that lies behind these facts. To juggle thus with barbarous Greco-Latin terms, when the facts are so simple, is the art of modern medical men lacking real science. No man who has faith in the infinite possibilities of Nature, can feel content to spend his life in a sham work which aids only that same pretentious medicine full of fallacies and superstitions. And when medical men would like to make the people believe that they have discarded the antiquated treatment of drugging, and misname their damnable administration of all kinds of obnoxious filth-poisons, called lymphs, serums, vaccines, and antitoxins, "drugless treatment," they may consider themselves very smart, but they will soon find out that the people are on to their cheap trick of masquerading an exploded medical drug fraud of the worst kind. Yes, people have learned something about real drugless healing, and the fact that over twenty millions of brainy Americans are patronizing the various drugless healing systems in this country speaks volumes in favor of the common sense of our liberty-loving people in matters pertaining to health. And the same people are ready to fight for medical freedom, to be sure.

Various systems of mental or psychic treatment take the lead in the drugless method of healing in this land of ours, today. In one sense, it is a good move in the right direction, in these days of materialism, although not everything that pretends to belong to psychology and the New Thought movement is genuine, we are sorry to state. Not all that goes under the name of psychology belongs to that grand science which just now is being very much misrepresented and abused by many miserable mercenaries and vile imposters, who are offering to a gullible public their "new psychology" in the form of "personal instructions," or some kind of "lectures," at so much per "lesson," which are but a hodge-podge of nonessential gush, and all kinds of catch-phrases, such as "dual mind," by which later they certainly betray their utter ignorance of the subject. Such is the fate of all true psychology in this world of deceptions and imitations with its selfish and irresponsible "teacher of psychology," and all kinds of "scientists," whose main "science" is money-making and humbuggery.

In order to be exact, psychology is the science of the soul, both as an entity distinct from the spirit, and in its relations with the spirit, mind and body. This is the conception of psychology held by true science. In modern medicine psychology relates only, or principally to conditions of the mind and the nervous system, and the psychical essence and nature of man are almost absolutely ignored. In fact, true psychology comprising all occult forces of the higher powers of man, is an unknown field to modern materialistic science which is powerless to explain that which proceeds directly from the divine nature of the human soul itself, the existence of which most of our scientific men deny, unwilling at the same time to confess their ignorance of the subject.

As a matter of fact, modern despiritualized science deals chiefly with the physical side of life, and too little attention is being paid to the spiritual side of life. Yet advanced science tells us that psychic or mental effort underlies all physiological conditions and organic functions, and may give rise to pathological conditions, by affecting the vital actions. That mental activity results in physical changes in our system has long since been recognized by science and daily experience. Thus we know that the state of mind, and our thoughts and emotions have an influence on internal secretions, on the condition of the blood, on our temperature, and the processes of respiration, circulation, digestion, nutrition assimilation and elimination. Emotions of fear, worry, anger, greatly interfere with the serous secretions, and produce chemical changes of a deleterious character, impairing other functions. While joy, cheerfulness, calmness, love, hopefulness, have a beneficent influence on all vital functions of our organism. In fact, our mind is the natural protector and physician of the body, and the poet expresses but a great truth of nature when he says: "It takes its mind to make the body rich." Hence it is well to pay attention to the controlling of our mind, the many sense-impressions, the impulses, desires and passions, and avoid all perverted mental and emotional states not conducive to health. But what controls the mind and will?

Life wants to express itself in perfection, and health is the normal state of physical life. But we allow environments and conditions to interfere with perfect expression of life, through our imperfect objective mentality. It is our mental attitude toward anything that determines its effect upon us; if we fear or antagonize a thing it will have detrimental effects on us, if we come into perfect understanding with it, by quietly recognizing and inwardly asserting our independence of, and our superiority over, mind and matter, no injury for us will follow from anything, and we will thus be able to master adverse conditions.

Some people evidently have peculiar ideas about the various new and old systems of "psychic" or mental and metaphysical healing that do need correcting. All true psychology is based on the fact that man *is a spirit with a soul, and has a mind and a body*, as a means to manifestation. Hence the "superiority of mind over body," through mastery of mind by the soul. The "power of mind over our body: is never manifesting itself in a way foreign to natural law, as some people think it does, but mind, like all forces of nature works through natural laws that are peculiar to its nature. However, mind force belongs to the finer or higher natural forces that are as yet but little understood by modern science.

Advanced science admits the fact that matter is not the beginning nor the end of everything; that there is something back of matter which appears to control or modify it, and for lack of a better word this something is called *mind*. And truly scientific men who have the courage and ability to think for themselves, and throw aside the fetish of school authority, just now venture to study mind. And they look at our physical organism as the instrument of the mind, and the temple of the soul, the indwelling spirit divine. For *man is essentially divine*, and by virtue of his triune nature is related to the spiritual, mental and physical worlds. Unless we recognize these facts and live accordingly, we do not lead a perfectly natural life conducive to health and happiness. As far as medicine is concerned, as matters stand today, it is a sad fact that medical men who have made their mark in this profession, are continuously showing the better informed observer, that they really know so little of psychology as to take up with any plausible scheme, or any clever pretender who comes their way, and so make themselves ridiculous in the eyes of the thoughtful student. It is no wonder that others who are eager to learn and to know are also taken in by the numerous fakes and grafters who, under some assumed Hindu or other Oriental names, fleece the easily beguiled general public. The fact that truly scientific psychology in its entirety has only been mastered in the Orient, where stood the cradle of mankind and of all science, does by no means imply that everything and everybody passing under an Oriental name is representing the genuine article.

Then there are those who pretend "to combine the Oriental and the Western ideas of psychology," but in fact can offer only an incomplete system of their own based on a mere smattering of science, as gobbled up from some doubtful Oriental authorities and from the current literature of the Western world which has hardly mastered certain branches of psychology. By all means, beware of the "psychologist" who sells you the "science" at so much per lesson. The true student knows where to find the true teacher. It is not to be wondered at that there are so many good people who are ignorant in psychological sciences, having studied only the rudiments of metaphysics, but they nevertheless are determined to fight these same metaphysics as well as psychology, of the one which they know as little as the other. Such is the fate of true psychology, which has the key to all truths and mysteries in nature. Indeed, it requires discrimination, efforts and time to attain the *true* science of psychology.

To refer only to the fundamentals, so many physicians ignore the fact that *man is a spirit soul*, and has a mind and body that are instrumental in his manifestations of life. Such are man's relations of the spiritual, mental and physical worlds, which the true physician must take in consideration. For health is but the result of perfect co-relation of the physical, mental and spiritual forces. Even the most materialistic physician of observant nature must admit that the physical conditions of men are greatly dependent upon the influence of the mind and the action of the will; and that disease is but the result or a condition of imperfect coordination of the spiritual, mental and physical. Hence it will never do to neglect the one or the other side of life in treating a patient. And that treatment is the best and most natural which takes *all* natural forces pertaining to man in due consideration. In fact, every successful treatment actually comprises the physical as well as the psychic forces of man either knowingly or unknowingly, as far as the efforts of the physician are concerned.

Indeed, the more of true psychology official medicine will take into its curriculum and practice, the better for all concerned. For true psychology has the key to all mysteries of life and no system of healing can attain to permanent success without this great science, comprising the essentials of all principal sciences.

REMOVE THE CAUSE

by Fred Kaessmann

The Naturopath and Herald of Health, XVIII(3), 158-159. (1913)

Undoubtedly many readers of this publication have tried various sug-gestions presented in its columns. Also, if their experience has been that common to many who have taken up rational methods of cure, they have at times been disappointed. Results have not come up to expecta-tions. They wanted much, and wanted it quickly, but, here is the rub, they did not stop to learn WHY they were sick. In other words they did not first REMOVE THE CAUSE.

Hereafter, before undertaking to cure yourself according to lines laid down in this and other similar publications, STOP, THINK, REASON. Find out first what you wish to accomplish.   Yes, that is it exactly, for unless you can see this clearly you are unlikely to score big and satis-factory success. No man would knowingly construct a house without being sure of the foundation, yet health culturists frequently undertake to construct physical human temples without giving the slightest thought to the foundation.

What would be a sound foundation? RIGHT HABITS and MODES of LIVING. Unless you lead a well regulated life, one based upon ways in accord with nature's requirements, all the physical culture work you do will help you little. The man who continually gorges himself with rich food can hardly be saved from the damnation of indigestion, dyspepsia, rheumatism, gout, and the like. The woman who, after copiously sweat-ing over a heavy weekly "wash", will run out doors without first taking means to protect herself from chilly winter blasts, is almost sure, sooner or later, to round up with rheumatism, neuralgia, pneumonia or some other fatal or painful illness. I know that some recommend these periods of "cleansing"—but they do not appeal to me as good, sound common sense. The body can be cleansed just as effectively, and far more agree-ably, by eating less, short fasts, or deeper breathing.

So it is throughout the entire category of diseases. Before you try to remove symptoms, REMOVE THE CAUSE. Do not aim at the removal of coughs by taking this cough cure or that. Keep your win-dows open, at least throughout the night, that you may have some fresh air. That will be more to the point. If your cough comes from too much knowledge of the red-light district, cut out the red-light district. The greatest lung specialist in the world cannot do anything for you until you do, for you will tear down quicker than he or nature can build. For the constant desire to urinate there is a reason. Just remove that reason, that cause, and the trouble will soon disappear, often without assistance of any kind. So, in fact, it is with many diseases. The cause removed—nature soon sets the house to order.

This is not the first article in which I have advocated REMOVING THE CAUSE. Nor will it be the last. My every effort is being bent along this line. It will be continued to be bent along this line. When people get to understand the value and necessity or RIGHT HABITS and MODES of LIFE, then there will be less sickness. In any event, I hope to see the day when people will try to cure themselves by first removing the cause of their sickness rather than by attempting continual patchwork, as nearly all remedial means are, drug or non-drug.

One thing I wish to impress upon all readers of this publication who are natural healers by profession, and that is this: When a patient presents himself for treatment who suffers from a complaint which later may become something more serious, be sure to point out to the patient the reason for his ailment—and also be sure to explain what it may lead to—AND WHY. For instance, many years before I knew anything of natural healing methods, I suffered from a liver trouble. Naturally, I went to the family M.D. for remedy. He treated me and for awhile I would be all right. Then I would have another attack. Finally, I had consumption. Now, had this M.D. told me that IMPROPER OXIDATION OF THE BLOOD was a primary reason for my liver trouble, and that, unless means were taken properly to oxygenate the blood other serious troubles, such as bronchitis, pleurisy, consumption would follow, the chances are that I should have done something to supply the deficiency. However, no such warning was given. I was told nothing except to go to the drug-store. As a result, I later put in many years fighting disease—at big expense. Therefore, I urge drugless healers to make plain to all patients to what any particular CAUSE may eventually lead.

In this connection, I will here make a statement to which some may take exception, but which I consider fundamental as to the ethics of the profession: Any physician, no matter of what school, who fails to tell a patient plainly as to what a certain line of conduct will eventually lead, IS A GRAFTER. Humanity certainly demands as much as this, and nothing but a DESIRE LATER TO PROFIT FINANCIALLY would deter a man from pointing out any dangers in this path. While well aware that patients will not, by any means, do all that is suggested, I am also well aware that where the explanation is given in good faith, and in an interesting and effective way that patients invariably listen—and often obey.

For instance, patients always manifest great interest in certain charts and books which I keep conveniently at hand. Surprising it is, too, to see how readily they grasp the full significance of any particular line of conduct, when clearly pointed out to them. Had I simply spoken to them, they might have listened and might simply have pretended to listen, but when they see the charts—that is a different matter. Then do graphic illustration and words work together for the benefit of the patient—and of humanity. Incidentally, I doubt if this course will ever injure the profits of any practitioner. His fairness and ability will be extolled, and ever a larger number of patients will flock to his office.

—70 Bennington Street, Lawrence, Mass.

Before you try to remove symptoms, REMOVE THE CAUSE.

When a patient presents himself for treatment who suffers from a complaint which later may become something more serious, be sure to point out to the patient the reason for his ailment—and also be sure to explain what it may lead to— AND WHY.

SYMPTOMATIC TREATMENT, A WASTE OF EFFORT AND TIME

by Dr. Carl Strueh

Dr. Carl Strueh's Health Resort, McHenry, Ill., near Chicago

The Naturopath and the Herald of Health, XVIII(3), 170-171. (1913)

The cure from disease can be brought about only by the great forces of nature, which in disease as well as in health, are bound to improve the function of every organ and cell of the body.

Any artificial treatment is merely *symptomatic* and as such admissible in *incurable* diseases in which the purpose of the treatment is to ease the patient's suffering, also in various temporary afflictions in which the symptoms require immediate relief and in which a speedy removal of the cause of the affliction is impossible.

However, to rely upon the symptomatic treatment in an established disease, as a great many patients are inclined to do, is poor policy. Symptoms are but the manifestation of disease, not the disease itself, and to direct our efforts toward the results, instead of the cause, is not a wise thing to do.

We can suppress most any symptom by means of a remedy, we can produce sleep in a person suffering from chronic insomnia by a dose of veronal, we can cause an evacuation of the bowels in chronic constipation by a laxative, we can suppress the symptoms of chronic rheumatism by administering salicylates, we can quiet a neurasthenic by means of a sedative, we can lessen the frequency of convulsions in an epileptic by administering bromides, we can relieve chronic headaches by a dose of aspirin.

But we do not cure in this manner. If we discontinue the symptomatic treatment, the former symptoms, as a rule, will reappear, and if we continue it we may cause the patient irreparable harm.

To *cure* a disease, our object must be to abstain from symptomatic treatment as much as possible, in order to occupy the entire cell action for the repair work which has to be done and not burden it with additional work which is incurred in the process of eliminating the drug.

A cure, in order to be a cure at all, must be fundamental, must go at the root of the evil.

Disease is not ordained by providence, but is the logical result of our irrational way of living, i.e., of our continued violations of the fundamental laws of nature.

Most all of us are living unnatural lives. We spend most of our time indoors away from sunlight and pure air and exposed to an overheated and impure atmosphere, we lack exercise or, on the other hand, overwork ourselves physically, or mentally, we do not eat the proper food or eat it in the proper way, we indulge in all sorts of excuses, deny ourselves natural sleep, we worry most of the time, in short live wrong in every way possible.

The stronger our constitution, the longer we may keep up under this unnatural way of living. But no matter how strong our constitution, the time will come when we will have to pay the penalty for our folly. Sickness will follow our disregard of nature's laws as sure as night follows day. And before we know it, some organic or constitutional disease makes its appearance.

In order to re-establish a state of health under such conditions it will not suffice to take a teaspoonful of medicine ever so often. It takes more than that. A cure from an established disease is not an easy matter, and unless the patient is determined to deny himself a great many things he has been accustomed to and to put up a stiff fight, he will not reach his goal.

It is absurd to expect to get cured with the causes which brought on the disease, allowed to continue.

The power which cures a disease is right within us. It is called the *vis medicatrix naturae*, i.e., the inborn natural healing power which exists in every living body: It is the power which in health as well as sickness, directs the action of every organ and cell of the body. It is the driving force which moves and regulates the circulation of the blood, the action of the lungs, the processes of digestion and assimilation, the function of the kidneys, muscles, nerves and every other organ of the body.

The purpose of the treatment is to act upon these various functions and thus increase and strengthen the patient's vital force, i.e., his healing power.

The agencies with which the purpose is accomplished consist of pure air, proper food, regular exercises, sunlight and baths.

These treatments are simple as such and still most powerful if properly applied. To *individualize*, i.e., combine these various agencies into a system which conforms with the condition of each individual patient, is the art of the physician.

> *Symptoms are but the manifestation of disease, not the disease itself, and to direct our efforts toward the results, instead of the cause, is not a wise thing to do. . . . A cure, in order to be a cure at all, must be fundamental, must go at the root of the evil. . . . These treatments are simple as such and still most powerful if properly applied. . . . To individualize, i.e., combine these various agencies into a system which conforms with the condition of each individual patient, is the art of the physician.*

PRINCIPLES OF ETHICS

by International Alliance of Physicians and Surgeons

The Naturopath and Herald of Health, XVIII(6), 376-379. (1913)

For Physicians of All Schools, Framed and Approved by the Members of the International Alliance of Physicians and Surgeons

The following principles of Medical Ethics were unanimously adopted and recommended to all physicians who desire to enter into fraternal relations with each other. The International Alliance of Physicians and Surgeons, anxious to put itself into an agreement with all physicians, has concluded it to be wise to adopt as far as possible the *Principles of Medical Ethics* already adopted by other medical associations.

In pursuance of this purpose, the following *Principles of Medical Ethics* are adopted from those promulgated by the American Medical Association and the American Medical Union, International Alliance of Physicians and Surgeons, with such changes as were necessary to reconcile them to the honest conviction and conscientious purposes of the International Alliance of Physicians and Surgeons.

CHAPTER I
THE DUTIES OF PHYSICIANS TO THEIR PATIENTS

Section 1

Physicians should not only be ever ready to obey the calls of the sick and the injured, but should be mindful of the big character of their mission and of the responsibilities they must incur in the discharge of momentous duties. In their ministrations they should never forget that the comfort, the health, and the lives of those entrusted to their care depend on skill, attention and fidelity. In deportment they should unite tenderness, cheerfulness and firmness, and thus inspire all sufferers with gratitude, respect and confidence. These observances are the most sacred because, generally, the only tribunal to adjudge penalties for unkindness, carelessness or neglect is their own conscience.

Section 2

Every patient committed to the charge of a physician should be treated with attention and humanity, and reasonable indulgence should be granted to the caprices of the sick. Secrecy and delicacy should be strictly observed; and the familiar and confidential intercourse to which physicians are admitted, in their professional visits, should be guarded with the most scrupulous fidelity and honor.

Section 3

The obligation of secrecy extends beyond the period of professional services; none of the privacies of the individual or domestic life, no infirmity of disposition or flaw of character observed during medical attendance should ever be divulged by physicians except when imperatively required by the laws of the State. The force of the obligation of secrecy is so great that physicians have been protected in its observance by courts of justice.

Section 4

Frequent visits to the sick are often required, since they enable the physician to arrive at a more perfect knowledge of the disease, and to meet promptly every change which may occur. Unnecessary visits are to be avoided, as they give undue anxiety to the patient; but to secure the patient against irritating suspense and disappointment, the regular and periodical visits of the physician should be made as nearly as possible at the hour when they may be reasonably expected by the patient.

Section 5

Ordinarily the physician should not make gloomy prognostications and should not fail, on proper occasions, to give timely notice of dangerous manifestations to the friends of the patient, and even to the patient, if absolutely necessary. This notice, however, is at times so peculiarly alarming when given by the physician, that its deliverance may often be assigned to another person of perfectly good judgment.

Section 6

The physician should be a minister of hope and comfort to the sick; since life may be lengthened or shortened, not only by the acts, but by the words or manner of the physician, whose solemn duty is to avoid all utterances and actions having a tendency to discourage and depress the patient.

Section 7

The medial attendant ought not to abandon a patient because deemed incurable; for continued attention may be highly useful to the sufferer and comforting to the relatives, even in the last period of the fatal malady, by alleviating pain and by soothing mental anguish.

Section 8

The opportunity which a physician has of promoting and strengthening the good resolutions of patients suffering under the consequences of evil conduct ought never to be neglected. Good counsels, or even remonstrances, will give satisfaction, not offense, if they be tactfully proffered and evince a genuine love of virtue, accompanied by a sincere interest in the welfare of the person to whom they are addressed.

CHAPTER II

THE DUTIES OF PHYSICIANS TO EACH OTHER AND TO THE PROFESSION AT LARGE

Article I. Duties For The Support Of Professional Character

Section 1

It is not inconsistent with the principles of medical science, neither is it incompatible with honorable standing in the profession, for physicians to designate their practice as based on an exclusive dogma, or any sectarian system of medicine; but the practice of an exclusive dogma or sectarian system of medicine furnishes no excuse of any honorable physician in withholding his fellowship or professional counsel from those whose practice is based on another dogma or adheres to a different sectarian system of the healing arts.

It is desirable that each physician should seek to maintain and honor his *alma mater*, and preserve the traditions and historic principles taught by his particular school granting to every other practitioner of the healing art, of whatever school, the same privilege, and for the sake of the growth and betterment of the medical profession as a whole, laying aside all prejudice on account of differences of opinion, associating themselves together in a common desire to heal disease, without any discrimination as to schools or methods.

Section 2

The physician should observe strictly such laws as are instituted for the government of the members of the profession; should honor the fraternity as a body; should endeavor to promote the science and art of *healing* and should entertain a due respect for those seniors who, by their labors, have contributed to their advancement.

Section 3

Every physician should identify himself with the organized body of his profession as represented in the community in which he resides. The organization of local or county (associations) societies where they do not exist should be effected so far as practicable. Such county societies, constituting as they do the chief element of strength in the organization of the profession, should have the active support of their members and should be made instruments for the cultivation of fellowship, for the exchange of professional experience, for the advancement of medical knowledge, for the maintenance of ethical standards, and for the promotion in general of the interests of the profession and the welfare of the public.

Section 4

All county (professional associations) societies thus organized ought to place themselves in affiliation with their respective State associations, and these in turn, with the international Alliance of Physicians and Surgeons.

Section 5

There is no profession from the members of which greater purity of character and a higher standard of moral excellence are required than the medical; and to attain such eminence is a duty every physician owes alike to the profession and to patients. It is due to the patients, as without it their respect and confidence cannot be commanded; and to the profession because no scientific attainments can compensate for the want of correct moral principles.

Section 6

It is incumbent on physicians to be temperate in all things, for the practice of healing requires the unremitting exercise of a clear and vigorous understanding; and in emergencies—for which no physician should be unprepared—a steady hand, an acute eye, and an unclouded mind are essential to the welfare and even to the life of a human being.

Section 7

It is not incompatible with honorable standing in the profession to resort to public advertisement or private cards inviting the attention of persons affected with particular disease, to make reasonable promises as to cures and remedies; to publish cases or operations in the daily prints, or to suffer such publications to be made (always concealing the identity of the patient except by consent of patient); to make truthful statements of cures and remedies; to adduce certificates of skill and success, or to employ any other methods decently and truthfully, and in a gentlemanly manner, to gain the attention of the public. But it is incompatible with honorable standing in the profession to invite anyone to be present at operations, surgical or other wise, other than the relatives or friends who desire to be at hand, or professional brethren in good standing in the profession.

Section 8

It is not derogatory to professional character for physicians to hold patents for any surgical instruments or medicines, or to dispense or promote the use of any medicines, secret or otherwise, provided only the physician's knowledge of the efficiency of such medicine is sufficient to warrant him in recommending their use. It is also perfectly respectable for physicians to adduce certificates attesting to the efficiency of any medicine, secret or otherwise, such certificates representing the exact truth, according to his best judgment. But it is derogatory and reprehensible in any physician to accept rebates on prescriptions, on surgical appliances, or to assist unqualified persons to evade any reasonable restrictions governing the practice of *healing*.

Article II. Professional Services Of Physicians To Each Other

Section 1

Physicians should not, as a general rule, undertake the treatment of themselves, nor of members of their families. In such circumstances they are peculiarly dependent on each other; therefore kind offices and professional aid should always be cheerfully and gratuitously afforded. These visits ought not, however, to be obtrusively made, as they may give rise to embarrassment, or interfere with that free choice on which such confidence depends.

Section 2

All practicing physicians and their immediate family dependents are entitled to the gratuitous services of any one or more of the physicians residing near them.

Section 3

When a physician is summoned from distance to the bedside of a colleague in easy financial circumstances, a compensation, proportionate to traveling expenses and to the pecuniary loss entrained by absence from the accustomed field of professional labor, should be made by the patient or relatives.

Section 4

When more than one physician is attending another, one of the number should take charge of the case, otherwise the concert of thought and action so essential to wise treatment cannot be assured.

Section 5

The affairs of life, the pursuit of health and the various accidents and contingencies to which a physician is peculiarly exposed sometimes requires the temporary withdrawal of this physician from daily professional labor and the appointment of a colleague to act for a specified time. The colleague's compliance is an act of courtesy which should always be performed with the utmost consideration for the interest and character of the family physician.

The physician should be a minister of hope and comfort to the sick; since life may be lengthened or shortened, not only by the acts, but by the words or manner of the physician.

There is no profession from the members of which greater purity of character and a higher standard of moral excellence are required than the medical.

Having been persecuted repeatedly by the Medical Trust of NY, Benedict Lust moved his school of Naturopathy to his Yungborn in Butler, New Jersey, in 1911.

BRIEF 7: NATUROPATHY

DR. CARL STRUEH

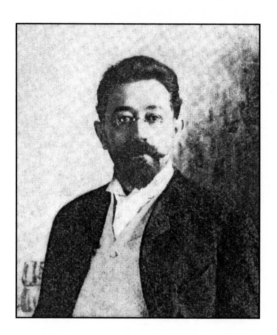

Dr. Carl Strueh.

BRIEF 7

NATUROPATHY

by Dr. Carl Strueh

The Naturopath and Herald of Health, XIX(4), 253-258. (1914)

There are many ways and means of *"treating"* the sick. There is the drug-method (allopathic and homeopathic), the electropathic method, the Christian Science method, the osteopathic method, and so forth. While these methods differ widely in their fundamental principles, all of them—including the numerous "fake cures"—boast of *"results"* which no unbiased observer can rightfully dispute.

We do not consider, however, that these so-called "results," to a great extent, are but accidental and quite independent from the applied treatment. We are too readily inclined to attribute to ourselves what, in reality, must be credited to that mysterious force which exists in every living being which we call the *vital* or *life force*. What this force consists of we do not know, not more than we know the secret of life itself. We only know that it exists and how it manifests itself. It is the driving force which from two minute cells develops a living being, knits together a fractured bone, repairs a lacerated skin, etc., and which also corrects, i.e., cures those numerous abnormal conditions which we call "disease".

The physicians of ancient times were well aware of the part the vital force plays in the cure of disease, and termed it the *vis medicatrix naturae*, i.e., the inborn faculty to cure. The better the physical condition of the patient, i.e., the more vigorous his vitality, the better his chances of recovery. A strong constitution may overcome disease under any sort of treatment, even under a harmful treatment, while a feeble constitution may succumb in spite of the most rational treatment. It, therefore, is unwise to form our conclusions merely from the "results" which often are but a matter of luck on the part of the patient.

It is the principles of the physician's method, which people must strive to understand. Ignorance in this regard may not be of consequence in one case, while in another case it may decide on life and death.

The vigor of the patient's vitality being the deciding factor in the cure of disease, it follows that any kind of treatment having a healthful, invigorating influence, will improve the chances of recovery, while any sort of treatment which is apt to diminish the patient's vitality, will naturally accomplish the contrary. For this reason the superiority of Naturopathy over the drug-method is undisputable.

Drugs are in their place in *incurable* diseases in which the sole purpose of our treatment consists in relieving, not *curing* the patient. It would not be humane to refuse a dose of morphine to a patient suffering from the pangs of cancer, for instance. Also in various unbearable or dangerous symptoms the causes of which we cannot remove speedy enough, the administration of a drug often is necessary.

However, when it comes to *curable* diseases, our policy must be entirely different. "Beware of drugs" should be the battle-cry in our fight against the conquerable diseases. The better chances for a cure, the more essential it is for the patient to abstain from the use of drugs almost all of which are more or less poisonous and injurious. Apart from the disturbance they cause in the digestive organs, they get absorbed into the blood-serum which contains the nourishing elements for the blood-cells, the "carriers of life." If these blood-cells receive a poisoned food, they will be enhanced in their normal function, and this disturbance again will bring on further commotions in the complicated cellular functions of our body.

Thus, a patient who relies upon drugs, will sooner or later have to cope with two or more diseases, instead of one. "Medicine is capital which is constantly increasing." Every honest physician will admit that there is not a single disease which we can cure by means of drugs. The effects of drugs are merely symptomatic, not curative. A person being afflicted with chronic constipation can affect a movement of the bowels by the use of a laxative, but the latter while giving temporary relief, will not cure the weak condition of the intestinal organs which is the cause of constipation. On the contrary, the continued irritation will make the condition worse and, in the course of time, destroy the function of the intestinal organs completely and lead to all kinds of complications.

In a case of insomnia the physician can put the patient to sleep by means of veronal or other dopes, but he cannot cure the insomnia. The longer the patient continues the use of these drugs, the nearer he gets to the mad-house. A person suffering from headaches may relieve the pain by a dose of aspirin, but let him continue this hazardous treatment and he will see where he lands.

And thus it is with all chronic diseases, such as rheumatism, neurasthenia, diabetes, gout, etc., etc. Most of these diseases consist in so-called "auto-intoxication," i.e., retention of toxins (poisons) which are formed in our system and, for one reason or other, are not eliminated.

Instead of suppressing the various symptoms which such a condition produces, we must try to eliminate the auto-toxins, for only by removing the cause can we remove the effects, i.e., the symptoms.

One more word about the drug-method. People not familiar with it imagine that it possesses a high scientific value. It is a mystic to them, and anything mystic is attractive to some people. Actually, the drug-treatment is and always will be a very poor science. What do we know about the action of drugs? That a dose of calomel will affect a movement of the bowels, a dose of sulfonal cause sleep, a dose of bromide relieve a pain, etc? If that is all, it surely is not much.

In the first place, our knowledge of the normal chemical processes going on in our body is as meager as it was at the times of Hippocrates. What we know in this regard is very superficial and of little practical value. Still less we know about the combinations the various drugs undergo after entering our body.

It is a fact that an examination of the eliminations, i.e., the urine, stool, expiration and exhalation, does not reveal their presence. Consequently they must have formed combinations and alterations in the chemism of our body, which escape our knowledge. Without such knowledge, however, it is absolutely impossible to form any conclusions as to the effect upon the body-cells, which these new combinations may produce.

And how about the proper dose? Not more than we know how much alcohol a man can imbibe before he becomes intoxicated, how many cigars a person may smoke before he shows signs of nicotine-poisoning, or how many cups of coffee a woman may drink before she becomes nervous, not more do we know how much strychnine or any other poisonous drug a person can take into his system without being harmed. To wait until so-called toxic symptoms, i.e., symptoms indicating a beginning of poisoning, appear and then reduce the dose or discontinue the drug altogether, is a policy more humoristic than scientific. It reminds of the midwife who when asked how she could tell whether the baby's bathing water was too hot or too cold, replied that if the child after being placed into the bath turned red, the water was too hot, and if it turned blue, the water was too cold.

Prescribing is mere experimenting. Two people may be of the same age, the same weight, the same build, etc., and yet one may show toxic symptoms from a certain drug administered in a certain dose, while the other may not show any visible effect of the drug whatever. An infant may be poisoned by a single drop of opium, which in another baby may not produce the slightest effect.

With such scant knowledge of the action of drugs it certainly is not an unwise policy to keep away from them as far as possible and only use them in case of emergency. Christian Science has done an enormous amount of good by freeing thousands of good people from the bondage of the drug method.

There is no progressive physician who does not share the opinion we expressed and condemn the lamentable practice of seeking salvation from sickness in the use of drugs. The "A teaspoonful every two hours"—method is gradually losing ground and will soon be practiced by unscrupulous and ignorant physicians on ignorant people only. If we would only employ a little more common sense, we would progress much faster than we do.

But whether progress will be fast or slow, the future as regards the treating of the sick, belongs to Naturopathy, i.e., the method manipulating with natural means, such as proper diet, out-door life, proper exercise and rest, hydrotherapy, etc.

A splendid example of the change of tactics which is taking place, is the modern treatment of tuberculosis. Consumptives used to be treated with immense doses of creosote or arsenic, then followed the tuberculin-treatment. And what are we doing to-day? No conscientious physician nowadays will waste time in dosing a patient with drugs or tuberculin, but will send him to one of the open air Sanitaria, where no artificial and mystic treatment, but a simple "natural" method will enable the patient to regain his health, providing his sickness has not progressed too far.

And what is the secret of these wonderful successes? Is there anything extraordinary or specific about the treatment? None whatever. Pure air, proper feeding, etc., are very simple means. Simple, indeed, but mighty powerful and the only means by which we can improve the patient's vital force and thus accomplish a cure. The treatment does not attack the sickness directly, but indirectly by the proper action of each and every part of our complicated physique.

What applies to the treatment of tuberculosis, also applies to the treatment of tuberculosis, also applies to that of other chronic diseases, such as diabetes, neurasthenia, gout, rheumatism, etc. There is no fundamental difference in the treatment of the various diseases. The same simple principle, i.e., to cure by improving the entire cellular action applies to all of them, and the same satisfactory results are the outcome in the majority of cases.

More than with any other treatment, the physician practicing Naturopathy, must be well able to *individualize*, i.e., apply the treatment according to the conditions existing in every individual case. We must not treat sicknesses, but sick people. Because two people are afflicted with the same sickness does not mean that we must apply the same treatment in the same manner and dose.

It is a pity that people in general are not better acquainted with the Naturopathic Method and still allow physicians to treat them with poisonous drugs. There will come a time, no doubt, when a physician practicing the drug-treatment the way it is being practiced to-day, will expose himself to the danger of being prosecuted in the Criminal Court.

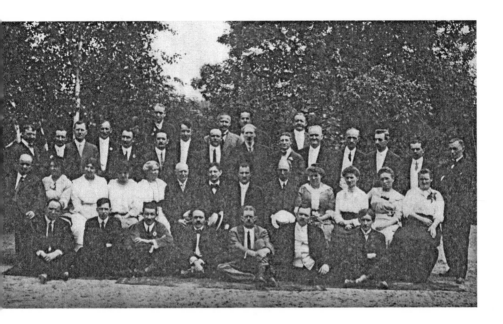

Graduates of 1914 Class of American School of Naturoapthy. The graduation took place on June 14th at the Yungborn Health Resort, Butler, N.J.

Instead of suppressing the various symptoms which . . . a condition produces, we must try to eliminate the auto-toxins, for only by removing the cause can we remove the effects, i.e., the symptoms.

There is no progressive physician who does not share the opinion we expressed and condemn the lamentable practice of seeking salvation from sickness in the use of drugs.

. . . the physician practicing Naturopathy, must be well able to individualize, i.e., apply the treatment according to the conditions existing in every individual case. We must not treat sicknesses, but sick people.

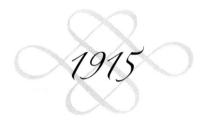

1915

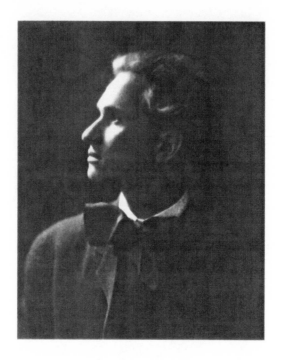

Edward Earle Purinton.

EFFICIENCY IN DRUGLESS HEALING, STANDARDIZING THE NATURE CURE

by Edward Earle Purinton

The Naturopath and Herald of Health, XX(3), 141-147. (1915)

What is Nature Cure? I don't know. Furthermore, I don't know anybody who does know. This fact, strange and unaccountable as it may seem, is easy of explanation, and in turn explains why the Nature Cure has not been legalized in America.

It is no disgrace, even for a drugless physician, not to know what the Nature Cure is. Few preachers know what Christianity is. Few teachers know what Education is. Yet they preach, and they teach, without molestation.

But they do not prescribe dangerous medicines, or give speculative treatments; they do not handle cases of life and death. The harm done by parsons and pedagogues through ignorance or prejudice, while considerable and unwarrantable, is of a mild, negative sort, without being immediately fatal. The harm done by ignorant physicians, whether old-school or new-school is violent, crucial, deadly. Hence the refusal of the Government to legalize the practice of the Nature Cure, prematurely. We already have enough licensed killers, in the ranks of allopathy, homeopathy, pharmacy and surgery.

The great trouble with naturopaths is an excess of emotionalism— they lack the courage or ability to look at cold facts in a cool, impartial, judicially-minded manner. I say this with an unholy joy, remembering how many readers of this magazine charged me, years ago, with being a mere poet. For a poet to be a poet is quite rational—however irrational the poet may seem; but for a doctor to be a poet is irrational, unscientific and unsafe. Most naturists need to take their brains out of cold storage, and to put their hearts in it.

An efficiency engineer is absolutely cold-blooded; thrills and throbs and sighs and sobs are nothing to him; facts are everything. I have been seeking facts; and to do so, have endeavored to place myself in the position of a State legislator, in the process of considering a bill to legalize Christian Science or Mechano-Therapy or Naturopathy. The job of simulation is a hard one—I wouldn't waste my life in a State legislature for a barrel of money, and a bevy of railroads thrown in. But my present, unanimous opinion is that, if I were afflicted with a job in a law-factory, I would positively refuse to sanction all bills to heal by drugless methods which have been drafted thus far. And in addition, I would refuse to look at any such documents in future, unless the framers of them assured me that they contained a rudiment of commonsense!

From a long acquaintance with Dr. Benedict Lust, I consider him one of the bravest men now living. Should he publish this article, I proclaim him the very bravest man now living. For in this article I am gently knocking out the underpinning of the whole Nature Cure propaganda as it now exists. Your tribute to the courage, honestly and sincerity of Doctor Lust might well take the form of complimentary subscriptions to this magazine, mailed at once for the benefit of your most valued clients or personal friends. In these days of policy and greed, the sight of an absolutely fearless man is a vision to enchant the gods.

I can prove my statement that nobody really knows what the Nature Cure is. For purposes of analysis and comparison, I recently obtained the descriptive matter issued by a dozen of the most prominent schools and sanitaria advertised in *The Naturopath, Physical Culture, Health Culture, The Nautilas,* and other advanced publications. The aforesaid literature includes booklets, pamphlets, prospectuses, personal letters, form letters, and all other printed or typewritten matter, aiming to secure customers, patients or students. I now have this collection before me. It is a rare exhibit.

The doctors and professors all agree that Nature Cure is the only cure, but no two of them agree in defining the term and describing the system. To get on the trail of a clear definition, from studying these printmarks, would require the allied services of a Philadelphia lawyer, a pack of old Virginia blood-hounds, a crop of New York detectives, and a posse of Wild West citizens in pursuit of a horse-thief. I give it up, and sadly and wearily hand the problem over to you.

Prior to analyzing the choice bits of literature now in hand, I wish to state a few reasons for obtaining the first-hand statements of the recognized leaders in natural therapeutics. I have been sorely puzzled for years, on many points of doctrine. Here are a few questions I have asked, and never had answered.

1. WHAT IS THE DIFFERENCE, LOGICALLY AND ETIOLOGICALLY, BETWEEN THE herbal remedies of Kneipp and the purely vegetable medicines found in a drug-store? The druggist on the corner, with whom I have had many a friendly argument, says that cascara, belladonna, certain opiates, and in fact scores of the medicines he sells are of strictly vegetable origin. He asks on what ground the Nature Cure apostles forbid the use of these, while prescribing tinctures, powders, and teas? How can such a position be defended? And is it not true that some of the herbal extracts in the apothecary of the German Nature Cure have a more violent effect than many of the milder forms of mineral drugs? Are *any* internal remedies "natural"? If so, which and why?

2. WHAT IS A "NATURAL" DIET? SOME ANIMALS ARE OMNIVOROUS, SOME herbivorous, some carnivorous. To which class do men belong? Birds and fishes have no meal-hours; should we therefore imitate the birds and fishes? Domestic animals, almost without exception, eat a regular breakfast, and vociferate loudly on being deprived or delayed in the matter. Does this invalidate the no-breakfast plan, followed with such good results by thousands of ambitious people, including the writer?

In the advertising pages of a popular magazine, a large and bold announcement of a certain school of diet affirms the everlasting injury of meat-eating; while, if you merely turn to another page, you read that brain-workers *must* eat meat, or become dyspeptic, morose, pimply and dull-minded. What in the name of all that is rational and honest can a layman think of reform diet? I know what he most likely thinks—but the answer is unprintable.

The editor of this magazine believes in sane fasting, in thorough mastication, in wholly natural foods. The editor of another health journal, as widely known as this, maintains we do not eat enough, calls Fletcherism rank folly, and declares white flour bread a much better food than whole wheat! Now where is the truth? Has either editor got it? Or has neither? When a legislator very properly asks us how foods cure, and what system of diet we prescribe for the sick and well, our answer is bedlam;—which induces a corresponding state of feeling in the weak-minded legislator. Foods will cure, safely and pleasantly, most of the aliments for which drugs are now employed unsafely and unpleasantly. But before we ask a State license to prescribe foods, we must present a solid, unimpeachable array of facts; instead of the loose, wild, conflicting theories that we now indulge, and scatter abroad with a rash and senseless virtue. A foolish virtue may be more unhygienic than a shrew vice.

3. DOES NATURE CURE PROPERLY INCLUDE OSTEOPATHY, OR CHIROPRACTIC, or mechano-therapy, or none of these methods, or all of them? The other day I talked with a chiropractor. He is a fine fellow and a remarkably successful practitioner. He was rational and sane upon all themes excepting one; but when I spoke the word "osteopathy," not knowing which form his unsuspected mania took, he immediately became wild-eyed, verbose and ugly, charging over the field of discussion with the recklessness of an escaped lunatic. It developed, after I quieted the unfortunate brother by agreeing with him, that he had formerly been an osteopath, but with his conversion to chiropractic had suddenly developed an unreasoning hatred of the former source of his bread-and-butter.

Marveling at this phenomenon, I sought the opinion of a famous osteopath—a man whose yearly practice yields $15,000 or more— and I asked him an explanation. He smiled a gentle, pitying smile, and he said, "When a man fails at osteopathy, he drifts into chiropractic, as a poor, discouraged medical doctor often drifts into the patent medicine field, or a 'Cure for Men Only'. We consider that the chiropractors owe all their possible cures to the principles of osteopathy, having merely added a sensational twist to their diagnosis and treatment." I wished to verify Brother Osteopath's opinion, therefore called up Brother Chiropractic on the telephone—deeming this a discretionary mode of communication under the circumstances. The reply scorched my ears, and was deafening in its detonations of wrath. "He is a liar, an out-and-out liar, that fool osteopath! Don't we know that the osteopaths took all they know from Bohemia, where chiropractic started years before A.T. Still was ever heard of?" And there you are. An interesting episode, characteristic of the perfect harmony and unity in the drugless ranks.

By a strict logic, there is no place for either osteopathy or chiropractic in the Nature Cure. Both depend upon a stimulation that is artificial, and extra-natural if not unnatural. Personally, I would class them as minor subdivisions of the Nature Cure, to be advised occasionally and employed judicially, but never to constitute a major system of healing. They are not massage, and have little in common with massage; but in relative importance they are little higher than massage considered with regard to healing as a whole. Medical men affirm that the successful osteopath or chiropractor depends really not on manipulation, but rather on suggestion, magnetism, the placebo-principle, and rational advice on bathing, eating, exercising, etc. This is probably true, save in those extreme cases where a pronounced "lesion" or "subluxation" does exist; therefore the osteopath and chiropractor may be voted natural healers in disguise. But I would not venture a final opinion, I would only ask that this point be somehow decided, conclusively and unanimously, by naturopaths in advance of pleading for a State license.

4.   WHAT FORMS OF EXERCISE BELONG IN THE PRACTICE OF NATURISM? ARE special devices needed—or are they unnatural? In studying the life of the "lower" animals, we observe that the muscular vigor of the young is derived largely from play, that of the adults from the daily search for food. Now contrast the involved systems of "physical culture" in vogue among men. Professor Jones invents a weight-lifting harness we must wear religiously, to retain our suppleness and strength; Trainer O'Toole prescribes a famous resort, where athletic stunts on the gymnasium style are all the rage; Doctor Pneumaticus vends a

wonderful breathing machine, into which we must solemnly blow so many breathes a day and Health Specialist Bumpaman superintends a lot of mechanical horses, wigglers and jigglers, that he guarantees will shake our ailments down and out.

We hesitate—not being able to spend all our time and money on gymnastic gyrations. Then comes Mr. Adonis Psychotherapy, declaring that all the foregoing methods are highly dangerous, tending to rupture the heart, the brain or the pocket-book, and the only natural scheme of exercise will be found to be his—without apparatus, but with a $30 fee for the magic lessons. Are we not now tempted to die of paralysis, rather than move a muscle ever again? Seriously, such a condition of things is a menace and a disgrace. If it is true, as I believe, that certain modes of advertised exercises tend to strain the heart; and other devices merely rob you politely; and that other patent schemes neglect the vital organs while demanding unreasonable waste of time and energy on superficial muscles;—then some recognized college, association, clearing-house or other tribunal should separate the good from the bad, affirming which is Nature Cure, and which is not.

5. SHOULD HYPNOTISM, MAGNETISM, OCCULTISM, AND OTHER MORE OR LESS intangible forces be admitted to the realm of Natural Healing? If not, we must avow that the human mind is not a part of Nature. This would be absurd, since even the snake charming the bird is a case of hypnotic influence, and the instinct of self-preservation warning certain animals of the approach of their foes cannot be explained on the ground of merely physical phenomena. Nature is an endless tale of marvels and mysteries; and the mystic element is the most powerful in human life, whether operating through pills of a secret nature or through prayers to an unknown God.

But is the violent imposition of a stronger will upon a weaker mind a natural, wise and ethical procedure? I know of ministers and doctors who state with every sign of omniscience that hypnotism was born of the Devil. And I know of cases where hypnotism has healed not only physical, but mental and moral diseases, that stubbornly resisted all other available modes of treatment. If hypnotism, magnetism and occultism are to be approved, taught and practiced in our Nature Cure sanitaria and schools, they must be confined and regulated with the utmost care and wisdom. Should they be so incorporated? If so, how and by whom and to what extent?

6. SHOULD THE NATURE CURE PLATFORM INCLUDE CHRISTIAN SCIENCE? YOU may smile at this question, but I assure you it is one of the most logi-

cal I ever asked. Anything logical in the vicinity of Christian Science is sadly out of place; but we are all a queer lot, anyhow, and must be prepared for strange happenings. My own firm conviction is that the principles of Christian Science should be taught in every sanitarium; and that the Christian Science mode of "treatment" is as much a part of Nature Cure as is diet, or massage, or hydrotherapy. The Christian Scientist and the Nature Curist will both disagree with me. But the only man everybody agrees with is a dead man; not being exactly dead, I am thankful to be able to stir up healthy opposition.

Christian Science is the gospel of concentration. As such it belongs in every health resort; where the poor inmates are now engaged in moaning over the ailments, comparing their feels-ifs, pitying themselves, and objecting to the food, the climate, the accommodations, the nurses, doctors, remedies, rules, and everything else in sight. The mental atmosphere of the ordinary hospital or sanitarium is a pall on the horizon. Midnight is a flare of luminosity, compared with it. I have often been obliged to urge friends, who were of a delicate nature and sensitive nervous organism, against planning a sojourn at a drugless institution, because I knew the mental, psychic and spiritual influence of the place were as bad as the physical methods were good. Until we can treat the sick minds, hearts and souls of ailing men and women as promptly and effectively as we not treat their bodies, we have no right to ask legal sanction as physicians of Nature.

7. WHAT IS THE NATURAL METHOD OF DIAGNOSIS? ARE THERE INFALLIBLE signs of detecting the presence of disease in the human organism? Do they record themselves in external areas and ordinary functions of the body, or must they be found in the deeper symptomatic states, from the blood-cell and plasmic change to the conditions of thought, emotion and etheric aura? How shall the tests of rational and complete diagnosis be applied? Is the practitioner of any single school of drugless healing adequately trained in the use of all the known tests for locating disease? The importance of such questions is fundamental and universal. Yet they have not received proper attention, so far as I know, in all the history of Nature Cure in America.

Go to any old-school doctor, whether allopath, homeopath, or eclectic, and he will diagnose your case in a definite, regular, unanimous fashion, thoroughly endorsed and solemnly applied by thousands of other old-school doctors. Medical diagnosis includes examinations of the pulse, tongue and temperature, with such local tests as the blood-count, urinalysis, nerve-reaction, minute inspection by the stethoscope, laryngoscope, or other similar device. Whether such methods are scientific, is not for me to say; the point is that every doctor knows what they are, and every doctor thinks he knows why they are.

Now observe the wild and irrational conflict of theory and usage in the drugless realm. No two practitioners follow the same plan of diagnosis; and as treatment depends on diagnosis, naturally no two practitioners prescribe the same schedule of treatment. One diagnoses by the muscles, another by the eye, another by the ligaments, another by the spine, another by the tissue, another by the temperament, another by the adipose, another by the aura, another by the state of mind, another by the intake of food, another by the astral conjunction, another by the hypnotic revelation of subconscious memory. The diagnostic method of A. T. Still, known as osteopathy and that of Professor Freud, known as pschyo-analysis, are utterly variant, if not antagonistic. Yet both may rightly claim a place in the scheme of non-medical practice.

How shall these disagreements be done away? How shall we arrive at a sane, comprehensive, mode of diagnosis that shall be error-proof? My own belief is that no practitioner should be allowed to diagnose the cases he treats; he is, consciously, or unconsciously, both ignorant and prejudiced. The time is coming when all the world's means of diagnosis—fifty or a hundred or a thousand methods—will be combined in one establishment. To this place, invalids will go, for diagnosis and perhaps nothing else. Then they will be sent to individual healers or doctors or teachers or ministers, as the need maybe be, for special prescription, advice and co-operation. We are now so far from this ideal state of things that the osteopath and the psychic are virtual enemies—each with his little grain of diagnostic truth, so proud and self-satisfied that no other grain can find lodgment for all the pride and prejudice that swell the minds of these gentlemen.

The foregoing questions and problems are but a few out of hundreds, propounded to me and by me in the last fifteen years—and thus far void of logical reply or solution.

Therefore I obtained, quite recently, the propaganda literature given out by the leading schools and sanitaria that seemed most influential and most modern. The discoveries here made bear a most interesting relation to the work of standardizing the Nature Cure; as will be shown in the next article of this series.

I would meanwhile suggest this one thought for you to ponder over: *Nothing can be legalized that has not been standardized. Hence the first step for drugless physicians to take is to decide among themselves what the Nature Cure is and what it is not, why it deserves legal recognition, and how its practice should be safely regulated.* To demand the approval of the law-makers at the present time is like summoning a party of dignitaries to a reception in a new house, not yet swept and dusted, furnished and put in order. The action is premature, and has failed simply as all things premature and rash deserve to fail. Our hearts may be of gold, but our heads have been of wood. And a head of wood is no head for a doctor.

P.S. On reading the proofs of the foregoing article, Dr. Benedict Lust informs me that he does not wholly agree with the article, and that he considers a few of the statement rather extreme and unnecessarily harsh. Doctor Lust knows a thousand times more about the Nature Cure than I do, therefore I am inclined to respect his opinion regarding its therapeutic administration. From the efficiency viewpoint I see no reason, however, to withdraw any statement here made.

Doctor Lust further claims that in Germany the Nature Cure has been standardized, the practice regulated, and the general criticism of this article satisfactorily overcome. I would suggest that if Doctor Lust or some other leading Naturopath would answer my questions in detail, the subject would be made clearer to us all. And if I am in the wrong, you will do me a favor by showing me how. Nobody knows very much anyway, and our wisdom lies chiefly in our willingness to learn.

What is the natural method of diagnosis? Are there infallible signs of detecting the presence of disease in the human organism?

No two practitioners follow the same plan of diagnosis; and as treatment depends on diagnosis, naturally no two practitioners prescribe the same schedule of treatment.

Nothing can be legalized that has not been standardized. Hence the first step for drugless physicians to take is to decide among themselves what the Nature Cure is and what it is not, why it deserves legal recognition, and how its practice should be safely regulated.

An Answer To Mr. Purinton's Article In March Naturopath

by Wm. F. Havard, Chicago, IL

The Naturopath and Herald of Health, XX(4), 211-215. (1915)

Before I attempt to answer the questions you ask in *The Naturopath*, let me say a little something for myself. I have studied and practiced Drugless Healing for the past ten years. When I first began I fear I was much like the Osteopath and the Chiropractor of whom you speak. With my one little "system" I believed firmly that I possessed the only key that would unlock the door to health. A short period of practice brought me face to face with the fact that practitioners of numerous other "systems" were achieving as much if not more success than was I. Realizing through many failures that I knew very little in regard to healing in its true sense I devoted my time to the study of all systems in regard to which I could gather any definite data. This included ancient as well as modern methods and my research has brought me to this conclusion:

Underlying all methods of healing there is a vestige of truth (even in Medicine) but that most of them are not basic truths, rather being founded on some particular phase of perversion which is often remote from the fundamental cause. For example in both Osteopathy and Chiropractic there is truth in the assertion that a correction of subluxated vertebrae will tend to restore the part affected to normal function, but the statement that all disease arises from this cause of even that all diseases are accomplished by subluxated vertebrae is absolutely false. Where the subluxation does occur it in itself is an effect produced by a more remote cause. The more I studied the more convinced I became that could I sweep aside all the complexity surrounding these various systems I would discover the simple principles underlying the treatment of perversions. I started on this quest with an absolutely free and unbiased mind. I have tested every subject with what logic and reasoning power I possess and have reached the following conclusions:

Every subject in medical teachings (except in some minor points) is fairly accurate up to the study of therapy. We do not dispute the word of the Anatomist; we can find little fault with the Physiologist or even the Pathologist and the Diagnostician is only limited by his own mental power, but when we come to the Therapist we must admit a decided failure to discover anything approximating accuracy or science. If all the material which is preparatory to therapy should be fairly accurate why should reversion to the shot-gun method be in order when it comes to the point of applying this knowledge? We are forced to admit that granting an accurate diagnosis, failure is due entirely to the misapplication of therapeutic measures.

Let us scan the laws and principles on which drug therapy is based. Drugs are classified according to the action which they have been known to exert by experiment on test cases. We find that drugs are employed mainly to counteract whatever symptoms are manifest—and there's an end to it. Homeopathy does the same thing—applies a remedy to counteract a symptom. Is that healing? If so, then it is scientific because it accomplishes the result it sets out to achieve. If healing is something more than the counteraction of symptoms, then it is not scientific. From the observation of final results we must admit healing is something far beyond the scope of drugs, although their use may be condoned in cases of extreme emergency.

No system of therapy is worthy of recognition, nor is it natural, which endeavors to heal by the counteraction of symptoms. It shows that the knowledge gained through the study of anatomy, physiology, pathology is thrown to the winds and the same principle of therapy is employed as was in vogue before man knew of the circulation of the blood, when disease was considered a devil and nasty mixtures were administered to drive him out of the body. Are their minds not running in the same groove today? Look at the germ theory. And I fail to see wherein their methods are any more refined.

What is disease and what is a symptom?

In the body there are two forces always at work to maintain normality—the negative and the positive. In health they are equal and opposite. Should the one overbalance the other trouble results. In the case of disease it is the negative which becomes the stronger and possibly I should say that the positive becomes the weaker. Physiologically applied this would mean that the balance between absorption and elimination had been destroyed. Elimination falls short with the result that the body accumulates waste products which in time turn to poisons through their decomposition. This is the conception of disease. Symptoms are the manifestations of this condition which are thrown to the surface or brought to the attention of the person afflicted. Symptoms manifest in accordance with the characteristics of the individual and may be of three kinds: Direct, Reflex or Sympathetic.

I have a very well defined idea of what Nature Cure is, but I am uncertain as to how well I can convey the idea in a few words to another mind.

I would define it as "The employment of every method which is in accord with the natural physiological action of the body in order to bring about the complete elimination of disease." It is largely "self cure" because it means the complete regeneration of the body. The body is an automatic machine and without abuse will be equipped to the task of properly carrying on its own functions. The trouble is

that we have too much interference with its action and too much bun-
gling-therapy. The Drugless Physician is just as much of a bungler as the
Medico and had he the same powerful means at this command would do
just as much harm. We are all lacking in commonsense and destroy our
reason by looking for things ultra-scientific. You are all trying to make
Nature Cure and Drugless Therapy as dogmatic a doctrine as legalized
medicine. Instead of fighting for legal recognition to add to the curse
we already have upon us, why not fight to have the whole matter put
upon an individual basis. Let whoever takes upon himself the responsibility of treating the sick be held responsible for the harm he does and
for all damage occurring through his neglect. You would soon find half
the Medical profession in jail or engaged in some more useful work.
Legalizing a profession shifts nine-tenths of the responsibility upon the
State and absolves the individual from risk. The Physician feels at liberty
to experiment upon his patients knowing that even in the event of the
patient's death he will not be held in slightest degree responsible.

Traffic in poisons should be placed absolutely in the hands of competent State or Government officers, and not even the medical profession
should be permitted to deal in them. No State has a right to favor private
colleges or other institutions. A college degree should not be required of
an individual who desires to practice Law, Medicine or any other profession. An individual's knowledge and ability should be respected irrespective of where it was obtained.

Examinations should be for the purpose of determining the appli-
cant's ability irrespective of the methods he uses rather than to determine
how much theory he has crammed in his cranium. He should be obliged
to diagnose and treat actual cases, using his own judgment as to materials,
methods and measures and his fitness should be determined by the results
he produces. Physicians should be graded and be compelled to exhibit
their grade upon their signs and cards. They would read somewhat like
this: Albert Underwood, Physician's Apprentice—or John White, Practical
Physician—or J.D. Smith, Master Therapist. Once a physician was admitted to practice as an apprentice under a master or a practical physician he
could from time to time present evidence of his progress and upon receiving a certain number of credits be advanced a grade. In this way all physicians would be classified according to their relative ability and each would
take upon himself the responsibility for his own acts. Of course incompe-
tent physicians are in the majority and this is the last state of affairs they
would desire to see. The medical profession should remember when it
wages war upon the drugless profession calling its members quacks and
incompetents, that there are more such in its own ranks than ever existed
outside of the practice of medicine! States should give the individual who
honestly desires to enter a profession, a fair chance to prove his ability.

I'm down on favoritism of any description. It is ridiculous and beneath the dignity of any State to stoop to it. I do not favor legalizing any system —drug or drugless.

Now let us return to the questions.

The Principle of Nature Cure is to increase the patient's power of resistance, increase elimination by opening up all channels designed to carry off waste products, increase oxygenation and the circulation of the blood, prescribe mainly eliminating foods and give the body its required rest.

You may say that this is general, vague and indefinite. We are led to error when we begin to particularize. One person can do no more than lay down the law and cite the principle for another. The individual must use his own intelligence in selection—and that is where the trouble starts. With the development of intellect and reason we have lost the keen instinct of the animal which leads him unerringly to select that which is in harmony with his being. However, had we our reasoning faculties developed to a high degree we would be able to guide our own affairs without the help of others. An ancient prayer in the Avesta says, in part, "May I conduct my life in such a way that the knife need never be resorted to and herbal medicines never need to touch my lips." They felt that the whole doctrine of healing was wrong or unnatural even in those days because disease was considered a sin and the diseased a sinner. The only means which they considered natural means of healing were fasting and exercise.

However, we make a grave mistake in looking for doctrines, for remember they are only opinions and interpretations of laws. Systems and doctrines have sprung up in answer to a demand and every race and nation have evolved that system which has proven to be the most effective in meeting the demands of the times. Wrong is the only right transposed or out of place. The reason we in this country are in such a state of confusion is because we have had imposed upon us the ideas and systems of numerous other nations and races which are out of place in this environment. We have not yet effected a compromise with the foreign element. The world of theory and principle is simple, but the world of application and action is complex and admits of many variations. It is said that circumstances alter cases—they do not change the law or the principle, they merely require a different application of it. I know you desire something hard and fast to pin your faith to and you may think that I am writing at random, but to answer you correctly and fully would require the writing of an extremely lengthy volume and all I am trying to do in this article is to give you a viewpoint.

What you particularly desire to know is what forms of treatment dare one person prescribe for or administer to another and remain within the sphere of truth when he terms it "natural." Omar Khayyam said, "A hair divides the false from true," so the individual must remain the judge of his own actions. This will remain a matter of individual concept, of individual opinion and will distinguish the Good Nature Curist from the Better.

But let me, nevertheless, give you some of my "opinions" since you have asked for them. All measures are arbitrary—you know that. No one but God Almighty can give you an absolute measuring stick, so you must consider me quite arbitrary.

Some internal remedies are just as natural as food. Food is divided into two general classes, Food proper—such substances as are designed for tissue building and heat production, and Eliminators or those substances which assist the natural action of the body in removal of waste products. Herbal remedies come under the classification of eliminators. They must be of vegetable substance in order to obey the laws of evolution. They must not be poisonous, nor must they act contrary to the normal physiological functions of the body. It is impossible to enumerate all these herbs and barks, but such as sage, jaborandi, buckthorn, chestnut leaves, sassafras, vanilla, gravel root, parsley, mint, dandelion, rhubarb and mustard are effective and natural. They are better in their natural state than made into tinctures. Extracts, active principles, etc., should be prohibited by Naturopaths.

I. In regard to what I consider a Natural Diet I am sending you a little by-me-written pamphlet in which I have endeavored to answer this question.

II. All forms of Mechanical and Manual Therapy belong to Nature Cure. As they are administered by the ordinary Osteopath and Chiropractor, however, I should hardly call the majority of such natural. Mechanical Therapy can be divided into three classifications:

  1. Those methods which aim to restore a balance to the nervous mechanisms controlling the circulation and the action of the viscera, this being accomplished by certain treatment to the nerve centres, controlling their action within physiological limits;

  2. Those methods which are employed for the correction of displaced vertebrae;

  3. Those methods commonly called massage which assist the circulation of the blood and lymph, thus relieving congested and infiltrated areas.

All cases do not need mechanical treatment, but it is one of the Naturopaths' most valuable measures in cases where indicated.

III. Exercise. From the standpoint of principle, special systems and special apparatus are necessary in Nature Cure. Breathing, stretching, movements and positions to counteract tension and restore suppleness is all that should be necessary. One can build strong healthy muscles without indulging in violent exercise. The athlete who overstrains inhibits brain development and lays the foundation for organic diseases. Athletes succumb quickly to pneumonia, Bright's disease, tuberculosis and intestinal disorders.

IV. Mental Therapy is decidedly in the scope of the Nature Cure. Disease can have either a mental origin with physical reflex, or a physical origin with mental reflex. It is the seat of the disease to which our treatment must be directed so diseases of mental origin must have mental treatment and in fact every mental reflex should receive attention.

However, I should place hypnotism in the same class with drugs and other methods which are not strictly Physiological, and not include it among Natural Therapies. I consider it exactly as I do an opiate—something which robs an individual of his will power and destroys his individuality.

V. Of course include Christian Science. It has its good points as have all other systems. By all means incorporate it in Nature Cure. Nature Cure is already too positive, so throw in the negative.

VII. Natural Diagnosis should incorporate every method which will assist the Naturopath in determining the exact condition of the patient. Do not try too hard to narrow yourself down to fine points—take it all.

I would define Nature Cure as "The employment of every method which is in accord with the natural physiological action of the body in order to bring about the complete elimination of disease."

The Principle of Nature Cure is to increase the patient's power of resistance, increase elimination by opening up all channels designed to carry off waste products, increase oxygenation and the circulation of the blood, prescribe mainly eliminating foods and give the body its required rest.

Eclecticism In Drugless Healing

by Wm. F. Havard

The Naturopath and Herald of Health, (1915), XX(4), 253-254

Eclecticism in Drugless Healing is not an amalgamation; it is not a mixture. It is more like a chemical combination (soluble and easy to take).

There is only one science of healing; there can be no more. There are, however, many forms of Therapy (and Pseudo-therapy). Eclecticism will tend to bring them all back to basic principles.

With the invention of one system of healing after another and the conflict of opinions and ideas attendant thereto the fundamental principles have been lost to view. Eclecticism will tend toward the restoration of Principle. It wages no war against any system of Natural Therapy, but rather takes from each system that which conforms to principle and law, discarding the superfluous and the unnecessary. Its object is to create order from out of the confusion of battle, to dethrone the complex and crown the simple.

The field of healing is one of chaos. Chaos preceded order. Order must precede sane thinking. Sanity is a gift of God. God has no use for dogmatic creeds and doctrines. God is law and principle. Creeds are ideas and opinions. Ideas and opinions are variable.

As the body follows laws of operation in health and as disease is caused by the reaction of these laws, so there must be some law and principle to guide the healing of disease. The principles of healing are extremely simple when stripped of all the superfluous material and the complexities of detail which have accumulated around them. The application of these principles is an individual one. And this is the rock on which all the systems ever invented have been wrecked. The fact that no two individuals are alike in all respects has been overlooked in the construction of "systems." The personal equation has been neglected. The system which does not first of all diagnose the individual under consideration is doomed to failure. They may all have their good points in treatment, but without the proper basis of operation they will not stand the test of universal application. "Good treatment" may prove ineffectual through wrong application.

To be a physician requires the mind of both a philosopher and a scientist. It requires the philosopher to know the law and to understand human nature and the scientists to make exact application of the one to the other. Medicine has always treated the disease, never the patient. Its rules consist in prescribing a remedy for a given symptom or set of symptoms.

The Laws of Healing deal first with the individual and secondly with the disease. Eclecticism builds its structure upon basic principles and fundamental laws. It is not an invention; it is not a discovery; it is not a "system." It is broadmindedness, liberality of thought, it spells unlimited application of the means and materials at hand. It lifts the lid—removes the limitation which systems have placed upon healing. It is not necessary for us to invent any new means of healing; goodness knows we have enough. We do not lack knowledge but the ability to apply it.

Eclecticism teaches us to know all and to use judgment and reason in selecting that which will be most effective in producing the best results in any individual case. It is not a special system; it is not a dogma. It teaches everything pertaining to Art and Science in healing, leaving the selection and the application to the judgment of the physician.

Principles are simple; the laws of application are complex. As no two individuals are alike, so no two cases can be identical. As the master builder selects his materials with thought and care so the master physician must select his materials to fit the case. A little knowledge is a dangerous thing, but false knowledge is criminal. The practitioner of any special system is limited by the dogmatic doctrine to which he adheres. The narrowness of his views prevents those entrusted to his care from profiting by whatever else might prove beneficial to them. Give any of these systems (and this includes Medicine) the sanction of the State, give their practitioners license and you place a block before the wheels of progress.

The Medical Trust is blockading Therapeutic Progress. But the cart of "Progress" is drawn by sturdy steeds and sooner or later the mangled form of "Medicine" will be ground into the dust of the past. The Medical Trust will continue to hold sway as long as Drugless Systems quarrel among themselves. United they would sweep everything before them. There are numerous Drugless Societies in the country; why does not someone try to unite all these Societies of Drugless Practitioners instead of forming new societies?

Drugless Physicians, you must become Eclectic in thought at least; broaden out; acknowledge the good in one another's methods and forget the bad. Let the people see that we are sincere in our attempt to displace the old worn out "Practice of Medicine" by something infinitely better "Healing."

The Medical Profession is giving up its whiskers. It's about time it gave up the ghost! Make way! Make way! Make way!

THE EDITOR AGAIN DIFFERS WITH MR. PURINTON

by Benedict Lust

The Naturopath and Herald of Health, XX(9), 538. (1915)

AN OPEN LETTER FROM BENEDICT LUST AND A REPLY THERETO

Mr. Edward Earle Purinton
July 22, 1915
Woolworth Bldg., New York City

Dear Mr. Purinton:

In reading the proofs of the August editorial, I have come to the conclusion that deserves a rectification from the editor. What you say about medicine and Nature Cure, may fit in with your conception of things, but not in mine.

In the first place when you were sick you did not have the Nature Cure facilities, you did not have a Nature Cure doctor or a Nature Cure institution to treat you. Your condition was such that you considered it best under the circumstances to go to a hospital under a medical doctor. On this point I cannot agree with you. Nature Cure is better than medicine in all cases and in every condition. I have had experience in treating sick people for over 20 years, and I know what I am talking about. The Nature Cure is applicable in more than a thousand ways. You have not yet the inside consciousness and are not familiar with the therapeutic possibilities of drugless methods, therefore you are no judge to give a final comparison of the two symptoms, Naturopathic and Medical.

You also accuse the drugless doctors of lack of intelligence and knowledge. You have not met all the drugless doctors, and you seem to form your opinion from what you have seen around New York. This is not sufficient. The fact is that drugless physicians are of a higher intelligence than medical doctors, a good many have studied medicine and got disgusted with it and dropped out, because their intelligence told them what is right and what is wrong between the truth and the untruth, and so they turned away from the medical school.

At several conventions, banquets and meetings recently, regular medical doctors were present, amongst them Naturopaths, and everyone of these doctors spoke about how long they were deceived and how long they were rooted in the system of medicine, and that they now have come to the conclusion that it is all wrong, that the Nature Cure is better in all cases and all conditions.

A Naturopath, very often a layman, has shown high intuitive understanding and reasoning power in adopting drugless methods instead of medicine on account of the advantages of Nature Cure.

Let me say also that if you had lived up to the Nature Cure principles, you would not have had so unnatural a trouble as appendicitis, and your statement about your hospital experience and surgical operation will discredit you as a Nature Cure writer. People always look for perfect health and strength in a writer on hygiene and therapeutics, and I am sorry you exposed yourself to the charge of weakness, by referring to your time in a hospital.

I can say conclusively that most people think you are a very good writer, but it is to be regretted that you are not a Naturopath. Dr. Carl Schultz, Dr. Lindlahr, Dr. Strueh, and others have expressed themselves in recent letters to me that in your efficiency articles you are not bringing out strongly enough the Naturopathic Physician's superior methods, intuitive powers, unselfishness and love for the sick. Tell me one doctor who does what a Naturopath does.

I hope that this lengthy letter will not in any way interfere with your vacation thoughts. I know you like to relax, but it is better not to cut loose from the world altogether. With kind regards, I am,

Sincerely yours,
B. LUST

The Nature Cure is applicable in more than a thousand ways. You have not yet the inside consciousness and are not familiar with the therapeutic possibilities of drugless methods, therefore you are no judge to give a final comparison of the two symptoms, Naturopathic and Medical.

1916

DRUGLESS HEALING
E. HOWARD TUNISON

The *Herald of Health and Naturopath* provided drugless practitioners a voice.

DRUGLESS HEALING

by E. Howard Tunison

Herald of Health and Naturopath, XXI(9), 371-374. (1916)

> *With Malice Towards None, with Charity for All.*
> —Lincoln

Blood-letting, or the periodic drawing of blood by cutting veins, a barbarism which in the early part of the last century was thought absolutely necessary for the maintenance and mending of health, has had its day. Dosing with calomel, a form of mercury, for all ailments, until patients' mouths became badly inflamed, an abuse which will make many people invalids by converting them into human barometers, sensitive to every slight weather change, is a memory of the past. Prescribing of alcoholics, whiskey and brandy, as medicines, as tonics par excellence, is a back number. Recommending of nauseous cod-liver oil as a matchless strength-builder has wellnigh ceased. These, as well as other silly and harmful old-time medical practices have been discarded and forgotten with the advent of a new century.

Many cherished medical notions and customs which are now in vogue will ultimately be classed as regrettable acts of malpractice. Rigid sanitation—enforcement of sane measures for the protection of the public's health, as clean living-quarters, clean surroundings, uncontaminated air, filtered water, and unadulterated, unrefined food, etc.—and strict personal hygiene—living close in harmony with and according to Nature's laws—will eventually reign.

In matters of medical concern the American public is beginning to think for itself. Drug remedies already are rapidly disappearing from the family medicine chests of intelligent folks. Continuous agitation by health reformers is gradually awakening people to the realization of "a better way."

A clerk, momentarily tiring of conventional chop-house fare, one day, about ten years ago, ate in a vegetarian restaurant. Its spotless linen, clean food, and abundant variety of seasonable, well-prepared non-meat dishes won his favor. The new patron, during his remaining business stay in that vicinity, continued to lunch there. In a short time his health had vastly improved. An aggravated case of chronic hives, which, because of intolerable itching, had long been a source of annoyance to him, vanished. He developed consequently an intense desire to learn something more definite about fleshless eating. So, buying a number of books, magazines, and pamphlets on the diet question, he read and re-read them until he felt he had absorbed their contents. Then, searching still further, he uncovered information and secured knowledge about other health agencies as fresh air, sunshine, water, exercise, and mind power. Thus one individual introduced himself to the fascinating study of Drugless Healing. Countless other individuals, a few through similar, but many through dissimilar, channels of experience, have developed and retained deep interest in the same study.

Drugless Healing or simply, healing without having recourse to drugs, means the same as Natural Hygeine, its scientific name; Nature Cure, its common name; and Naturopathy, its official and popular name. A Drugless Healer, then, whether he practices one branch, several branches, or all branches of the Drugless Healing System, is either partly or wholly a Naturopath.

Qualified Naturopaths, however, do not place exclusive reliance upon any one natural healing branch. They are eclectic (liberal and selective) in their choice of drugless methods of treatment. They use, in many different ways, all of Nature's common and accessible forces—air, light, water, food, motion, and mind.

Naturopaths claim that drugs, serums, and non-"first aid" surgery are not essential to the successful combating of either acute (short) or chronic (prolonged) illnesses.

From the Naturopathic standpoint, let us now consider two questions:

First, "What is Disease?"

The answer is; "Disease is an unclean and, nearly always, abnormal state of the blood-stream. Impure blood is caused by the gradual accumulation and continuous retention of body-waste or cell-refuse, and the steady absorption into the blood-stream of poisonous, putrid food products from the body's large bowel-sewer-pipe. Abnormal blood, as here meant, is blood which is wanting in certain vital tissue salts or cell-renewing substances." Read it again.

Second, "What will 'cure' Disease?"

The reply is "Disease can be 'cured'—or, better yet, 'good health can be restored'—by eliminating or getting rid-of blood waste material; by improving assimilation (power to use nutriment); and by supplying natural, wholesome nourishment (food) in proper amounts and in suitable combinations."

Thus, Disease in a bad blood condition co-existent with and inseparable from utter lack of hygiene—observance of "back to Nature" living habits.

Remove "the cause" of disease by establishing careful attention to hygiene, and Nature will do the "curing".

Satisfactory elimination—through disposal of waste or refuse—can be brought about only by natural means: not by saturating or inoculating the human system with additional foreign material in the form of drugs, etc. Complete cleansing of the human "river of life" is absolutely dependent upon the normal and harmonious working of the eliminative organs—the lungs, skin, kidneys, bowel (sewer-pipe), and liver; the detoxicating (rendering harmless) action of the ductless glands—small structures, without ducts or tubes to lead off their secretions, which are located in several parts of the body (for example, the thyroid gland, which lies in the lower forepart of one's neck); and the unending toil of the body's tiny, wandering white cells—phagocytes (eating-cells) or blood "street-cleaners".

A well-circulated supply of pure blood, and an undiminished flow of nervous energy to every remote body section constitutes health.

Nature Cure advocates admit the existence of germ life, but, unlike their worthy opponents, Doctors of Medicine, do not consider them to be "microscopic mad dogs" bent upon "snapping" at healthy and unhealthy beings alike. In the estimation of Natural Hygienists: bacteria are small friends in disguise; agents for good; in reality, small scavengers, place by Mother Nature on earth to remove dead animal and vegetable matter, by changing it "back to dust".

Any animal or human being that dies out in the heart of Nature, as in a deep forest or on a plain, if it remains unburied, is effectively removed by wolves (scavenger animals) or vultures (scavenger birds). The clean-picked bones mould, or bleach, crumble, and go back to Mother Earth.

Bacteria, then, are solely "the result," and not, as they are held to be, "the cause" of disease.

To illustrate the Naturopathic removal of "the cause": The backyard of a city dwelling is paved over with cement. In time dust, then dirt, and finally soil gathers in its fence corners, provided the janitor is lazy. Seeds finally blow onto the accumulated soil. The seeds are rained upon, sprout, take root, and grow into weeds. The problem confronting us is, "How shall we remove the weeds?" Shall we pull them up, roots and all? No! there is a better way. Get a spade and broom. Dig out the soil, and the weeds along with it, and throw them both into an ash-can. Then sweep the corners until they are fully clean. Thereafter keep the corners swept, and no more weeds can grow in them. So simple! Is it not?

Drugless Healers, like diligent janitors, believe in keeping all (body) "fence corners" clean. When germ "seeds" alight upon blood "soil" and sprout into disease "weeds," they apply their therapeutic (curative) "spade and broom"—methods of the Drugless Healing System—and clean out the body "fence corners"—the entire human body. Clean "body corners," in the opinion of Naturopaths, are the only sure health basis. If a patient after once having had his "body corners" well cleaned for him by a Naturopath, will keep them "well-swept" by continuing to live correctly, there will be no need for him to fear germ "seeds" sprouting into disease "weeds".

An unhealthy mortal, one who in the accepted sense cannot be considered "sick," but who is on the verge of being "sick," has a blood-stream which is very much befouled with waste or "garbage". Unless he cleanses his blood-stream by natural means, germs in time will "wade in" and dispose of its refuse for him. Then, during the sojourn of these human "cesspool renovators" he will be "laid up for repairs," or actually be "sick" until the overhauling has been finished. His sickness will derive its name either from the type of "renovator" that "lands the contract," or from the "site" (particular body organ) where the "cesspool work" is localized. If his blood should be too morbid, or if his body has become an almost useless mass of material, the mortal will not recover from the ordeal.

Here is a brief outline of the Drugless Healing System:

AIR

Ventilation
Heating and Humidity (moisture)
Deep Breathing
Air Baths

LIGHT

Sun Baths
Focused Sun Rays (through a lens), used as cautery or local stimulant

WATER

Water Drinking
Water Applications
Steam Applications
Wet Earth (mud) Applications
Bowel Flushing

FOOD

Fleshless Diets
Food Combinations
Milk Diet
Fletcherism (correct mastication)
Fasting

MOTION

Outdoor Labor (gardening, wood-chopping, etc.)
Physical Culture (gymnastics)

Sports (running, swimming, etc.)
Swedish Movements and Massage
Mechanical Vibration
Osteopathic and Chiropractic
Rest and Relaxation

MIND

Sleep
Suggestion

Each of the six main headings just tabulated could be used as a separate topic upon which to write and interesting and a detailed discussion. The subdivisions under the main headings could be further and more specifically divided, but economy of space prevents. However, one example of continued subdivision will be given:

FOOD

Fleshless Diets
Vegetarianism (use of vegetables, cereals, milk, cheese, and eggs)
Uncooked Food (use of salads, fruits, nuts, milk, and cheese)

Cooked Food
Its Preparation
Use of Low, Slow Heat in Cooking
Saving of Vegetable "Waters" (Casserole cooking)
Use of Vegetable Waters (as soups)

Fruitarianism (use of fresh and dried fruits, nuts, and milk)

Food Combinations
Action Upon the Blood of Acid-forming and Base-forming Foods
Action in the Stomach and Intestines of Improperly Mixed Sugar, Starchy, and Acid—or Sour-tasting Foods

Milk Diet—the exclusive use of milk, in large quantities, during periods varying from one week to a month.

Fletcherism—chewing food until its taste disappears and it virtually "swallows by itself"

Fasting—abstinence from food, with the allowance of water: a measure which gives the eliminative organs a chance to work without hindrance.

Qualified Naturopaths, however, do not place exclusive reliance upon any one natural healing branch. They are eclectic (liberal and selective) in their choice of drugless methods of treatment. They use, in many different ways, all of Nature's common and accessible forces—air, light, water, food, motion, and mind.

Remove "the cause" of disease by establishing careful attention to hygiene, and Nature will do the "curing".

1917

The Poison Of Lake Erie Water
Ferdinand Muckley, N.D.

Disease, A Transimission Of Morbid Matter
Louis Kuhne

Cold Hand And Feet, Hot Head: Their Cause And Cure
Louis Kuhne

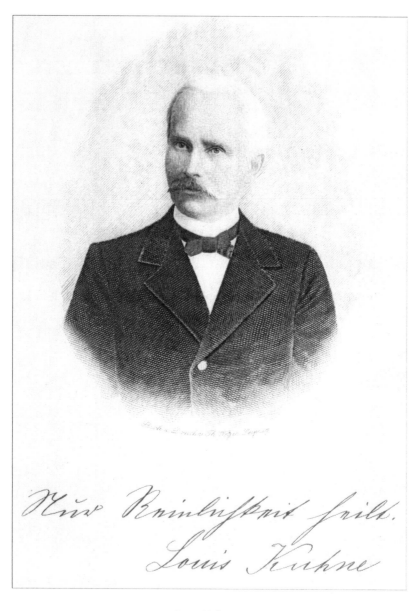

Louis Kuhne.

THE POISON OF LAKE ERIE WATER

by Ferdinand Muckley, N.D.

Herald of Health and Naturopath, XXII(6), 335. (1917)

The south shore of Lake Erie consists of immense deposits of shale, disposed in horizontal layers, which are heavily charged with deleterious chemical substances that are being continually dissolved by the water of the lake, so as to practically poison same. The water in consequence is so harmful to life that even the fish migrate to the Canadian shore during the summer months to escape death.

In spring, when the ice breaks up on the lake, the stench from the mushy ice is almost unbearable. The waterworks in the different cities along the south shore are doing the best they can to purify the lake water, and by the use of alum, chlorine, and other poisonous chemicals, they manage to prevent typhoid and other malignant disease which afflict the public.

Such chemicals unfortunately add to the virulence of the lake water, with the consequence that those who use such water suffer from a catarrhal condition of the mucous membrane. In men, acute and chronic stomach and bowel troubles prevail, while in women, goiter and other throat gland troubles predominate, even girls of ten being subject to these afflictions.

The native Indians refused to drink the lake water, and depended on rain water for their needs. The Moravian and other Pennsylvania Dutch pioneers also depended on their cisterns, as did also the Connecticut Yankees that settled the Western Reserve, and many of their descendants use only rain water until this day.

While the upper strata to a depth of 125 feet contains these poisonous minerals, in the deeper strata, a thousand feet below, a wise Providence has deposited the very antidote for the superficial poisons. From this artesian source, in God's own laboratory, comes the Water of New Life that is such a powerful remedy in all blood diseases.

The stomach and bowel troubles that affect the male residents of the Lake Erie region are so severe that every tenth individual dies from cancer of the stomach, bowels, or rectum.

The prevalence of goiter among females is very marked and spreads so severely that every fifth female is afflicted with this throat affliction, which later spreads over the rest of the gland system, then to the ovaries, and after years of suffering, a useless operation is performed which consequently ends in cancer.

In all cases, it is absolutely necessary to obtain rain water exclusively for drinking and cooking. Olive oil is necessary for soothing and healing the corroded surfaces of the mucous membranes. The diet should be bland and non-stimulating. Fried food should be tabooed, also pork, and onions and tomatoes, which only add to the irritation of stomach and liver.

To remove goiter, we advise a pack, steeped in a strong solution of borax, around the throat the first night. On the second night, use a plain Norwegian oil bandage. For the third night, the pack is steeped in A.N.V., "the Water of New Life." On the fourth night, rest. Always cover the pack with oiled silk and pack cold wet towels over that. If the throat is sprayed night and morning with A.N.V. solution, recovery is hastened. Three months of faithful treatment as suggested will, as a rule, remove goiter.

DISEASE, A TRANSMISSION OF MORBID MATTER
(The New Science of Healing*)

by Louis Kuhne
Herald of Health and Naturopath, XXII(6), 337-342. (1917)

Excerpts from the *Universal Naturopathic Directory, Drugless Year Book and Buyers' Guide*; published by Dr. B. Lust, 110 East 41ˢᵗ Street, New York City. Vol. I., 1918 Edition.

In all these forms of disease, we always observe one of two things: either increased warmth (heat), or increased chill (cold). Both of these symptoms, as we have seen, are fever, whence it follows that they are both cured by the same treatment, a fact which I have proved in thousands of cases. All forms of disease are to be traced back to encumbrance of the system with foreign matter; or in other words: There is only one disease, appearing in the most various forms; and therefore—as regards essentials—only one method of treatment is necessary. All the various forms of disease are, as we have seen, only efforts of the body to recover health. They must not, therefore, be suppressed and rendered latent, as the orthodox medical school teaches, but the body must be assisted to effect these curative crises as quickly as possible, in the least dangerous manner. Only in this way can the body really recover. Disease if repressed or rendered latent, leads slowly but surely to severe and wholly incurable conditions of health. For the morbid matter in such a case, does not remain inactive in the body, but is subjected to continual changes and transformations.

One word now, concerning the diet in all cases of disease. This must be such that no new foreign matter is introduced into the system and the fermentation thus increased. As vigorous action is going on in the body, it should be burdened with as little additional work in digesting as possible. The first point, therefore, is: Give the patient but little nourishment, and never urge him to take food and drink when he does not call for such.

And here I desire to add a few remarks concerning the danger of contagion by the sick.

No acute disease (fever) whatever is imaginable, which has not been preceded by a chronic stage, consisting in the encumbrance of the system with foreign matter. For this reason the chronic condition is the most

---

* Louis Kuhne first wrote his book, *The New Science of Healing*, in Germany in 1892, which was then published in English in 1899 as *The New Science of Healing*, (The International News Co., New York). Then in 1917, Benedict Lust translated and published Kuhne's books as *Neo-Naturopathy, The New Science of Healing*, (Benedict Lust Publishing, Butler, New Jersey).

dangerous. True, a transmission of this morbid condition takes place only from parents to children; but it occurs in every case where the parents are encumbered with morbid matter, and is therefore a sure way of such matter being propagated. When we see how children inherit the outward bodily form, the color of the eyes, even the mental characteristics of their parents, it is easy to conceive that foreign matter, too, is transmitted, especially from the mother. The direct proof is found in the fact, that the same forms of disease usually show themselves in the children as in the parents.

Infection has hitherto only been supposed to take place in the case of acute diseases; but as I have shown, the transmission of foreign matter from parents to children is nothing else than a transmission of the disease, that is infection. The transference of this foreign matter, signifies the transference of the cause of the acute illness. As I have already stated, disease of children are only to be explained by assuming the inherited encumbrance of morbid matter.

The question may be asked whether acute diseases can be transmitted, and it may be answered both with "yes" and "no". Perfectly healthy persons—persons whose bodies are free from foreign matter—cannot catch an illness by contagion, even were they to swallow or inhale any number of bacilli, bacteria or microbes. In the case of persons whose systems are encumbered with morbid matter, however, such products of fermentation can act as the exciting cause to fermentation, especially if the temperature favors this. If there is only little encumbrance, there is little danger of infection.

In the course of acute disease, foreign matter is continually fermenting and being expelled by the system. This is especially the case while the patient is recovering, i.e. when he is expelling the morbid matter by secretion. Hence the danger of infection is greatest from convalescents. How the infection itself is brought about, I will try to explain clearly by a familiar illustration.

If we set an easily fermenting substance in fermentation, like yeast or leaven, and add it in this state to any other readily fermenting substance, as dough, milk, etc., everyone knows that fermentation will also quickly begin in the latter, if warm enough. Thus, the yeast, itself a product of fermentation, produces again a state of fermentation when added to dough or milk. We say the bread rises, or the milk curdles. In acute diseases the process is similar. The fermenting foreign matter passes into the air from the breath or exudations of the sick person, or from the stool. Should it now enter into the body of some other individual encumbered with foreign matter, and be retained there, that is, not be immediately secreted, it works upon the foreign matter already present, exactly like the yeast in the dough or leaven in the milk, i.e. as a ferment. Thus there arises in the second body, the same fermentation, and therefore, the same disease, as in the first. This whole process of infection is, properly speaking, nothing but an inoculation of the fermenting morbid matter into the body of another person in natural dilution. Such matter can, however, only work as a ferment when it finds sufficient foreign matter in a latent state in some other person. Only those are in danger of infection from an acute disease, whose systems are already sufficiently encumbered with foreign matter; or, as commonly expressed, who are predisposed to such disease. Up till now it has not been known where this predisposition consists. The difference in operation between this natural inoculation of morbid matter, and the unnatural process of inoculating it by vaccination with the lancet, lies in the difference in the inoculated matter and in its dilution. Homeopathy teaches that all substance are most effective in a state of dilution, for which reason the fermenting morbid matter is so highly efficacious in its natural dilution, when it finds a suitable soil. In allopathic doses the vaccine virus, like all allopathic remedies, has a paralyzing effect on vital power; that is, it deprives the body of the vigor which it needs to throw off the foreign matter in it by acute disease (curative crisis, fever). It increases, also, the quantity of the morbid matter and thus produces a far more chronic state, as clearly proved by the steady increase of all chronic diseases since the introduction of vaccination. All the other remedies against fever, such as quinine, antipyrin, antifebrin, morphia, etc., have the same effect. They simply paralyze the efforts of the system to regain health, and reduce, or even stop, the fermentation of the foreign matter, but never eject it. Hence arise the diseases which were formerly rare, as cancer, intense nervousness, insanity, paralysis, syphilis, consumption, scrofula, etc. The system becomes more and more encumbered with foreign matter, but is without ability to summon up strength to throw it off by some acute curative crisis. The encumbrance reaches its highest limit in the above diseases, and full relief is then usually no longer possible. Precisely those medicaments which possess the property of most speedily suppressing fever, as quinine, antifebrin, antipyrin, phenacetin, etc., have become the favorite remedies of the physicians against fever. It is our firm conviction that such are precisely the most dangerous means of injuring the health.

We have all had experience how medical science daily seeks for new remedies to apply, because the old are no longer effectual. Recollect the blind enthusiasm for tuberculin inoculations before a single patient was even apparently cured; such a spectacle the world has surely never seen before. At first, each new medicament paralyzes the vital powers; but in time, the system grows so insensible to it, as no longer to react. A new and more potent remedy is now required to paralyze the vitality further, until finally the fermentation of foreign matter cannot be longer prevented by any means at all, and the destruction of life is the result. An illustration will render this plainer.

Anyone who is learning to smoke has to battle with his stomach until the latter grows insensible to the poisonous nicotine. At first, the stomach is vigorous enough to defend itself successfully against this poison, but very soon its strength is weakened, and complete insensibility to the poison is the consequence. We now require a stronger poison than before, to produce the first effect on the stomach.

Those who are beginning to smoke and cannot immediately bear it, usually tell us, to our astonishment, that their stomachs are still too weak, they must get used to it, they cannot stand smoking as yet. The very opposite is the case: as long as the stomach resists smoking, it proves that it still possesses enough vitality, that is, it is strong enough to forcibly expel the poison. When it offers no resistance, the former natural activity is gone, it has become weaker.

The body, thus encumbered with this latent foreign matter, requires a far more powerful external exciting agent, if it is to be roused to expel the matter, because its vitality is diminished. I have already pointed out wherein such excitant consists. It is generally a change in the weather which is the direct cause, for which reason we always have great epidemics after unusually cold winters.

I will add a few mental illustrations. If you carry a bottle of beer into a dark, cold cellar, fermentation will not easily set in. But on exposing the bottle to sunshine and a warmer temperature, fermentation begins at once, even if the bottle is tightly closed. This fermentation is caused neither by bacilli nor by microbes, but merely by light and warmth. At the same time, the outward appearance of the beer is changed; at first clear, it has grown turbid, and if bacilli are now contained in it, they are the product of fermentation.

We observe the same thing in the air. One day we have a glorious clear summer day; then next, the sky is overcast. But every one knows that the watery vapor floating invisibly in the air is condensed to clouds by a change (in this case a fall) of temperature. We also perceive here, how each specific degree of cooling produces its own kind of precipitation (dew, mist, rain, hail, snow); yet there is no difficulty in recognizing them all to be simple products of water.

In marshy, tropical regions, the atmosphere is constantly filled with fermenting matter from the swamp, so that a short stay suffices to bring on a fever (that is fermentation) in a person encumbered with foreign matter. The marshy ferments act upon the foreign matter in the system like yeast in dough, producing fermentation (fever). All stagnant water acts similarly, but not so violently. Only notice the difference between clear mountain lakes, the stony bottom of which admits of no fermentation, and other muddy land-locked pools.

Sometimes the latter are also fairly clear, but with every change in the weather, fermentation takes place in the water, starting from below and making the entire lake turbid, so that one can often recognize what bottom the water rests on. Standing water on a muddy bottom is often set into a sort of fermentation by a change of weather, just like marshy water, and it then operates as a ferment on the other substances. This process of fermentation may be clearly seen by comparing the estate in summer and winter. In winter, even standing marsh-water is comparatively clear, because the cold prevents all fermentation, but in hot weather it is nauseously foul and muddy.

The only question is, what may be the cause of an epidemic when direct contagion seems impossible, for we see the same disease appearing today in one place, tomorrow in another.

Without the presence of foreign matter in the body, epidemics are, as already stated, quite out of the question. On closer inspection, we find epidemics every year, though not always so wide-spread as the influenza at the beginning of 1890. But who is not aware that every year at certain times measles, scarlet fever, diphtheria, whooping-cough, colds, influenza appear epidemically? It follows, in view of the general, uniform mode of life of the masses, that their encumbrance with foreign matter, whether regarded quantitatively or qualitatively, likewise displays a certain uniformity. Now, if one and the same exciting influence affects this matter, i.e. should the weather exert a similar external excitement on the vital powers of the body, the latter will also make similar efforts (fever) to regain health by expelling the foreign matter. And where the encumbrance in a number of individuals is pretty uniform, the like cause will at the same time produce a like effect in many of them, thus creating an epidemic. But one should never forget that even in epidemics, individual cases of sickness are never quite similar, always differing somewhat in their symptoms and course. When an epidemic, such as we saw in the case of the influenza, appears here today and there tomorrow, the cause is simply the weather. In this respect such diseases resemble thunder-storms, which also at times appear "epidemically," today in one region, tomorrow in another. When an epidemic once breaks out in a place, direct contagion does the rest, as before described, in spreading the disease, just as in the last influenza epidemic.

Widespread epidemics have been rarer in recent years. But as observed above, the sole reason of this is, that the medical profession has learned so far to paralyze the vital powers of the people, that in all sweeping, epidemic curative crises, the system can only rally the requisite vitality when compelled under particular stress. The necessary consequence of this, however, is a far more serious and general, chronically (latent) diseased condition; and we doubt not that the time will come when this will be universally recognized.

Summing up the result of these remarks, we find:

1. That in the transmission of diseases from the chronic state (i.e. from parent to child), the foreign matter alone is the cause of the transmission. Whoever is desirous of preventing such transmission must, therefore, first of all take care to get rid of this matter. Such transmission is the worst propagator of disease, because it takes place in all cases; whereas infection through an acute disease, occurs only when there is predisposition.

2. In the case of infection by acute diseases, the latter pass from one person to another by the transmission of fermenting matter, usually through the medium of the air. But infection is impossible without the presence of foreign matter (predisposition) in the system of the other person, as disease arises only from the fermentation of such matter. Pure air is, therefore, the first condition in the sick-room. This is obtainable in no other way than by opening the windows, or using proper ventilating apparatus. All the perfumes and disinfectants so often employed, do no carry off the foreign matter, but simply help to pollute the air. At the same time they dull the sense of that guardian of our health, the nose, making it indifferent to even the most ill-smelling exudations of the patient; they operate exactly like the remedies mentioned above, not for the better but for the worse. All possible attempts may be made to destroy the ferments in the air by poison, but they will never succeed; and as a very little morbid matter suffices to set up fermentation in the system, disinfection is but a vain endeavor. The only proper remedy is one which cleanses the system and drives out the foreign matter, the source of predisposition. You already know it—the friction hip and sitz-baths and the steam bath. In the treatment of patients I have often been obliged to inhale their frequently disgusting exhalations. At the next friction sitz-bath which I took, just the same horrible odor was often given off by my own body, only it was less intense. Here we have a plain proof that the vital powers of the body were so much increased by the bath, that it could expel the virus of disease.

3. This simple remedy also protects us from infection in all epidemics, because the foreign matter (predisposition) is thereby removed from the system, and without it, no disease, and thus no epidemic, is possible.

I have thus shown that the transmission of disease and infection by it, are only possible when foreign matter is present in the system. Without this no disease, and without disease no infection. But any encumbrance of the body with foreign matter means nothing else than its inner defilement. He who knows how to keep his body clean inside and not merely outside, is safe from all infection. It is only cleanliness that cures. One always imagines that different forms must conceal new and various causes, quite forgetting that nature very often exhibits one and the same thing under most varied forms. This we see in the case of the caterpillar and butterfly, and of rain, snow, hail, dew, and mist.

The extent to which the system is encumbered with latent foreign matter can be ascertained by the *Science of Facial Expression*.

If now, considering these principles, we think of the preventive measures which the medical profession takes against contagion in the case of acute diseases, e.g. diphtheria, small-pox, cholera, one must really be almost moved to pity. We see whole houses carefully isolated from all communication, and everywhere in the dwellings, the odor of carbolic acid and other useless disinfectants, which are supposed to destroy the contagious matter. One loses all patience when one reads again and again in the newspapers, of ships being kept without purpose for weeks, or even months in quarantine, in order to prevent contagion. Whoever has been so long engaged as I in the practical treatment of the sick, must, if he is not blind, get quite a different picture of the dangers of infection. I have seen children suffering from diphtheria, scarlet fever, measles, small-pox, sleeping in the same bed with their brothers and sisters, the family circumstances not admitting of other arrangements. Yet there was no contagion, for there was no predisposition on the part of the other children, i.e. they were not encumbered with morbid matter, which would form a nutritive medium for the development of the disease. On the other hand, I have seen in some fever, diphtheria, and small-pox, notwithstanding that all the directions of the physicians regarding disinfectants had been most scrupulously observed. In such cases, too, I have often informed the parents beforehand, that although only one child was attacked at the moment, the others would probably catch the illness also, because the *Science of Facial Expression* showed me that there was predisposition to such. We see, then, how utterly absurd the preventive measures of the medical profession against contagious diseases are. We only have to turn to nature to see that this is the fact. In the forest we find the stump of some old tree, eaten up by worms and insects and overgrown with fungi, whilst close beside it a young tree is sprouting up proudly, quite unconcerned, notwithstanding the dangerous foes around it. Were the young tree already infested by the germs of disease and filled with morbid sap, it would certainly not be proof against the fungi, insects, and worms. As it is, however, it shoots up with vigor; no worm or insect attacks it, no fungus can take root upon it, because for all, the appropriate nutritive medium is wanting.

May the importance of what I have said about infection be grasped by the masses of the people, so that the superstitious and false teachings of medical orthodoxy may be broken down! The public would then no longer so easily lose its head at the outbreak of an epidemic, but cool and collected set about the cure.

All the various forms of disease are, as we have seen, only efforts of the body to recover health. They must not, therefore, be suppressed and rendered latent, as the orthodox medical school teaches, but the body must be assisted to effect these curative crises as quickly but the body must be assisted to effect these curative crises as quickly as possible, in the least dangerous manner.

At first, each new medicament paralyzes the vital powers; but in time, the system grows so insensible to it, as no longer to react. A new and more potent remedy is now required to paralyze the vitality further, until finally the fermentation of foreign matter cannot be longer prevented by any means at all, and the destruction of life is the result.

He who knows how to keep his body clean inside and not merely outside, is safe from all infection. It is only cleanliness that cures.

COLD HANDS AND FEET, HOT HEAD: THEIR CAUSE AND CURE
(The New Science of Healing*)

by Louis Kuhne
Herald of Health and Naturopath, XXII(6), 354-355. (1917)

Let us now consider the origin of *cold hands and feet* and a *hot head*. We all know that the head ought to be cool, and the hands and feet warm, yet we very often meet with just the contrary state. Now let us see how these symptoms of disease arise. I said in one of my former lectures, that there is no disease without fever, and no fever without disease. Therefore, according to my assertions, this condition must also be a feverish one. That this is so in the case of a hot head, no one doubts. Cold feet and hands are less likely to be regarded as indications of fever. I maintain, however, that both—the hot head, and cold hands and feet—are caused in one and the same manner. How can that be? Every disease is occasioned by the presence of foreign matter in the system. By fever—fermentation—this matter is transported from the abdomen into the remotest parts of the body. Some is deposited in these remote points, that is, in the head, feet and hands. If the fermentation matter enters the feet and hands, it finds there but very slight resistance. The foreign matter first accumulates in the toes, then in the feet, and thus spreads gradually upwards into the legs, obstructing the circulation and consequently lowering the warmth. It is the same with the hands. With many people only the finger *tips* are cold at first; with others; only *one* foot; later on, in the course of years, they begin to complain also of the legs, which are cold up to the knee. Warm stockings are tried, but they, too, will not help for long. Even fur boots afford but temporary relief; there comes a time, when no warm clothing will suffice. The feet can no longer be warmed. This makes it very evident, that, as is well known, the clothing does not warm the body, but the body the clothing. And if, in the beginning, the warm clothing does protect one against the feeling of coldness, the reason is that there is still a certain amount of warmth in the limbs, which is communicated to the thicker clothes and retained by them. But this protection given by the warmer clothing does not long avail. Whenever the secretion of the skin and the regular circulation of the blood gradually decrease, the warmest clothing becomes useless.

---

* Louis Kuhne first wrote his book, *The New Science of Healing*, in Germany in 1892, which was then published in English in 1899 as *The New Science of Healing*, (The International News Co., New York). Then in 1917, Benedict Lust translated and published Kuhne's books as *Neo-Naturopathy, The New Science of Healing*, (Benedict Lust Publishing, Butler, New Jersey).

With the head it is quite a different matter. The brain, with its abundant supply of blood, is far more capable of offering resistance to foreign matter pressing upon it than the hands or feet. Hence, strong friction results, and as a consequence, warmth. Thus the riddle is solved. Exactly the same thing which makes the hands and feet cold, renders the head hot at first. But even the *heat* in the head terminates sooner or later. In my practice, I have met with patients enough in whom the head had already grown quite cold. Thus there is a limit here also. When the foreign matter presses on to the head in great abundance, the resistance here also ceases after a while, and the head likewise grows cold. A proof of the correctness of this supposition can be given only in the cures resulting from a treatment founded upon it. If a patient would be relieved from the chilliness in hands and feet and the burning feeling in the head, he must commence his treatment at the place from which the fermentation started, *i.e.*, the abdomen. The digestion must be regulated, and then the hands and feet will grow warm and the head cool. A cold head will at first grow warm again and then attain its normal coolness. And this has been observed in a thousand cases, fresh instances occurring daily in my practice. Here I will add, that sufferers from cold hands and feet are always especially liable to rheumatic attacks.

There is no disease without fever, and no fever without disease.

By fever—fermentation—this matter is transported from the abdomen into the remotest parts of the body.

The digestion must be regulated, and then the hands and feet will grow warm and the head cool.

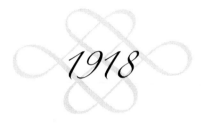

1918

Am I My Brother's Keeper?

By WM. F. HAVARD

*I*F *you saw a woman or child about to be robbed, beaten or abused, would not your conscience prompt you to go to that one's assistance? Or if it happened to be a man who looked well able to take care of himself, would you not at least call out a warning?*

The advocates of Natural Healing are sometimes criticized for the severe manner in which they condemn medical and surgical practices. But how shall an abuse ever be rectified if those who know the truth do not cry out against that abuse?

For centuries there has been built up, under the guise of science, a practice of medicine which has come to be an abomination.

It has lured countless thousands of human beings to their destruction by lending a false sense of hope and security. By allaying symptoms and suppressing nature's healing efforts, medicine creates the "chronic," and there leaves him to his fate, at last acknowledging that it can do nothing to save him.

Medicine has contributed to immorality by relieving the individual of personal responsibility for his disease and blaming the cause on external conditions over which the individual has little or no control. It has invented the germ theory to replace the old devil, and promised salvation through vicarious atonement, thus leading humanity to a false belief that health can be attained and maintained by artificial means.

Not one tenet of medicine can be proven in the last analysis. Its centuries of demonstrations point to nothing but dismal failure.

Is it not time, then, that someone braved the authorities, and dared to tell the truth?

It is criminal to withhold the truth. We are each and every-one morally bound to promote the welfare of our fellows, and the man who withholds knowledge which would benefit his brother, is as much of a criminal as he who commits a crime.

Naturopaths are bound by conscience to tell the truth. They realize their responsibility, and in spite of organized opposition, in spite of governments and courts, they are continuing their activities in the interest of humanity.

May their noble efforts prosper, and continue to find favor in the minds of the more intelligent until mankind shall follow nature and obey her laws, and disease shall be known no more.

William Freeman Havard acted periodically as Editor of *Herald of Health and Naturopath* between1918-1919 and submitted prose to address important issues that the Naturopathic community faced at the time.

Affirmations

by Edward Earle Purinton

Herald of Health and Naturopath, XXIII(1), 33. (1918)

An affirmation is a mental exercise which, when sufficiently repeated, strengthens the good, and crowds out the injurious thoughts. It is easy to say, "I am strong" when the body shows forth perfect health, or "I am happy" when everything goes right, but we must learn to make these statements in spite of present conditions, realizing that by so doing we are helping to bring about the desired results.

A few affirmations are hereby presented to the reader which may be changed to suit individual needs:

I am master of myself.

I can and will do whatever I desire to do.

I am moulding my mind and my body now.

I am bright, cheerful and happy this minute.

I am growing each day in health, strength and power.

I am looking forward, not backward—upward, not downward.

I am reaching out to the source of power for help to overcome.

I am at peace with all the world, and realize more the Great Love which enfolds me.

I am a part of all that exists, and live, move and have my being in Infinite Life.

I am letting go of all thoughts of sickness, sorrow and anxiety.

I am selecting only the thoughts which shall create harmony within.

I am given dominion over all things, and will make this body a temple of health.

I am looking on the bright side of every event, and evolving power to get good out of each.

I am avoiding all irritability, impatience, and pessimism, and growing amiable, so everyone likes me.

I am refraining from censuring, criticizing and condemning my fellow traveler along life's journey.

I am attracting to myself the friends, the work, and all that I need to make my life happy, useful and prosperous.

I am becoming receptive to the inflow of Divine Life, power, health, knowledge, success and plenty.

I have no fear of the future, of disaster, sickness, disease or poverty, for I live in God, and am supplied by His bounty.

By affirming these and other vital truths, you will fill the mind with new thoughts and crowd out accumulated rubbish.

The majority of the people need to pass through many bitter experiences before they are aroused to think and live according to the new light which is given them. They refuse to die to the old, hence can not live in the new, and realize the happiness and satisfaction it brings.

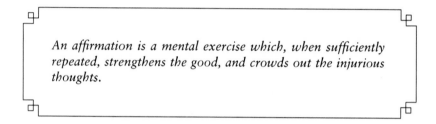

An affirmation is a mental exercise which, when sufficiently repeated, strengthens the good, and crowds out the injurious thoughts.

How I Became Acquainted With Nature Cure

by Henry Lindlahr, M.D., N.D.

Herald of Health and Naturopath, XXIII(2), 122-130. (1918)

The Law Of Periodicity

Nature Cure, for the first time since the days of Hippocrates, has definitely applied the law of periodicity to the occurrence of healing crises in chronic diseases under natural treatment. Dr Buchanan, in his little book, *Periodicity*, reveals the manifestation of this great law in "sevens" in many domains of life and action, in the processes of birth, growth, maturity, fruitage, decline and death. But he failed to perceive its application to the development of healing crises in chronic cases. In fact, he was only very dimly aware of the existence and true meaning of healing crises.

In accordance with this law of periodicity, if conditions are favorable and the treatment is "natural," the crises manifest counting from the beginning of natural treatment, on the sixth day in the sixth week, sixth month, sixth year, and in periods of seven thereafter.

Treatment Of Acute Disease

Many people who know that we can and do cure all kinds of so-called "incurable," chronic diseases, such as tuberculosis, cancer, tertiary syphilis, locomotor ataxia, infantile paralysis, et cetera, et cetera, seem to think that we are unable to cure acute diseases such as measles, scarlet fever, diphtheria, etc. Incidents like the following are of frequent occurrence: Some time ago I met a lady in a street car who had been one of our patients. Before she came to us she was suffering with a disease of the lower jawbone. Under surgical treatment the bone was scraped and shaved half a dozen times. But, as usual, the old trouble re-appeared in aggravated form. Then the surgeons told her it was cancer, and in order to prolong her life, the lower jaw would have to be removed entirely. Frightened by this terrible alternative, she was ripe to listen to Nature Cure talk from one of her friends, who had attended my lectures. She placed herself under our care and treatment, and in six months the jawbone was sound, after another three months she had false teeth fitted, and has not had any trouble since.

When I made the usual inquiries after the health and the welfare of her family, she told me tearfully that she herself had been getting along fine, but that she had lots of trouble with her children. One of them had been taken with diphtheria. The child was getting along fine until the attending allopathic physician administered the diphtheria antitoxin. Then within twenty-four hours that child became paralyzed from the hips down, and died two days afterward.

When I expressed my astonishment at the treatment, and asked her why she had not called in a Nature Cure physician to treat the case, she seemed greatly surprised and said, "Why, Doctor, I did not know that you could cure such diseases as that." The trouble with her was that she came to us for treatment on the transient plan, and had not had the opportunity of attending our lectures, nor had she read the Nature cure books; like many others, she did not know what cured her, and therefore had to suffer again the penalty of ignorance and of violation of the law.

As a matter of fact, it is in the treatment of acute diseases that Nature Cure works its greatest miracles. In our sanitarium practice, in the treatment of chronic diseases, we cope with the hardest phases of the work. Most of the sanitarium patients do not come to us for advice and help until they are "down and out"—until there is nothing more to spoil," and then if Nature Cure cannot make good within a few weeks or months, they grumble and complain "because it is so slow". I sometimes meet such complaints with remarks like the following: "Nature Cure is the fastest cure on record, because there is nothing else that does cure chronic diseases. It is the Twentieth Century Express in healing. You just have the choice of two things: either get cured by slow Nature Cure or keep your chronic disease until the undertaker finishes the job."

Priessnitz, the pioneer of Nature Cure, replied to one of these impatient ones, "To cure you quickly, I should have started with your grandmother."

I realized from the first that I could have acquired greater fame and more money, with much less work and trouble, if I had confined myself to the treatment of acute diseases. The only reason why I took up the sanitarium work, in spite of the advice of my close relatives and best friends, was that I wanted to demonstrate to suffering humanity and to the medical profession that possibility of curing chronic diseases.

I also wanted the opportunity of teaching and training as many young people as possible in this great work of curing chronic ailments. It has been a very slow, arduous, and from the worldly standpoint, a thankless work but a few years more of growth at the present rate of development will see the realization of my fondest ideals.

THE UNITY OF DISEASE AND CURE
. . . as taught in Nature Cure Philosophy, and practically demonstrated with the greatest possible efficiency in the treatment of all acute diseases is undoubtedly the most valuable contribution of Nature Cure to medical science. It marks the greatest of all revolutionary advances in the art of healing human ailments.

Briefly, the idea of the Unity of Disease and Treatment is based on the following propositions:

Barring injury by accident (trauma), and conditions uncongenial to life and health, there is but one primary cause of disease, namely, violations of nature's laws in our habits of living, and in our treatment of the acute diseases resulting therefrom. Violations of nature's law in our habits of living result in:

(1) Lowered vitality.

(2) Abnormal composition of blood and lymph (mainly through wrong eating and drinking).

(3) Accumulation of waste, morbid matter and poisons in the system.

(4) Mechanical lesions: pressure, tension or strain on nerves and nerve centers, caused through luxations of centers, caused through luxations of bony structures, or straining of muscles and ligaments.

(5) Abnormal, that is, discordant or destructive mental and emotional attitude.

When through these primary causes of disease the vitality has become lowered to such an extent that the morbid and poisonous encumbrances, (Pathogen), begin to endanger health and life, then the organism reacts to these disease conditions through acute healing efforts in the form of inflammation and fever.

These inflammatory processes, if properly treated and assisted, are therefore always constructive, that is, purifying and healing of nature, always run their course through the same five stages of inflammation, and if allowed to do so, always result in effecting better conditions; that is, they leave the system purer and more normal than before they started their salutary work of house-cleaning.

While readers of Nature Cure readily accept in theory this principle of the Unity of Disease and Treatment, they find difficulty in applying it practically at the sick bed. It sometimes happens that those to whom *Nature Cure and Practice* has been sent on approval return the book because no specific treatment for their particular disease is given. They have failed to grasp the great fundamental principles of Nature Cure.

The greatest achievement of *Nature Cure Philosophy and Practice* lies in the fact that it has reduced the treatment of acute and sub-acute diseases, as well as of chronic ailments, to the greatest simplicity.

Allopathy lists hundreds of different diseases, each one to be treated with different "specific" drugs, serums, antitoxins, vaccines or surgical operations.

Compare with this the marvelous simplicity of *Nature Cure Philosophy and Practice* which reduces the treatment of all acute and sub-acute diseases to a few simple principles and methods.

The truth of this we have proved in daily practice for 15 years. Just think what this means! It means that anybody with common intelligence and ordinary good sense can treat any and all acute diseases in a most efficient way with the best possible results, though he has never seen a medical college.

It is the wonderful simplicity of *Nature Cure Theory and Practice* which for the first time in human history makes medical science an exact science.

The fundamental Law of Cure, the Laws of Crises and of Periodicity, will do for medical science what the laws of gravitation and of chemical affinity have done for physics, astronomy and chemistry. Before the discovery of these natural laws, astronomy, chemistry and physics were a mass of superstitious beliefs and contradictory opinions, just as medical science is today. Nature Cure Institutions, comprising all the schools of natural therapeutics, work side by side with those who practice magnetic, mental and spiritual healing.

Nature Cure Philosophy has done original and revolutionary work in the discovery and practical application of the fundamental principles underlying the vital processes of health, disease, and the cure of disease.

THE NATURAL TREATMENT OF WOUNDS AND OPEN SORES

Ever since the author publicly began to teach and practice Nature Cure, he has maintained in his lectures and writings and demonstrated in his daily practice that the natural and most efficient treatment for wounds and open sores consists in exposure to air and light, and that the best of all antiseptics is lemon juice diluted with water.

The efficiency of this treatment, which flatly contradicts the most firmly established doctrines of medical science, I have demonstrated for many years even in the germ and dirt-laden air of Chicago. We have cured through this simple treatment many wounds which under heavy coverings of antiseptic bandages and under continuous soaking with poisonous antiseptics and germicides had entered into advanced stages of malignant, necrotic, degenerative processes.

For many years I have been denounced as an ignoramus and a dangerous fakir, for thus contradicting and opposing "the most important discoveries and practices of modern medical science as to surgical cleanliness and antiseptic treatment." The editor of a magazine foremost in the ranks of scientific and philosophical publications in this country had to discontinue a series of articles from my pen because hundreds of protests came in from old-school physicians on account of my uncompromising stand against the use of antiseptics, serums and antitoxins in the treatment of wounds and of inflammatory, febrile diseases.

But *tempora mutantur, et nos mutamur in illis*, which in our beloved United States vernacular means, "Times change and we change with them." Some time ago, Chicago dailies announced in a leading article, *The Most Recent Wonderful Discovery of Surgical Science.* They related that, thanks to the discovery of a prominent surgeon in one of the great West Side hospitals, wounds were now being treated with uniform success without antiseptics and germicidal agents, and that this revolutionary treatment consisted solely in exposure of the wounds of light and air. The article concluded by saying that such a revolutionary discovery could be made only by a great and learned surgeon.

Until recently I was in danger of arrest and trial for malpractice for teaching and practicing this "recent wonderful discovery of surgical science."

I do not bring out these facts from a desire for vain boasting, but in order to point out the fact that many of the teachings of Nature Cure Philosophy are being gradually adopted by orthodox medical science, which gives hope that other Nature cure ideas and practices may also in time receive due recognition.

In this connection, it may be of interest to call attention to the fact that the open air treatment for tuberculosis and the hydropathic treatment in typhoid fever were adopted by the medical profession from the Nature Cure people in Germany. For more than thirty years, Ignatz, Priessnitz, Father Kneipp, Kuhne and other pioneers of Nature Cure, were dragged to the courts and tried for mal-practice for using hydropathic treatment in the cure of acute and chronic diseases, until Dr. Brand, of Berlin, began to notice that his own typhoid fever patients died at the rate of 50 or 60 per hundred, while the typhoid fever patients of the Nature Cure "quacks" made uniform recoveries. He tried the water treatment, found it eminently successful, and then gave his "discovery" to the medical profession in an essay, in which he described the wonderful efficacy of hydropathic treatment in typhoid fever.

Since that time, this treatment has been adopted with great success by advanced physicians all over the earth. But they have not yet awakened to the fact that the same simple cold water treatment and fasting will cure every other acute disease with exactly the same efficacy as in the case of typhoid fever.

When they do grasp the full significance of "the unity of disease and of treatment," as demonstrated in these pages, they will cease to waste millions upon millions of dollars in the creation of medical foundations and research institutes which serve no other purpose than to experiment upon helpless sufferers with concoctions of poisonous drugs and disease products in the form of vaccines, serums, and antitoxins. A rather useless and superfluous waste of money, time, energy and human lives, when the problem of curing all acute and sub-acute diseases has been solved by Nature Cure Philosophy and Practice.

This awakening will sound the death knell of the darkest superstition that over obsessed humanity—the belief that health can be created and maintained by saturating human bodies with disease-creating agents.

The Treatment Of Chronic Diseases

In the treatment of chronic diseases, Nature Cure undertakes and accomplishes "the impossible." "Chronic," in the vocabulary of the old school of medicine means "incurable." If the reader should doubt this statement, I advise him to read any standard work on medical practice. He will find that the medical authorities divide diseases into two stages or types, the acute and the chronic. The acute stages of disease they attempt to cure by the ordinary medical methods. When it comes to the treatment of the chronic stages of disease, we find invariably expressions like the following: "When this disease reaches the chronic stages, you cannot cure it. You may advise the patient to change occupation or climate, to rest or to travel; aside from this, treat the symptoms as they arise." These symptoms arising in chronic diseases from our viewpoint are Nature's feeble efforts to purify the system. To treat them from the medical viewpoint means to check and suppress them with poisonous drugs and surgical operations.

To illustrate: Suppose a chronic patient develops a healing crisis, as we would call it, in the form of a vigorous diarrhea, acute catarrh, leucorrhea, boil or fever, under medical treatment these purifying efforts of Nature would be promptly "treated," that is, thoroughly suppressed, and the disease poisons driven back into the system. How, under such treatment, in the name of common sense, has the chronic patient a chance to recover? Is it not clear that the very "treatment" of the symptoms makes the cure an impossibility?

Nature Cure, on the other hand, through natural methods of living, as before explained, builds up the blood, purifies the system, adjusts the mechanical lesions, harmonizes the mental and emotional conditions so that the organism can once more arouse itself to a cleansing, healing effort in the various forms of acute elimination. Anybody endowed with common sense should be able to decide which is the natural way and which the unnatural and destructive way.

Natural Dietetics

This is another science of vital importance to the welfare of humanity, created by the founders of the Nature Cure movement. I first became acquainted with the principles and practical application of rational vegetarianism during my search for health and knowledge in European schools and sanitariums.

When I returned to this country, I was naturally anxious to learn what progress vegetarianism and natural healing methods had made on this side. I found that the leaders of vegetarianism in England and America had built their systems of meatless diet on the teachings of the allopathic schools of medicine, according to which protein, fats and starches are the most important food elements, in fact, the only ones worthy of consideration in the daily dietary or in the treatment of diseases.

About that time, E. P. Mills, one of the leaders of vegetarianism in England, published a book entitled, *Why Vegetarians Fail*. The gist of his argument was that they fail because their diet does not contain enough protein to remedy the deficiency caused by excluding meat and eggs. To supplement the protein in vegetable foods, he recommended a preparation called "plasmon," made from fresh cottage cheese, consisting mainly of concentrated protein and fat.

We know, now, thanks to Nature Cure, that the failures of vegetarianism, which Mills observed, were due to an **excess** of protein, starches and fats in their diet, and to a **deficiency** of the positive alkaline mineral elements.

Another reason why many vegetarians in his day, as well as in our day, failed to be benefited is because they did not combine with the vegetarian diet other necessary methods of natural living and treatment. What they gained through a meatless diet they lost through hot bathing, wrong breathing, lack of exercise, smoking, drugging and suppression of acute elimination.

Others fail, or think they fail, because they do not know of the existence of the fundamental law of cure, and of the laws of crisis and of periodicity. They follow a rational, vegetarian diet, and practice faithfully cold bathing; they exercise systematically, breathe deeply and rhythmically, and think and feel constructively and harmoniously. As a result of these rational and natural habits of living, they improve in health steadily up to a certain point. Then suddenly all their old aches and pains and other troubles come back. Then they believe that vegetarian diet is a snare and a delusion, and return repentantly to the flesh pots of Egypt, and to the good old pills and potions.

The editor of *Vim*, whose "cure-all" and sole hobby is deep breathing, is, or was, a rabid anti-vegetarian. In his magazine he published a few years ago a series of letters from readers of *Vim*, "who had tried vegetarianism and failed utterly." Most of these letters ran about as follows:

"I had been suffering for years from chronic rheumatism. I tried many doctors and remedies without relief. Finally, yielding to the urgent pleadings of a dear friend, I tried a strictly vegetarian diet consisting mostly of fruits, whole grain bread and dairy products. I also practiced systematically cold bathing, deep breathing and other health exercises.

"For a while I seemed to improve splendidly, but after a few months suddenly all my old rheumatic aches and pains and other symptoms came back in aggravated form. Then I realized that my friends were right when they told me I was making a fool of myself by following this starvation diet and by continually chilling my body with cold bathing. I then returned to the ordinary, good, nourishing food and dropped all fads."

If this wise one and many others like him had known the laws of cure they would have rejoiced at the arrival of these healing crises and would have assisted Nature's cleansing, healing efforts by even stricter adherence to the natural regime, thus laying the foundation for perfect health in the future.

In the largest and best appointed sanitariums in this country the law of crisis is unknown, or, if known, flatly denied and ignored. Quite frequently, I meet with people who tell me they have tried the same treatment we are giving in this or that big sanitarium. The story usually runs like this: "I seemed to improve splendidly for a while, but then I got worse again; all my old troubles came back as bad as ever, and then of course I realized that this natural treatment was not good for my trouble." So of course they packed their trunks and went back to their old diet and medicines or had an operation performed.

It is a fact that down to this day the best known and most luxuriously appointed sanitariums in this country which are supposed to educate and practice (more or less) natural methods of healing, favor a high protein diet, rich in proteins, starches, fats and sugars. Their large factories and food stores offer to the health-seeking public nothing but foods prepared from cereals, nuts, legumes and olives. The menus in their institutions give the amounts of heat-producing units (calories) of the various foods and the patients are told that they need so many hundred food calories per day in order to supply the necessary fuel for the production of animal heat and energy. They are taught to select and figure out the kinds and quantities of food required to supply their needs.

On these menus and food tables supplied to patients, nothing is said about the functions of the positive mineral elements in the human organism, nor about their importance in a well balanced diet.

Soon after my return from Germany I met Otto Carqué in Doctor Lahn's Sanitarium near Lincoln Park, which at that time was the favorite rendezvous of the few Nature Cure "cranks" in Chicago. Carqué had caught the infection and published a booklet entitled, *The Foundation of All Reform*, an interesting treatise on the virtues of a meatless diet. After reading the book, I called the author's attention to the fact that he, the same as all his predecessors in this country and England, had entirely missed the true and only solution of the problem, the mineral salt aspect of the food question.

I called his attention to the classics of German vegetarianism, to Hensel's *Bread from Stones*, to his *Makrobiatic*, to Dr. Lahmann's

Dietische Blutentmischung and to Dr. Haig's *Uric Acid*. Friend Carqué eagerly followed the new lead with much benefit to himself and to the cause of vegetarianism in this country.

Soon after this, Arthur Brisbane, the gifted and versatile literary editor of the Hearst newspapers, published one of his strong articles against vegetarianism. I have always admired Mr. Brisbane for his wide erudition. He is well informed on the most varied subjects of philosophy, science, history and sociology. But when he writes about vegetarianism, vaccination, serums, drug treatment and surgery, he moves in the old ruts, and hits way off the mark.*

Otto Carqué seized the opportunity and answered Brisbane's article in a pamphlet entitled *The Folly of Meat Eating*. In this treatise, he emphasized the importance of the positive mineral elements in the metabolism of animal and human bodies and consequently in food, drink and medicine. This was the first essay written in the English language dealing with the mineral salt problem in nutrition and medical treatment. I followed up the subject in a series of articles in the *Nature Cure Magazine*. These articles on *Natural Dietetics* appeared monthly covering a period of two years. Since that time (1907-1909) practically all advanced food reformers in this country emphasize the importance of the positive mineral elements in their writings and in their diet prescriptions.

An example of this is Alfred McCann. The title of the book which brought him into public notice is *Starving America*, which means America starving for the mineral salts while over-feeding on starches, proteins, fats and sugar. The book deals with the mineral salt problem in straight Nature Cure fashion. Since McCann was not a Nature Cure doctor and therefore not an offense to the regular medical profession, a New York daily published his articles and established his fame as an authority on food chemistry and dietetic subjects. Then the *Chicago Daily News* began to publish his writings and advertised them in all the big Chicago newspapers in full-page advertisements which must have cost a thousand or more dollars each.

Not many readers of these writings are aware of the fact that they are based strictly on Nature Cure philosophy and practice, which proves once more that sometimes good does come "out of Nazareth".

DIAGNOSIS FROM THE EYE

I have already mentioned so many original discoveries and revolutionary scientific achievements in the art of healing given to us through

---

* "The Jack of all trades is master of none"; so, also, the dabbler in all sciences cannot be well instructed in every one of them.

Nature Cure Philosophy, that it seems to become monotonous. But the end is not yet by a long way.

The Diagnosis from the eye is a very valuable gift of Nature Cure to diagnostic science. Dr. von Peckzely, of Budapest, Hungary, discovered Nature's records in the eye, quite by accident, when a boy ten years of age.

Playing one day in the garden at his home, he caught an owl. While struggling with the bird, he broke one of its limbs. Gazing straight into the owl's large, bright eyes, he noticed, at the moment when the bone snapped, the appearance of a black spot in the lower central region of the iris, which area he later found to correspond to the location of the broken leg.

The boy put a splint on the broken limb and kept the owl as a pet. As the fracture healed, he noticed that the black spot in the iris became over-drawn with a white film, and surrounded by a white border (denoting the formation of scar tissues in the broken bone).

This incident made a lasting impression on the mind of the future doctor. It often recurred to him in later years. From further observations he gained the conviction that abnormal physical conditions are portrayed in the eyes.

As a student, Von Peckzely became involved in the revolutionary movement of 1848 and was put in prison as an agitator and ringleader. During his confinement, he had plenty of time and leisure to pursue his favorite theory, and he became more and more convinced of the impor-tance of his discovery. After his release, he entered upon the study of medicines, in order to develop his important discoveries and to confirm them more fully in the operating and dissecting rooms. He had himself enrolled as an intern in the surgical wards of the college hospital. Here he had ample opportunity to observe the eyes of patients before and after accidents and operations, and in that manner, he was enabled to elaborate the first accurate Chart of the Eye.

The discoveries of Von Peckzely have been elaborated and verified in their details by many conscientious and able investigators who have devoted their whole life to the study of this new method of diagnosing human ailments and their causes.

This method has been tested and used successfully by many Nature Cure physicians in Germany and by a few homeopathic doctors, but so far it has been entirely ignored by the representatives of the regular school of medicine. This is not strange since Nature's records in the iris reveal the destructive effects of poisonous drugs and of uncalled-for surgical mutila-tions.

Diagnosis from the Eyes, or Iridology, was first introduced in this country, about 15 years ago, by Doctor H. Lahn and by myself. Now it has become widely known among drugless healers in this country and has proved its value as an important addition to diagnostic science.

While we do not claim that Nature's records in the iris disclose all pathological conditions in the human body, they reveal so much of great interest and real value about the internal processes of health, disease and cure, especially about the underlying causes of disease that we cannot afford to do without this new method of diagnosis.

What makes Iridology of especial interest and value to the followers of drugless healing systems is the fact that the signs in the iris verify all the fundamental laws, principles and teachings of Nature cure, Philosophy and practice.

Dr. Lahn wrote the first book in English dealing with this subject. I followed him with articles in the *Nature Cure Magazine* which appeared every month, covering a period of two years. I hope to find sufficient time to re-edit and publish the substance of these articles in an additional volume of the Nature Cure series.

The Nature Cure Attitude Toward Mental And Metaphysical Healing

While Nature cure realized to the fullest extent and endeavors to apply practically in the treatment of disease all that is good in magnetic, mental and spiritual healing methods, it cannot accept and subscribe to all the teachings advanced by the various cults, schools and systems which deal with these all-important branches of natural healing. Nature Cure Philosophy has brought out certain weak points and errors in these systems which never before have been clearly recognized and brought to public attention.

Nature Cure cannot accept the dogma of the unreality of matter and of disease. Matter is just as real and substantial in the highest spiritual and celestial spheres as it is on this earth plane. **Acute disease, whose existence Christian Science tries to deny in theory and to ignore in treatment, is in reality the cure.**

Another weak point in this system is the prohibition of all physical, material methods of treatment and self-help. In my books, I call attention to the wonderful discoveries of modern science which reveal the fact that matter in the final analysis is nothing but particles of electricity in vibratory motion, that these modes of motion are intelligent or controlled by intelligence, and are therefore an expression of an intelligent mind, of that which we call "Divine Mind". While it is true that these revelations of physical science in a way confirm the Christian Science doctrine of the unreality of matter, we cannot approve of Mrs. Eddy's deductions and dogmas based on this fact.

When she says that matter, sin, disease, and evil are in general errors of mortal mind she contradicts herself while formulating the fundamental proposition of her creed. An erring mortal mind is an abnormal mind, and an abnormal mind is a **diseased** mind. Whereby she admits the existence of disease.

Disease, evil, sin, are real enough; as a matter of fact **they are not figments of a diseased imagination** (errors of mortal mind), **but the results of violations of Nature's laws.** If this conception of Nature Cure Philosophy is the right one, then we are responsible for disease and evil, and then it is up to us to study the laws of our being and to comply with them,—the only way to prevent disease and evil in general. If the Christian Science conception is true, if there is no sin, no disease, no evil, then we are not responsible (for things which do not exist), then there are no laws for us to study nor to obey. Then this does away with personal responsibility. If there is no personal responsibility there cannot be a normal obligation. Thus the Christian Science conception of sin, disease and evil does away with the basic law of morality, which is personal responsibility. Thereby it does away with the necessity for individual inquiry into the causes of our troubles, and benumbs and paralyzes personal effort to prevent them. This will prove the weakest point in this philosophy of disease and cure, and will prevent its general adoption by the progressive intelligence of the present and coming generations.

We must admit that Mrs. Eddy is absolutely consistent in the treatment of disease based upon these dogmas when she prohibits her healers and followers, under threat of expulsion from the church from reading anything concerning and pertaining to the physical, material conditions of the human body in the way of anatomy, physiology, chemistry, etc. Prohibition of rational inquiry and self-help through personal effort however, must inevitably lead to mental and moral stagnation and atrophy. No fanatical creed or tyrannical government has ever endeavored to exert such absolute control over human minds and souls as this system, which is not Christian and is not Science.

The good and the bad points in mental and metaphysical therapeutics from the viewpoint of Nature Cure are clearly brought out in another illuminating chapter of this helpful and healthful volume.

That which makes some of these teachings so attractive to the multitudes, and the reason why intelligent people submit to such mental tyranny which stultifies reason and paralyzes will-power and self-control, is the innate tendency of human nature to get something for nothing, to make short cuts to health, happiness and success. Christian Science is the most alluring "get-rich-quick" system every devised, but every-day experience shows that the devotees of this cult cannot cheat nature forever. Sooner or later, she will exact her equivalent. Every day we see "scientists" succumbing to acute and chronic diseases in just about the same proportions as those who do not subscribe to their beliefs.

Omnipresent Life

by Helen Wilmans

Herald of Health and Naturopath, XXIII(2), 168-171. (1918)

[That the world of the mind dominates the world of materiality is a universally admitted fact. Some metaphysicians believe that our senses deceive us and that all matter is only a phase of mind and that what we call matter has no existence as such. This and that other ideal that man is a god, are illustrations of the human mind overleaping itself in its desire to control its destiny. While we are anxious to afford a free arena for the discussion of all kinds of metaphysical subjects, we do not endorse such extreme doctrines.

We take pleasure in announcing that we have secured the rights to publish the Twenty Lesson Course in Mental Science by the founder of Mental Science, the late Helen Wilmans, of Seabreeze, Fla. These famous lessons were sold for Twenty Dollars, but our readers will have the benefit of receiving one or part of one every month, which will greatly enhance the value of the magazine. As we commenced to publish the Herald of Health and Naturopath monthly with the January, 1918, issue, this means that the entire Course of Lessons will extend from the present issue to the December, 1919, issue. No greater argument for the supremacy of the human mind and will has ever been formulated.

Besides these Lessons, there will be published in this Department, from time to time, articles on Psychotherapy, New Thought, Therapeutic Suggestion, and every phase of Spiritual and Metaphysical Research.—Benedict Lust, Editor]

Devoted to Mental Science, New Thought, Therapeutic Suggestion, Psychotherapy, Spiritual and Metaphysical Research

Home Course In Mental Science
Lesson 1

Emerson says there is but one mind, and that we are all different expressions of it.

The Mental Science student means the same thing when he says there is but one Life, of which we are but individual manifestations.

If there is but one Life, then life is omnipresent—it fills all space. There is nothing outside of it. Indeed, there is no outside. There is but one Life. This Life is the universal Principle of Being that men call God.

But God is a word which is not used in Mental Science, because it is unscientific and misleading. The personal meaning which is attached to the world by the churches has become so universally accepted, that it is impossible for any one to hear it and not have his thoughts at once begin to shape that strange personality of old theology, the God that the race has made out of its ignorance and set up as a bugaboo—ostensibly to love—but really to frighten itself into better behavior; thus creating a master for itself which stultifies its intelligence and prevents its freedom.

Therefore, in the very beginning of these lessons, I state boldly that there is no such God, and I cannot use the term.

But there is a Life Principle, and it is unlimited; it is one. It holds the visible universe in place, though it is invisible. It is a self-existent principle. It is law. It is the one Law—the Law of Attraction—and beside it there is no other law. It is also the very essence of love; and the recognition of it as love is expressed by us in love for each other.

All the races of men have felt the presence and the power of this Law of Attraction, whose ultimate expression is love, or life, in a myriad of different forms. Feeling it and not comprehending it, being governed by their own narrow and childish ideas, they conceived a personality for it, and said it was somebody who made things, and they called it God.

God, they say, made all things. He first made the world out of nothing; after which He had material to make other things of, and so He made man and the animals out of the dust of the earth.

This idea belongs in the early intellectual awakening of a baby race. The race had grown to a place, mentally, where it had begun to ask questions of itself; and its answers were suited to its infantile development.

But to retain answers now, at a time when the great body of the thinking world has outgrown them, and to bolster them up by every system of popular education in vogue, is a fearful thing and must be ended, so that truth shall have her say and be glorified, even as error has been glorified in the past.

But the Life Principle exists. The undeviating Law exists. It has never been violated, and never will be. And this is our hope. It is unchanging, diseaseless, deathless; and a knowledge of it **conforms us to it in a way that renders us diseaseless and deathless.**

For the law does permeate all visible forms. It is one with all substance. And no doubt that an expanded and spiritual interpretation of the word "God" has been the foundation for the expression that "God and man are one."

For in spite of the person, and, therefore, limited interpretation of the word "God", there have been in all ages of the world a few thinkers who were not so entirely confined to its narrow meaning, but they were able to see it in an enlarged, in a spiritual sense; in a sense that proved it to be the moving impulse of all visible life. And these men have said, "God and man are one."

A more scientific statement of the same truth would have been this: The Law and man are one; or, man and all the visible universe are one with the law of their being—one with the indestructible Life Principle, or the Law of Attraction; the Love Essence.

Now, the object of Mental Science, as I teach it, is to rescue man from his beliefs in his own limitations by showing him his true relations to the Universal Law; this demonstrating to him the unlimited possibilities of his being.

Unlimited, I say, because he is in the image and character of the omnipotent Law. He is an exponent of the Law, and cannot divorce himself from it, except by his own false and foolish beliefs.

He has made for himself a personal God on whom he has bestowed such powers as his own limited intelligence has been able to suggest. But even from this God—such as He is—he has divorced himself by imagining It (the personal God) to be in every respect his own superior. So much so, indeed, that it has seemed sacrilege for him even to aspire to be like Him—not to mention the idea of being one with Him.

And so he has believed that his chief duty, in order to augment the glory of this imaginary being, was to abase himself; to call himself humble, and weak, and powerless, and worthless—unworthy of even the small amount of vitality that infused him.

If any one doubts that this imaginary God was the creation of an infant race, he has but to examine His character in order to believe it. What but a baby race could imagine that a great being would be pleased with an unfailing stream of the most obsequious praise, poured constantly into His listening ears? What but a baby race could suppose that this unbroken deluge of flattery was a necessity to the happiness of a great being, or that it would turn the tide of His wrath away from the unfortunate wretches He had made on purpose to curse, if they failed to render Him the proper amount of praise?

That this personal God was the creation of the baby chieftains for the baby clans of a baby race is to be seen by its resemblance to its creators. The chieftains loved power and praise and spoils and were unmerciful to those who refused to render them their demands. The God they made was no larger than themselves. (No man can create a God larger than himself.) But having made a God of their own size, they could supplement His deficiencies by giving Him some supernatural power either to destroy or bless. And this is what they did. And this, with some improvements added by the growth of the race, is the God of theology today.

And because the word God does really and truly mean, in the eyes of the public, just what I have described, I cannot use it in a series of lessons that are scientific in the highest sense.

If the word God was universally accepted as meaning the Principle of vitality, or the Law of Attraction, that runs through and infuses with life every atom in the universe, I would use it. But there are only a few who so understand it; and it is not to this few that these lectures are addressed; or at least, not to them alone.

To be divorced from this personal God—if such a being could exist—would be no great matter. Indeed, we could get along better without Him than with Him.

But to be divorced from the Universal Spirit of Life would be instant annihilation. On the other hand, to know more of this Universal Spirit of Life than we now know would be to have more life, more health, more strength, more intelligence, more beauty and more opulence. Or, rather, it would be **to be these things**, instead of **having** them. To truly mental creatures, such as we are, **knowing** more is **being** more.

The crying want of the race is a remedy for present conditions of sickness, poverty and death; and the whole strength of my effort in these lessons is to furnish a clue to this remedy. Now is the time to be saved. Tomorrow will not only bring its own needs, but its own remedies.

In Mental Science the great principle laid down is this: Man is conjoined to the Eternal Life Principle. He is that Principle—its very self in objectivity—and in proportion as he becomes intellectually conscious of this tremendous truth, he finds an unfailing supply to all his needs, and grows more into a knowledge of his own mastery.

We are manifestations of the unchanging Life Principle; of the Universal Spirit of Being; the inextinguishable I AM. It is the soul to nature—the body. It is internal Man. Man is the eternal of it. And the seeming two are one.

This Law, or Principle, is Man in subjectivity.

Visible man is the Law, or Principle, in objectivity.

When the race knows this great truth, it will appreciate its own dignity and worth and power, and then there will be no more (so-called) sin and sickness and death; no more shedding of tears; no more want or sorrow or the feebleness of old age. We shall know that we are one with the deathless Law of Being, and that our progression through the realms of the universe will be by constantly knowing more and more of the power and beauty and opulence of the Law, which is the vital spark within us.

A condensed expression of the principles of Mental Science would read as follows: There is but one substance. This substance is both seen and unseen. On its unseen side, it is the Universal Spirit of Life, or the Law of Attraction, which is love. On its seen side, it is Intelligence, or mind—falsely called dead matter.

All is real. All is transitional. All is perpetual. The universe yields its substance to man in proportion as he comes into an intellectual understanding of it.

There is no limit as to the supply you may receive; there need be no limit to your demand. But unless you demand aright, you may as well not demand at all. Mental Science will teach you how to demand; and in so doing, it will unlock the store-house of the universe to you.

An advertisement of *The Home Course in Mental Science* offered by Helen Wilmans and Edward Earle Purinton.

The universe is one mighty magnet, having its positive and negative poles. In Mental Science, the two words 'positive' and 'negative' explain the whole. And yet these words are used to describe **relative** and not **absolute conditions**; and the words themselves are relative in their application. There is nothing absolutely positive. The whole—everything we can see or get any conception of—is one grand, sliding scale; the negative growing into the positive, and the positive into the more positive throughout all time. The words which will best explain negative and positive are "unintelligent" and "intelligent," or "unripe" and "ripe". Let me illustrate. The rocks are extremely negative as compared with my hand, and my hand is negative as compared with my brain, and my brain is negative as compared with that essence which it generates, and which we call "thought".

And yet it is all one substance through and through the great whole. Thought is substance just the same as rock is; the endless variety of objects and conditions to be met with everywhere **is this one substance in many different degrees of positive and negative development, the difference in the manifestation being due to different degrees of development,** and not to difference in substance. We can think of nothing that is not substance. This one substance is apparent in all the different forms of life, both animate and inanimate—in the minerals, animals, plants, and in man, it expresses itself in different degrees of positive and negative (or intelligent and unintelligent) development. The rocks are not so intelligent as my hand, and my hand is not so intelligent as my brain, etc.; but the rock is not absolutely negative, not absolutely devoid of intelligence, or vitality, because it contains the possibility of all development, and it does develop. The possibility of all life is in it. It bides its time for incorporation into these bodies of ours and its evolvement into the highest thought.

And where is the dividing line between positive and negative? In strict truth there is no dividing line; but for the sake of convenience in making these lessons clearer we will establish one; and it shall be at that point in development where we begin to be consciously intelligent; where we begin to reason on things, and to investigate ourselves and our surroundings. In short, it shall be as nearly as possible at that point where the intuitive life of the lower order of animals passes into the **consciously intelligent** life of man; though it must be remembered that even inanimate things have intelligence, but their intelligence is unconscious; by which I mean, that it takes no thought of itself; does not reason on itself. Man is the highest expression of conscious intelligence. It is the **consciousness** of intelligence that makes him the creature of power that he is, and that gives him the authority to rule over all things. I have said that the universe is one mighty magnet. It is all one. It is not hard to understand that all the varied forms of life—seen and unseen—are composed of this one mental substance when we consider that steam, now and ice are all different conditions of water. "Uni" means one. This idea of oneness must have had firm lodgment in the minds of those who first began to formulate our language; hence the name **universe** as applied to the whole. The universe is a **universe,** and not a **diverse.** Bear this in mind, for if the student loses sight of this point in these lessons, his bearings will be gone, and from that time on, he will find nothing in them that he can clearly understand.

Now, the object of Mental Science, as I teach it, is to rescue man from his beliefs in his own limitations by showing him his true relations to the Universal Law; this demonstrating to him the unlimited possibilities of his being.

"Uni" means one. This idea of oneness must have had firm lodgment in the minds of those who first began to formulate our language; hence the name **universe** *as applied to the whole.*

Editorial: The Point Of View

by William F. Havard

Herald of Health and Naturopath, XXIII(5), 419-420. (1918)

"How Science is Saving Life and Making Men Immune to Disease" is the title of a full-page article in a recent issue of the *New York Sunday World*. It is a medical defense of vivisection, vaccination and serum inoculation. It gives facts and figures, showing how the death-rate from smallpox and typhoid has been reduced by the latest scientific discoveries.

We wish the case were as good as our medical friends try to make it. But, unfortunately, the truth has been perverted. They do not state the facts as they are. Furthermore, it is useless to try to refute them. We are not arguing from the same standpoint. Medicine persists in looking upon every disease manifestation as a separate entity in itself, and with their germ mania rampant at present, they turn a dead eye on basic causes. They fail to realize that acute diseases, such as typhoid, smallpox and the host of other healing crises, are but the outbreak of accumulations of morbid matter. It is true that their serums, antitoxins and vaccines may prevent the disease taking that particular form. But there is nothing to prevent its assuming another character. For example: diphtheria was an unknown condition before the introduction of vaccination as a preventive for smallpox. And if the morbid matter does not come out in some acute form, it lays the foundation for chronic ailments. Serums do not prevent disease; they merely cover them up.

Never will our medical profession realize this, in spite of the fact that their own pathologists point out to them that disease is not an entity, but a process. The form it takes is in accordance to both internal and external conditions. Change the internal condition by introducing another foreign substance in form of serums, or what not, and you change the form in which the disease will manifest.

Hippocrates, the father of medicine, pointed out this truth, and medicine has made no progress since. Improved sanitation has done more to prevent contagion and epidemics than all the inventions of medical savants.

Medicine is a long, long way from its starting point, to which it must return before it can progress. At present, it concerns itself only with the counteraction of symptoms and the suppression of nature's curative efforts. Cure is an entirely different process from counteraction.

Medical statistics look fine in print, and we wish that disease could be eliminated by so simple a procedure as a squirt in the arm; but time will prove that serum therapy is another medical bubble like all the others that have gone before.

Whether or not one is to consider serums a preventive for this, that or the other, depends on our point of view.

We are not arguing from the same standpoint. Medicine persists in looking upon every disease manifestation as a separate entity in itself, and with their germ mania rampant at present, they turn a dead eye on basic causes.

Serums do not prevent disease; they merely cover them up.

NATURE'S SAFETY VALVE

by J. W. Wigelsworth, N.D.

Herald of Health and Naturopath, XXIII(8), 731-732, (1918)

A baby was born into the world—and what happened?

When it had been here a little while it developed, we'll say, an intestinal disturbance.

Mothers—what was the diarrhoea for? Did baby's intestines go off in a rampage for pure and simple cussedness, or was there a reason?

Why did Nature want to get the morbid mass from the little one?

Can you imagine health and such material in the same body?

That's the "Why."

Baby's body was not pure, so Nature tried to purify it.

But when baby had the blessed eliminating spell, what happened?

Didn't every neighbor and even the doctor tell you how to suppress it? If they were the average of their kind, they did,—if you followed their advice, it worked, and you congratulated yourself that you had done a good job.

But did you?

Baby's food then did not seem to agree with it, and it became feverish and peevish, and the doctor, your friends and yourself blamed it on the poor child's teeth or some other unoffending member.

But was it the teeth, or the tonsils, or the bowels?

No. In the average case it was just another attempt of Nature to get rid of the poisons. The kiddie's little liver, his bowels, his lungs, and every part of him saw a chance in a period of great activity to again do the natural thing, namely, get rid of inherited taints and other poisons.

Again some medicine was poured into the little one, the morbid matter dammed back, and the body called upon to neutralize it instead of getting rid of it.

Taking medicine for such a condition is like the little boy whose mother had punished him for spilling gravy on the table-cloth. The next time he spilled a drop, he poured salt on it so that it would not show. He covered the evidence of his carelessness, but when the maid came to brush the crumbs, the salt came off and the gravy showed up worse than ever. The little fellow was punished more severely than if he had not attempted the deception.

The argument is not that drugs do not work—they do—but that they are not the best things under the circumstances. Drugs do stimulate the eliminating organs, but they do not prepare the poisons for elimination. Most drugs are given to suppress rather than eliminate, however.

Drugs taken into the body must be eliminated themselves and thus added strain is put on the system.

Each succeeding child's disease (including colds, etc.) is the same story, an attempt of Nature to purify the body, and all our good, old-fashioned remedies and doctors balk Nature at every turn and we grow up weak, sickly and "resistanceless" mortals.

Don't say "stuff and nonsense!" But think.

Can you imagine good Mother Nature putting a curse on a wee, innocent baby and causing distressing symptoms for nothing?

When you see such morbid matter coming from a child, can you imagine any good reason for damming it back and allowing the tiny body to be poisoned?

Can you see a grown man lying with typhoid fever or pneumonia and think that he is condemned to suffer to satisfy a ravaging nature?

No. Away with pessimism and superstition.

All acute diseases are great eliminating crises. They occur when Nature springs her safety valve.

They do not spring into being in a moment or without cause.

They come to cleanse a body laden with morbid matter accumulated through changes in structure which interfere with functional activities, wrong living, inherited tendencies, or any one of a dozen or two other causes.

Up to a certain point, the body will manufacture materials which attach themselves to the poisons and render them inactive, but when "the last straw that breaks the camel's back" is added, then up pops your eliminating crisis, no matter whether it strikes most severely in the intestines as typhoid, the lungs as pneumonia, or the tonsils as tonsillitis.

If these are eliminating crises, or attempts at elimination and neutralization (and what else can they be?), why should we suppress them? We should not. Nature must be helped.

The first crises seldom kill. It is when repeated crises in early childhood or later in life have been suppressed, or checked, that danger enters, or when suppression has been practiced on the immediate and remote ancestors, and the inherited tendencies are too great for the child to overcome.

Infant mortality is due more to the prevention of Nature's performing her normal function of elimination than to any other cause.

What about getting the germs and catching the disease?

If you do not supply the morbid matter for the germs to thrive on you need have no fear of them. Disease germs do not thrive on healthy bodies. If they did, none of us would be here to tell the tale, which perhaps is the most conclusive argument which can be advanced in favor of this theory.

Think that over for a while. It's worth it.

To sum it all up, acute disease is a beneficial thing when correctly treated, for it is an effort on the part of Nature to throw off that which goes to cause chronic disease. It's the "Safety Valve".

Chronic disease is the result of checking these eliminating efforts of Nature and of lowered vitality. To effect a cure, the vitality of the patient must be increased, and an acute eliminating process produced.

This does not mean that acute diseases do not need treatment, but it does mean that a doctor should be in attendance who will help Nature to make the best of her violent efforts to cleanse the system and thus to make health.

Chronic disease must be treated to bring it to an active eliminating stage, or it can never be cured. The poisons must be forced out of the body.

The cause must be removed, not simply glossed over.

Now you ask what is the natural method of treating disease?

First, correct the connective tissue abnormalities in the region of the spinal nerves which are present in all chronic and most acute diseases.

Second, stop putting wrong food mixtures, poisons and drugs into the system.

Third, assist Nature in every possible manner to get rid of the accumulated morbid matter.

Fourth, prevent the acute manifestations exceeding the body's limitations.

Bad after effects do not come from properly treated acute disease. Wrong treatment is what causes them.

The folks who will have pneumonia or other diseases next winter are laying the foundation **now.** Think that over.

The progressive Naturopath helps Nature to restore health.

You can be cured of any ailment if you have enough vitality to force elimination and support reconstruction, provided you employ a doctor who will direct this vitality to the greatest possible extent in harmony with Nature's efforts.

This the progressive Naturopath does.

Drugs do stimulate the eliminating organs, but they do not prepare the poisons for elimination.

All acute diseases are great eliminating crises.

Chronic disease must be treated to bring it to an active eliminating stage, or it can never be cured. The poisons must be forced out of the body.

"Rational Healing" Address
Dr. Wm. F. Havard

"Rational Healing" Conclusion Of Address
Dr. Wm. F. Havard

Nature

By WM. F. HAVARD

IT is hard to write on disease or other unnatural things when the aromas of Spring are in the air and Nature is waking from her winter sleep. It is hard to keep one's mind upon the ills and ailments of human kind when Nature exercises all her wiles to call us into the open. Even the affairs of nations pale into thin mist and the reports of the peace conference fail to arouse our interest. The boys are at their games on the vacant lots and the little girls are coming forth in garbs of brighter hue, forerunners of Nature's season of joyousness. The Spirit of the Earth is preparing her for a new birth.

Today I saw some shrubbery putting forth its first tiny leaves. I heard a robin chirping on the lawn and had a bee light upon my arm. Nature calls in many tongues. "O Man, put aside for the moment all your boasts and fears. Listen while I speak. Learn now from my gentler moods, that I may never again be called upon to use more forceful measures to impart my knowledge. Put aside your petty squabbles over this and that. Stop fighting over possessions—there is plenty and to spare. No one shall be in want who will obey my laws. For you I produce an abundance and nine-tenths of my efforts are wasted upon you. Come with me to the fields, the woods, the mountains, the brooks, the streams, the rivers, and learn from me the lesson of life. Let me be your teacher. Heed my word and you shall suffer no more."

Do you not hear the call? We who preach about Nature, talk Nature, write Nature, do we live Nature? Do we know Nature and her works, or are we merely clumsily repeating somebody's interpretation of Nature's phenomena? Why take things second-hand when, by putting ourselves in harmony with Nature, we can commune with her spirit and know the truth? Take yourself in solitude to Nature's abode and there let her permeate your being with ennobling thoughts and lofty ideals. Then come back to your everyday affairs with hope renewed, with faith restored, and a heart filled to overflowing with love for your neighbor. So in a world of strife could strife be made to vanish and peace and harmony be made to reign upon earth.

Address On The Subject Of "Rational Healing"

The Twenty-second Annual Convention of the American Naturopathic Association, held on June 6th, 7th and 8th, 1918 at Hotel Winton, Cleveland, Ohio

by Dr. Wm. F. Havard

Herald of Health and Naturopath, XXIV(6), 272-274. (1919)

DR. HAVARD:

I believe the subject which has been given me is Rational Healing.

Very much like the average drugless physician I began the study of this work by taking up the so-called newer systems of drugless healing, largely the manipulative systems.

My first experience with the healing art was with a system known as neuropathy, or what was originally called by its founder or founders mechano-neural therapy. It was a mechanical treatment designed to control the nerve action within certain limits, I wouldn't exactly say control it, but to influence nerve action and particularly the nerve action which related to the animal functions of the body; the nerve action which we know is incorporated in the sympathetic nervous system. It was largely a spinal treatment by the application of certain mechanical, or I should say manual, measures to the spine and thermal applications. The application of heat and cold with the idea of either raising or lowering the sympathetic nerve activity and so bringing about the necessary changes in circulation and effecting a cleansing of the various tissues of the body, and a purification of the blood.

Like all of the rest of those systems, when it was first inaugurated it was hailed as a cure-all. It took three years of practical experience with this work to teach me where its shortcomings lay. Hearing of some of these other systems at that time, particularly chiropractic, and having had already some acquaintance with osteopathy, I found they were up against practically the same obstacle in bringing individuals back to a state of health. I found that these treatments, while they gave benefit, while they gave relief were not capable of carrying an individual through all of the processes of cure; that there were certain essentials that these systems failed to take into consideration. They failed to make any distinction between acute and chronic diseases. Any deviation from normal was looked at from the same angle, from the same standpoint. Anything, I might say, in the nature of a disturbance of function, was considered to be a disease. I found this out, that in the course of treatment of diseased conditions by these mechanical measures, before I knew anything about diet or hydropathy, I found that inevitably the individual who was being treated for some chronic condition would develop in the course of his treatment an acute condition. Of course, at that time we were influenced to a large extent by medical conceptions of disease. We had accepted medical symptomology. We had accepted medical diagnosis, we had accepted the germ theory as to the cause of disease, we recognized that the germ was a primary irritant which was introduced into the body from the outside, and at the moment it got in there it disturbed function and raised havoc. I found after a time that this conception of diseases, or of the cause of diseases, was to a large extent erroneous; that the poor germ was really maligned, that he was not, even in these acute conditions, the primary cause of the disease. I went on studying, taking up one system after another and practicing them until I became thoroughly discouraged and disheartened. The results were not up to the claims of any of them, they all fell short. And I said to myself, drugless healing is attempting the impossible, it is attempting to relieve the individual of the natural consequences of his own acts, carelessness or ignorance, in other words, it is striving at vicarious atonement.

I had studied the various systems of philosophy and I came to the conclusion that there were certain principles in nature which were absolute and that there were certain laws in nature which were largely timely or circumstantial.

I came to the conclusion there were definite laws regarding the health or the normal operation of the body and I came to the conclusion there must be definite laws regarding the unnatural operation of the body or the operation which took place during the process of disease. I concluded that these two phases were expressions of the laws of action and reaction.

I said to myself, disease cannot be a haphazard matter, it must have some foundation. And it was about that time that there fell into my hands a book, a very old book, a book which was written in the year 1861 originally, a book called the *New Science of Healing* by Kuhne, and I got just one fact out of that book. I overlooked a great deal that was of value, but my mind was searching for something, and when I stuck on that one fact everything else in the book was obliterated, so I just carried the memory of that one thing, and that is the unity of disease and the unity of cure— that disease at the foundation is all one, that these things which are called diseases are all nothing more than the manifestations of a primary cause. And Kuhne pointed out that primary cause. He said it is the accumulation of morbid matter, waste products within the body. Kuhne was not very scientific, we have to acknowledge that, and I mean by that, he did not go ahead and explain in detail every step in the production of disease. I forgot my former discouragement and went back to the problem with a new enthusiasm.

It was about that time I became acquainted with Dr. Lindlahr in Chicago, and read his book on Nature Cure, and then I made up my mind that I had the essence of the whole thing, that I could now explain scientifically, in accordance with our knowledge of anatomy, physiology and pathology, every step in the process of disease and every step that is necessary to be taken towards the cure of disease.

Now you think with that knowledge (of course, I am not the only one that has it, there are thousands of people in this country that have same thing) and the ability to put in into operation cure would be a simple thing. But these curists overlooked the personal equation in this proposition: they overlook the fact when they believe they treat diseased conditions they are in reality treating an individual, a person. They are not treating the disease. We have now certain men who are endeavoring to combine all of the physical methods of therapy. They are using all of these so-called natural agents, trying to put them into operation from exactly the same standpoint as the medical man prescribes his drugs, largely for counter-active purposes. They are treating symptoms only, and that is the difference between physiological therapeutics and Nature Cure. The physiological therapist employs all or most of the measures which are used in nature cure, but he has not the fundamental conception of disease and its cure. He only has in his mind the immediate symptoms, while the nature-curist has a plan in mind, and he employs these various methods of treatment with the idea of producing two effects, and then he leaves the rest to nature. His first object in the rational treatment of an individual suffering from some diseased condition, is to produce greater elimination. Now, you heard a very splendid talk last night from Dr. Pratt, and Dr. Pratt told you that the blood stream was the keynote to the whole situation. In the blood are either the products which will tend towards destruction of right physiological action, and ultimately to changes of structure of the organization, or it has within it those products and energies which will maintain the right and proper balance within the body, which will promote harmonious action and which will keep the individual in a state of health.

I wish I could review the whole system of pathology with you. I wish I could start in with the very inception of disease and carry it right through to its ultimate conclusion, where it either renders the body absolutely incapable of performing its functions, resulting in death, or where it results in the culmination of a healing crisis which produces complete elimination of all waste products and of all disease products from the body.

The nature-curist, besides having in mind the increase of elimination, or the draining out of the body or out of the blood stream of those products which are at the foundation of the disease, works on another principle, and that is of raising the individual's power of resistance to a point of establishing a reaction. Now, Dr. Pratt told you another thing. He told you it was not the immediate effect of any measure or method which you employ for the cure of disease that really did the work, but it was the body's reaction to what you did for it, or to it, that in reality brought about the changes, physiological changes, which would result in changing the process from one of disease to one of cure.

I came to the conclusion there were definite laws regarding the health or the normal operation of the body and I came to the conclusion there must be definite laws regarding the unnatural operation of the body or the operation which took place during the process of disease. I concluded that these two phases were expressions of the laws action and reaction.

Kuhne pointed out that primary cause. He said it is the accumulation of morbid matter, waste products within the body.

The nature-curist, besides having in mind the increase of elimination, or the draining out of the body or out of the blood stream of those products which are at the foundation of the disease, works on another principle, and that is of raising the individual's power of resistance to a point of establishing a reaction.

"Rational Healing" Conclusion Of Address

The Twenty-second Annual Convention of the American Naturopathic Association, held on June 6th, 7th and 8th, 1918 at Hotel Winton, Cleveland, Ohio

Stenographic Report Of Dr. Wm. F. Havard

Herald of Health and Naturopath, XXIV(6), 272-274. (1919)

DR. HAVARD:

Now, under these circumstances the cell is taken up entirely with this manner of performing its internal function and stops contributing to a large extent to the general operation of the body, and as a consequence the individual becomes weak; he has to take a recumbent position because of the tendencies of the blood pressure to fall. But remember this, that every individual cell in that body is more active than in the ordinary state of health, much more active. Do not ever think under an acute condition that the cells of the body are weak and inactive. There is a revolution going on in that body. Here comes your other compensation. Under these circumstances the heart action must increase, and we all know how high the heart action is likely to run in a case of pneumonia.

What are you going to do with this case? Are you going to treat him in such a way as to knock down the fever, are you going to literally hit him on the head with a club and stop his activity, are you going to give him a dose of medicine that will stop this reaction in the body or destroy all compensation, or are you going to nurse him along and let nature work the thing out? What can you do? The best you can do in your treatment of any acute disease is first to get rid of the idea of trying to counteract symptoms and nurse the case. It does not require so much treatment as it does nursing so that you will not interfere with the natural reaction which is taking place in that body. If you try to increase the respiration or try to decrease the heart rate or try this or that with your various methods of psychological therapies, you are only delaying your case. You are delaying your case and instead of the individual recovering from that attack of pneumonia and being built up into a healthier and stronger individual than he ever was before, by getting out of his system all this accumulated morbid matter, your individual is liable to go into a chronic state of the disease, and we have so many pneumonia cases terminating in an accumulation of pus in the pleura, which has had to be drained off and the individual is sick and in bed sometimes for months where, as matter of fact he ought to be back on his feet within three weeks at the most.

Furthermore, every medical man knows that a pneumonia patient who recovers after medical treatment has to be watched for the development of tuberculosis. Every doctor watches his pneumonia recoveries very carefully to see if they are going to develop any of the symptoms of tuberculosis. Why? Because the process that was going on there has been interfered with, and these poisons have been thrown back into the system and bottled up there to again cause trouble instead of begin allowed to pour out at the proper time. Do not concern yourself with the reduction of the fever, do not concern yourself with the reduction of the heart action. That body is doing everything it possibly can to throw off those conditions itself. Do not interfere; do not place yourself above the intelligence of that body by attempting to counteract its reactions. Some of us have a very hazy conception of the physiological functions of the body or the normal reaction to disturbances and the compensatory actions which occur in that body. Your treatment of this case must be in such a manner as to help the body to increase its elimination.

Now, suppose I give you a prescription for the treatment of pneumonia. Would it work in every case? No, only from a general standpoint. You always have to use your own judgment, use your thinking apparatus in every individual case. The outcome of a great many of these conditions does not depend on the methods you employ because some individuals have such a strong power of reaction that they will get better in spite of anything harmful you may do to them. But I am going to give you a prescription for the treatment of pneumonia, and I might say it applies to almost any acute condition. The first thing is to clean out the alimentary tract and keep it clean during the entire process. Put nothing in there that will ferment or decompose, because remember the process of digestion cannot go on while this reaction is taking place in the body. Any food you place in there simply increases decomposition, putrefaction, and helps to poison the body all the more. The old idea of the treatment of pneumonia was to feed the patient with the idea of building up his strength, and it is coming back into being in the medical profession, even in the typhoid fever. Some of the doctors are beginning to recommend feeding a typhoid patient. But the first thing is to cut out food. Then what are you going to give the individual? Nothing but water, the broth from vegetables (made without meats or fats), which contain a high percentage of organic salts, which are so necessary to the body in helping render crystalline all of these colloid waste articles, or give him the juice of citrus fruits. You will have to use your judgment about that. Usually the pneumonia patient craves clear fruit juice like orange juice, grape juice, grape-fruit juice or lemon and water. All of these fruit juices must be fresh, do not use canned fruits, do not use prepared or bottled preparations, give fresh fruits, and the citrus fruits are the best. What does that do? It helps promote elimination, it keeps the kidneys open, keeps the bowels open, it helps to neutralize and render crystalline waste products so that the lungs will be relieved of this enormous burden that has been imposed upon them. In other words, you will not have such a great pouring of your waste material into the air sacs, or as the case may be into the space between the cells around the air sacs, or wherever that condition manifests itself.

What is another factor in this treatment? To make the skin active. You heard a little talk on the skin last night and I hope some of you took it to heart. Think of the skin as an enormous sewage system. Think of the miles of pipes that we have in the skin. Now, here is your best friend—your best friend in the treatment of acute diseases is the skin. What do you want to do? Why, we have a body where the temperature has been raised several degrees above normal. There is an acute reaction going on. In the beginning, in order to maintain that reaction and keep up that temperature, there must be some compensation upon the part of the vasomotor mechanism, and we have all the blood vessels of the skin contracting, and in contracting they cut down the blood supply and consequently the activity of the skin is decreased. That condition maintains for a certain length of time, it may be hours or days. It is a compensatory action, but here is the thing: you have a great internal generation of heat now with very little radiation, so that your temperature is likely to go too high unless some relief measure is employed—unless you use some means to increase the radiation and elimination by increasing the skin action: so we now endeavor to open up the pores. Now, you can do this by heat, can't you? You know you can bring the blood to the surface of the body by the application of heat, but we have found—and that has been known for a few centuries—that the application of heat has an immediate effect and it is quickly over, and so we have to turn to the other practice. Remember I told you that thermal measures were irritants, and that they only worked or acted through their power of bringing about a reaction in the body; they were only effective to that extent. So what do we do? We use cold to the surface of the body. Now you say, "Oh, do you approve of throwing a pneumonia patient into a tub of ice water?" Not by any manner of means. That is criminal, barbarous, you are likely to kill your patient, the shock is too great. How about cold sponge baths and alcohol rubs? Alcohol through its rapid evaporation draws out a certain amount of heat, and reduces the temperature temporarily, but it is not our concern to reduce the temperature without getting at the cause of the rise of the temperature. Approve of cold sponge baths? No. How are you going to apply cold? We are going to envelop that individual in a sheet which has been dipped in cold water. In order to prepare your patient for this you put down a rubber sheet, put on top of that two blankets, usually two are enough, two heavy blankets, and on top of that upper blanket put your wet sheet; place the patient on the wet sheet and wrap him carefully in it so that only his head is exposed and you bring over that the blankets and pin them fast so that individual is obliged to remain encased like a mummy. The first effect is to create constriction; reaction of constriction is dilation, and you have the circulation drawn to the surface with increased radiation and elimination. The pack keeps drawing off heat until after an hour or so of such procedure you have the temperature down two or three degrees. The effect of the wet pack is to draw the circulation to the surface, thus increasing elimination, and when that individual is taken out of the sheet pack you will find that sheet is stained with waste products which have been drawn out of the blood. I have seen sheets of that sort taken off a typhoid fever patient that were almost brown. Please study use and application of packs.

What else do we do? But very little, very little else. Simply watch your case, keep your patient in that pack for a certain length of time; it may be an hour or two hours. It is never advisable to reduce the temperature too much. If the temperature is 106, be satisfied for the first time when it falls to 104, take him out and dry him thoroughly—there must be no draughts in the room—and let him rest. Renew your pack after an hour or so if your temperature shows a tendency to rise again.

Now remember the cleanliness of the alimentary tract. Keep it clean throughout the entire proceedings, by not introducing anything, any food at all, which will undergo decomposition. The body doesn't need it. Don't feed proteins or starches. While the cells of the body are eliminating to a great extent, they are not taking in very much besides oxygen, salts, and water. Their process of rehabilitation comes after the acute attack is over. You cannot carry on the two processes at once. While the cell is tearing down, throwing out waste products, cleaning its house, it doesn't want to eat and won't eat. Don't try to feed the patient; the patient doesn't want it in the first place.

I may say that process, that prescription is good for the treatment of any acute disease. Just recognize these acute conditions as the natural reaction of the body, and instead of trying to treat them and counteract the symptoms, let nature do the work she is seeking to do.

How about the chronic case; what about him? An individual suffering from chronic disease, or from some chronic disease process, is only an individual whose power or reaction and whose power of resistance has been incapable of rising to that point where it will produce a reaction in the body. In other words, if the individual had an acute attack of some kind, his body would have been relieved of the poisons, but here we have certain conditions which go on accumulating year after year, these things that we call auto-intoxication, and the body never makes a reaction, because our habits are such that we keep down the natural resistance of the body, we lower our vitality either through not taking sufficient rest or through overstimulation of the body by these various habits, and things that we have contracted which are contrary to nature, and we slip into this state of chronic disease and ultimately die due to the fact that the organs have become so encumbered, so overloaded, that they are not capable of relieving the body of these irritants, and our life functions are in reality prematurely worn out through the action of foreign agency.

Now, that is what we call rational therapy: the treatment of chronic patients—mind you , I don't say disease—the treatment of chronic patients or patients chronically diseased, for the purpose of increasing their elimination, increasing their power of resistance to the point where the body will of its own accord react to those conditions.

Now, I have been asked this question often, so that I am going to anticipate you in this matter. I know it is going to occur to somebody's mind. Is it necessary to produce this reaction? Does the individual have to go through those crises in a case of a chronic disease? I will say this, that if the cure is to be complete the individual must go through the crisis, there must be a reaction. Only acute conditions are "curable." Things cannot be normalized, cannot be stabilized, unless there is a revolution in that body. And why? We hear the blood stream is a great carrier, consists of the healing properties as well as the disease properties. Now, suppose through doing a lot of natural treating we succeed in stimulating the organs of elimination, neutralizing and helping with the elimination of waste products, and we practically clean the blood stream. You say that is all that is necessary. The blood is clean, nature will do the rest, the body will return to a situation of health; a process of reconstruction will set in. Did you ever consider this factor? That disease is in the cell? You all know the principle of osmosis, and how the cells feed. How many have studied cellular physiology? It is not a long story, but at the same time I fear I am taking up too much time here. The contents of the cell and the contents of the blood stream are about the same specific gravity. There is about the same osmotic pressure in the blood that there is in the cell, which is subject to certain fluctuations like the tides of the ocean. There is a rise and fall of osmotic pressure. In the cell there is a rise and fall in the pressure and in the blood stream. But these changes are so small that we say that this pressure is practically a constant, but it is not. (The mean pressure is constant.) If it were every operation of the body would stop; it can never be allowed. Conditions on the inside of the cell and outside of the cell can never be permitted to thoroughly equalize on another. But there is a tendency to equalization as well as a force to prevent it. What is the force which swings the pendulum; what is the action in the body that prevents it? Why, it is the chest action, the breath function, the rise and fall of the chest, that is the thing that keeps the pendulum swinging from side to side, it changes the pressure, the osmotic pressure. That changes even the density slightly in each case, just enough to keep the products flowing in two directions, on the expansion the products into the cell, on the contraction the surplus and wastes flow out of the cell. (Don't confuse this with the expansion and contraction of muscles.) This expansion and contraction of the cell keeps things moving so that there is a flow of renewing material, oxygen, and all of the food products into the cell and there is a flow in the other direction of the waste products out of the cell. So you have a continuous change going on which spells l-i-f-e. Life is a continuous change.

Now, suppose you have the same products in the cell as you have on the outside of the cell, and suppose these products in the blood stream surrounding the cell are, say, disease products, and they get into the cell. You notice that disease products within the cell cut down the activity of the individual cell.

In the chronic disease process you have the same disease product within the cell as in the blood stream and as a consequence there is very little exchange, or change in the constituents of the cells through the process of osmosis, and the cell holds much accumulated matter and its own waste. If you cleanse the blood stream, you disturb the balance which existed between the blood contents and the cell contents. What does the cell begin to do? When it finds a clearer, purer blood stream; when it becomes surrounded by products which are health giving instead of disease giving, then it begins its reaction to throw out of itself all morbid matter. It is the cleansing of the individual cells of the body which brings about the acute reaction. Otherwise all of your acute reaction would only be local manifestation. Every one of these healing crises, as we choose to call them, are general manifestations. They involve the whole organization, throw the whole organization into a hyperactive state. What I call rational therapy, is to treat your chronic, because therapy only applies to chronics, in such a manner as to bring the condition to an acute stage. The body is its own therapeutic agent when it comes to the acute condition. In the chronic conditions we have to employ certain methods of therapy in order to induce the body to react. Now, what will they be? That is up to every individual who undertakes to conduct the cure of a patient. The methods and the measures and the means he will select, are largely in accordance to the conditions which he has to deal with.

Now, do you blame us when we hesitate a little about endorsing these different systems that claim to be complete in themselves, that make such exaggerated claims? When a hydropath comes along and says he can do everything with a hose and a towel? The hydropath can do a great deal, but not everything. Do you blame us when we cannot sanction the use, excessive use of one little method for the cure of all kinds of diseases? We cannot conscientiously do it. But we say this, we recognize this much: that every one of these systems is doing a good work in one respect, that it is giving the people a new conception of health, a new conception of life. They are getting the people out of the ruts; and in time it will remain for the more liberal ones, for those who recognize the fundamental principles of things, to educate these men who have started with their one little system, just as I said I had started, in the same way, and I think if every one of us were honest we would all say at some time we had some little bug working in us that directed us into and held us in a certain narrow little groove.

It is all a matter of education, of development. It is all in our evolution for us to learn and realize one thing after another. But suppose you just went along learning this thing and that and the other thing, one method and system of healing after another, and you had no common foundation for all these things; you do not recognize any laws or principles, but apply these measures separately and independently, why, then you are a physiological therapist; but if you put all of these things on a fundamental basis and recognize the natural physiological actions and reactions of the body, and you work with the idea of completely cleansing that body of its disease producing elements through its natural actions, then you are a naturopath.

The best you can do in your treatment of any acute disease is first to get rid of the idea of trying to counteract symptoms and nurse the case.

Do not interfere, do not place yourself above the intelligence of that body by attempting to counteract its reactions.

Does the individual have to go through those crises in a case of a chronic disease? I will say this, that if the cure is to be complete the individual must go through the crisis, there must be a reaction.

An advertisement soliciting Naturopaths to join the A.N.A. membership.

Naturopathy Versus Medicine
Per Nelson, N.D.

Can The Mind Heal All Diseases
E. Dickenson

Benedict Lust's publishing company, renowned for its large selection of Nature Cure classics, also published books by Helen Wilmans on mental culture.

Naturopathy Versus Medicine

by Per Nelson, N.D., Harford, Conn.

Herald of Health and Naturopath, XXV(2), 78-82. (1920)

One need not use lanterns or field glasses to discover the many defects of the so-called science of medicine; neither does one need to waste any time in constructing arguments against the drug system, for the reason that this system itself furnishes us with the best of arguments, —living arguments, if you please.

Look around in any community and what will you find? You will find hundreds, yes, thousands of so-called incurables or chronics—men, women and children. You will meet them on the street, in the trolley cars, churches and everywhere. You will see thousands of crippled and defective people, thousands of nervous wrecks,—yes, and their dull eyes, their bent backs, their deformed bodies, their shaky limbs and their pale faces will tell you a story, not only of the inefficiency of the drug treatment, but of **malpractice, the thousand time damnable malpractice that is going on.**

Visit the hospitals, the insane asylums, the institutions for dope fiends, the colonies for epileptics, the homes for defective children.

Do you wish for any more evidence? Do you want any sharper arguments against the system of medicine? Can you help wondering why we have so many defectives? Haven't you read in the Sunday paper about the advance in medical science? What is the matter with this crazy world, anyway? Why all this suffering?

Haven't we got health boards in every city and town? Haven't we a dozen doctors,—highly educated, college-bred and dignified men—in every city building? Haven't we a drug store on every street corner, each one with barrels of specific drugs?

Let us calm ourselves. Let us stop asking questions. Let us try to reason out what is wrong with medicine, and also what we can do to alleviate all this suffering. The history of medicine will help in this respect, and we will therefore consult her pages. She tells us, among other things, that there was a time when disease was looked upon as something mysterious or supernatural that no human being could explain; something frightful that had to be fought with all kinds of weapons. Yes, the belief at that time was that evil spirits entered the bodies of persons who were sick and that these had to be driven out by forcible means for driving out evil spirits, such as, for instance, prayer, temple sleep, etc.

The very same idea, but in somewhat modified form prevails in the science of medicine of our day. The evil spirits of today are the germs, and the whip that is used in driving them out is the drug; and these germs, according to medical science, are lurking around everywhere to find those "whom they may destroy." In other words, medical science attributes the various diseases (to the presence of specific disease—producing microorganisms, some of which have been discovered and classified into "family groups," others, again, that have escaped the eyes of the bacteriologists, and who, therefore, work on our destruction like thieves at night. These germs, according to medical science, are carried around by flies, mice, mosquitoes, dogs and cats, and also, according to the latest fad, by "human germ carriers."

Germs are supposed to be equally dangerous to each and every one of us, and no matter how strong and healthy we are, if it should happen that they get into our systems, they will at once begin to raise "cane" with us, especially so if we haven't had all of the 59 varieties of artificial antitoxins injected into our blood.

With the above conception of disease, we can readily grasp the reason why practically all of the research work conducted in medical circles today is concentrated on the discovery and production of serums of antitoxins that will kill off these germs, and, as shown during the recent influenza epidemic, they have succeeded in this respect so remarkably well, that not only the lives of the germs, but in many instances also the lives of the patients were taken.

In contrast to the medical men, the Naturopaths do not blame disease on external causes, which are not under our control, but claim that disease is merely the result of bad habits or wrong modes of living, which have to be corrected before a cure is possible. We claim that all persons born from healthy parents have a certain amount of vitality. This vitality or force controls and enables all organs and parts of the body to functionate. If the vitality is good, the skin, bowels, kidneys, lungs and every organ in the body will functionate properly. The food we eat will be transformed into heat, energy and tissues, and the gases that are set loose in this chemical process, as well as the waste materials given off from the cells, will be expelled from the body through the four channels mentioned above (the skin, kidneys, bowels and lungs). But should we abuse ourselves in any manner, so as to lower our vitality, (this can be done in hundreds of ways, such as, for instance, through sexual abuse, over-eating, lack of sleep, overwork, etc., etc.,) the organs of excretion will at once become impaired, and poisonous gases and waste products that under normal conditions would leave the body, will begin to collect. When this has been going on for some time, Nature will be forced to try a housecleaning, and this she performs in the form of an acute disease. Thus it will be seen that acute disease is nothing more than an outbreak of morbid matter that has accumulated in the system, hence the bad odor you will always find in the sick-room.

Acute disease may be compared with a thunderstorm on a hot summer day. When the air is loaded with foreign substances, the thunderstorm is bound to come and clear the atmosphere. But what would happen if we, through some artificial means, could suppress or hinder the thunderstorm from breaking? Simply this: The air would become so foul that we could hardly breathe. And this is just what takes place when we suppress the body's thunderstorm, the acute diseases, and here lies the terrible crime that has been, and is being committed daily, and the very cause that has produced our chronics, our invalids and nervous wrecks. Here is the cause that has filled our hospitals, insane asylums and homes for defective children.

The recent influenza epidemic has probably more than anything else proven the Naturopathic conception of disease to be correct. What was the cause of the so-called Spanish influenza? Let us see. We all know that the American nation is a wheat-eating nation. Being wheat-eaters, our systems have been accustomed and are quite able to neutralize and to get rid of the waste products of wheat; but, owing to war conditions, the government deemed it necessary to substitute wheat with barley and corn-meal. Now, everybody knows that barley and corn-meal ferment very readily, and as our systems were not used to handling these "sticky" substances, their waste products began to clog our cells and tissue-spaces. Well, everything went fine until the leaves started to fall from the trees and ferment. During that time of the year the air is always full of fermentive substances, and as we inhaled these substances, as the air in the sick-room of those who had this disease, the barley and cornmeal products, which loaded our systems, were set into fermentation, and here is the whole "mystery" of the Spanish influenza, which seemed to puzzle especially our medical men so very much.

As a contributing cause, we can mention that early in the fall, we had a short spell of very cold weather, which scared a number of people into heavier underwear. After this short spell of cold weather, we had about two months of very warm weather, but many of those who had put on heavier underwear during the short cold spell, continued to wear it during the two warm months that followed, and in this manner interfered with the skin elimination. Sorrow, caused by loss of relatives and friends in the Great War, also undermined the body vitality, and in this manner made the population more susceptible to disease. Overwork, which was very common during the war, may also be regarded as a contributing cause.

The causes of other acute diseases are identical with influenza, in that they always constitute Nature's efforts to eliminate waste material from the system. An individual description of each and every one of them would be superfluous. We will, therefore, leave the subject of acute diseases in order to describe chronic disease.

What is a chronic disease? A chronic disease is a condition where the body is so loaded with waste material that Nature can not arouse herself in an active reaction, or produce the "thunderstorm" that would rid the system of poisonous waste material, and this accounts for the heavy, draggy feeling always connected with chronic disease. The cause has already been explained; it was simply due to the suppressing of the acute diseases by means of strong drugs, which rendered the poisonous waste material in the body latent, instead of expelling it through the body's natural channels. These waste products, after being sealed up in the body, inhibited Nature's functions, and attacked the cells and structures, sometimes only causing functional disturbances, but more often causing pathological changes in the tissues themselves.

Insanity and mental diseases are but another form of chronic disease, and very similar to all other chronic ailments. One need not be a philosopher to understand that if a human brain is built up on pure blood alone, and if only pure blood is circulating through its vessels, that no insanity can exist unless same is caused by external traumatic conditions.

If, on the other hand, the brain is built up on abnormal and poisonous blood, and if only poisonous blood is circulating through the vessels, constantly irritating the cells and structures, then, of course, insanity or other mental diseases must necessarily be the logical outcome, and here again the blame is to be placed on the suppressive methods used by the medical profession.

When knowing the nature of disease, i.e., that acute diseases are simply Nature's way of expelling poisonous waste matter from the system, and that chronic disease is caused by the sealing up in the body of these same substances, it is easily reasoned out that elimination must necessarily be the keynote to the treatment of all diseases, and here is where the Naturopath comes in with his hydrotherapy and massage, his light treatments and electricity, his chiropractic stimulation and concussion, his diet and mental suggestion, his herb and bio-chemical remedies. In other words, the Naturopath simply assists Nature in her efforts to eliminate waste material through the body's natural channels, by improving and equalizing the body fluids, and by stimulating the lungs, kidneys, bowels and skin to normal activity, and this is the reason why Naturopaths are able to cure diseases after all other systems have failed to do so.

But the Naturopath goes even further than to merely cure disease. Knowing that transgression of Nature's laws lies at the root of all human ills, he also considers it his duty to teach humanity how to follow these laws, thereby making it possible for them to avoid disease. The Naturopath is, therefore, not only a healer who is able to cure disease, but also a reformer and preacher in the true sense of the word, and he believes in his system not only as a science and an art, but as a religion that will, if followed, lead humanity to the heaven of health and happiness.

As I have not, in the above description of disease been mentioning the germs at all, some one may ask: What about the germs? Is it not possible that they cause disease, or if they do not, what then is their function, and in what way are they related to disease?

In order to answer these questions, it is necessary to make a comparative study of germs and their functions in all Nature, not only in the bacteriological laboratories, and perhaps if we find out what their function is outside of our bodies, then we can probably be in a better position to draw our conclusions as to their function in our interior during acute disease.

As far as we can make out at the present time, and as we will try to prove in the following, the function of germ life in all Nature is to split up complex chemical compounds into simpler ones. Let us begin with a few illustrations from farm life. When the farmer or gardener sows his vegetables seeds in the ground, these seeds are at once attacked by thousands of germs, and their albuminous matter is through this germ action softened and broken up into simpler chemical substances, which the young seedling is able to use for its nourishment.

The same happens when fertilizer is put into the ground. Here again the germs have to split up the complex material of the fertilizer into simple substances, which can be used as a food for the plants. Indeed, manure which has not been acted upon by bacteria is practically useless. The up-to-date farmer knows this. He therefore always puts the manure in heaps for ripening, as he calls it. During this ripening process, the manure is attacked by billions and billions of germs, and all complex materials are thus converted into simple chemical substances.

Let us take another illustration from germ life, which will perhaps be a little different from the previous two. We all know that when a tree falls in the forest, it does not forever stay on the top of the ground. After a short while we find that its bark loosens from the wood and falls off. A while longer, and we find that the whole tree has been reduced to a powdery mass, which is finally absorbed by the soil. What has happened in this case? The same as happened to the vegetable seed and the fertilizer. Here again the germs have been at work and reduced its solid mass into substances which can again be used in Nature's cycle.

Hundreds of illustrations, similar to the ones spoken of above, could be given to prove our assertion that the function of germ life in all Nature is to split up complex matter into simpler chemical substances, but they would in the main be the same story repeated, and as my article has already lengthened to a greater dimension than was intended at its start, I shall give just one more example, taken direct from the greatest laboratory in the world—the human body.

We are often told that millions of germs are lodged in our intestines, but we are very seldom told what their function is. Needless, however, to say that their function there is the same as everywhere else in all Nature—to split up complex chemical compounds into simpler ones. Foods that have escaped the digestive fluids are thus acted upon by various kinds of bacteria. Proteins are broken up into peptone amino-acids and ammonia, starches into sugars, fats into valeric and butyric acid, cellulose into carbonic acid and methane, etc., etc.

Now, if we use a little logic and reasoning, what conclusions can we form from the foregoing? Must we not necessarily be led to the belief that if the germ-function everywhere else in Nature is to split up complex compounds into simpler ones, that that most likely also is their function during acute diseases, and when we furthermore know, as stated in the beginning of this article, that acute disease is merely an outbreak of morbid matter, then it seems so much more logical that the germs must be present during an acute attack in order to split up or decompose the complex colloid material which otherwise would remain too complex to be eliminated.

The Naturopath, therefore, holds the view that the germs are the result of the disease, and not its cause, and that germ action during acute disease (the splitting up of complex pathogenic material into substances which the body is able to eliminate) is beneficial, not harmful.

Now, someone may ask: "Is it not possible that there are harmful germs also, as well as useful ones, inasmuch as in animal life we have poisonous snakes and reptiles, and in vegetable life poison ivy, etc., and if that is the ease, is it, then, not proper to kill off these dangerous germs with strong drugs?"

To this we answer: Yes; it is quite true that there are a few species of dangerous germs—for instance, the tetanus germ (Bacillus tetani); but these dangerous germs are in a very small minority compared with the thousands of different species of useful germs, and do not affect the body unless there is a medium in which they can live—an accumulation of foreign matter, in other words. But in the treatment, the Naturopath again holds the trump card, as the danger from these germs lies in the fact that they produce poisonous toxins which affect the body structures. It, therefore, stands to reason that elimination, the great principle on which Naturopathy is founded, is again the proper measure to employ—indeed, elimination is the only salvation in these cases, as pathogenic germs show a very high resistance to poisonous drugs. The problem of killing pathogenic germs inside of our bodies with strong drugs is identical to killing our selves, and has, therefore, no therapeutic foundation whatsoever.

But the world slowly but surely keeps on moving, and old theories everywhere are forced to make room for new and more advanced ones, and this holds true in the science of medicine also, despite all efforts, conscious or unconscious, to hold back the wheels of progress; and as a result of this, we find broadminded men in the medical profession also—men who dare to think for themselves, and who are not afraid to let the world know their thoughts.

In contrast to the medical men, the Naturopaths do not blame disease on external causes, which are not under our control, but claim that disease is merely the result of bad habits or wrong modes of living, which have to be corrected before a cure is possible.

In other words, the Naturopath simply assists Nature in her efforts to eliminate waste material through the body's natural channels, by improving and equalizing the body fluids, and by stimulating the lungs, kidneys, bowels and skin to normal activity, and this is the reason why Naturopaths are able to cure diseases after all other systems have failed to do so.

We are often told that millions of germs are lodged in our intestines, but we are very seldom told what their function is. Needless, however, to say that their function there is the same as everywhere else in all Nature—to split up complex chemical compounds into simpler ones.

CAN THE MIND HEAL ALL DISEASES?

by E. Dickenson

Herald of Health and Naturopath, XXV(3), 140-143. (1920)

An address given before the People's Forum of the Llano Colony, Leesville, La., the largest Socialist colony in the world, Tuesday evening, June 18, 1918.

To the question, "Can the mind heal all diseases?", there can be but one correct answer in the light of the proved facts of the time.

The Mind can and does heal all diseases. It has done so from the dawn of history. But it is doing so today on a larger scale than ever before, and anyone who takes the trouble to honestly and sincerely investigate a few of the hundreds of thousands of cases of permanent mental healing, must acknowledge this.

The Christian Science church with its two million members or more, the New Thought centers and societies with about an equal number of members and believers, and the multitude of other cults and organizations which practice mental healing in one form or another and under one name or another—faith curists, Swedenborgians, adherents of the Emmanuel movement of the orthodox churches, "Divine" healers, Dowieites, etc.—furnish undeniable evidence of the practically unlimited control of the mind over the body. These organizations are composed of people of exceptional intelligence and judgment. To say that they are falsifying would be ridiculous. What would be their object in pretending they have been healed when they have not been healed? Even if they had an object, they could not "get away with it" and cursory investigation would quickly expose the misrepresentations. Granted, then, that they are not falsifying, it is equally as preposterous to assert that they are deceived. They might with much more justice say that believers in drugs and doctors who continue to be sick, are deceived, and they—the believers in mind cures—are right in their beliefs, since they are daily demonstrating their faith by their physical conditions.

To say that persons receiving mental treatment have died, is no answer to the statement that the mind can and does heal all diseases. Believers in the efficacy of medicine do not blame the medical science for the death of patients under the care of physicians. They assume that the death took place because the physician did not know and apply his own science as thoroughly as he should. The same is claimed by advocates of mental healing and the claim is an entirely reasonable one. They assert that as believers in the power of the mind over the body, learn the higher laws of nature more fully, and comply with them to greater extent, they will be more and more successful in both healing and preventing disease.

It should be borne in mind that a majority of cases that are brought to mental healers are cases which have been given up by physicians, as "incurable". If mental science can heal such ailments—as it has done and is doing all of the time—what can it do when the world generally comes to believe in it and practice it, first-hand, instead of going to medical doctors first and mental healers afterward?

Even under tests which were and are manifestly difficult, mental healing has more than held its own. It has healed hundreds of thousands of people who were scheduled for the cemetery in short order by orthodox doctors and hospitals. And this as the result of New Thought or scientific thinking, applied, in most cases, for first time in a whole lifetime, when the accumulated thoughts of fear, worry, evil passion, anger and expectancy of sickness and old age, had crystallized into diseased cells and decomposing tissues, which the healer was expected to transform in a few days or a few weeks.

If the mind can restore the body to health in such cases, counteracting the wrong living and wrong thinking of many years, it certainly can build up a body which will never be sick, just as mental scientists claim, if it sends its energies of thought into right channels regularly and consistently, all of the time.

If you say, "Oh, yes, the mind can heal some diseases, but not all diseases, for that is impossible", I will reply by referring you to the countless cures that are being made all over the world every day of our lives. They are facts. They can be verified easily. They are found almost entirely among people who have hitherto been unbelievers in New Thought, mental science and allied beliefs, so the cases are the more convincing. I venture that there are many right here in this meeting who have been cured or have friends who have been cured by mental methods. And I venture that even in so small a number as the few hundred people living in this colony, the diseases healed by mind, include most of the known physical ailments.

For a few instances which I personally know about, I will mention that I know a woman who had been a cripple for years; a young man who had tuberculosis and was pronounced by several doctors as sure to die within a year; a man who had a long standing case of stricture, extending over several years; a woman who had suffered from both insomnia and constipation for a long time, and a man who had been subject to asthma from childhood, all of whom were absolutely healed by New Thought healers. There is no guesswork about these cases. I know them, for I know the persons, knew their former condition and know their present condition. In each case no medicine was used and the patient was healed solely by mental methods.

Bear in mind, mental healing does not confine itself to slight affections such as headaches, nervousness, insomnia, etc. It is just as effective in dealing with functional and organic ailments. In fact, it is by curing serious diseases in so-called "incurable" cases, that the science of mental healing has gained so many adherents.

In magazines like the *Nautilus*, published at Holyoke, Mass.; *Unity*, published in Kansas City, Mo.; *The Christian Science Journal*, published in Boston, Mass., and other journals of the cults which practice mental healing, hundreds of testimonials may be read each month, testimonials which are signed, and in which the addresses of the healed persons and the names of corroborating witnesses are given. Skeptics who have written or called on some of these persons have been astonished to find the overwhelming testimony in favor of mental healing that has been quickly laid before them.

Dr. Thos. Jay Hudson, author of the great work, *The Law of Psychic Phenomena,* and generally considered one of the sanest, most level-headed writers on psychology in his time, declared that out of 100 cases of absent treatment, he failed in only one, and in that one case the patient was strongly prejudiced against mental treatment.

Helen Wilmans, called the "mother of mental science", in her long fight with the post-office department and government officials who tried to send her to prison for healing without medicine, proved in open court that she had healed persons in her presence and persons at a distance, simply by the power of thought. The only claim she failed to prove, was that she had healed a child through the mind of its mother, but that has since been proved in numerous cases and prominent educators nowadays use mental methods to a large extent in eradicating weaknesses, diseases and bad habits from children.

The Weltmer Institute of Suggestive Therapeutics at Nevada, Mo., which was founded more than 20 years ago, has performed some of the most marvelous cures which history records. Its founder, Prof. S.A. Weltmer, cured himself of tuberculosis after physicians had told him he could not live longer than a year.

Science has positively proved that by directed thought, the cells of the body may be healthy and vigorous and that special faculties may be strengthened. Prof. Elmer Gates of the Smithsonian Institution at Washington, D.C., proved by his scientific experiments that in a few months' time he could train dogs to discriminate between 7 shades of red and 6 of green, besides manifesting unusual mental ability in many other ways. Their brains, upon examination, showed a far greater number of brain cells than any animal of like breed ever possessed.

Prof. Gates, who is one of the leading scientists of the day, said, speaking of mental suggestion:

"This system of development can be applied to regulate the assimilative processes, the diseases of which are dyspepsia, alcoholism, etc. A woman unable to eat fatty or greasy substances, even in the smallest portions, was by this system trained to take them in normal quantities. *** My experiments prove that the mind activities create the structures which the mind embodies or manifests".

In his book, *The Mind and the Brain*, Prof. Gates shows the definite chemical effect of various emotions of the body. He shows how constructive, harmonious, optimistic thinking strengthens the heart, stomach and other organs, makes the blood circulate more freely, helps in assimilation and excretion, and makes the body remain young and supple. He shows how fear, worry, expectancy of sickness, and evil passions poison the blood, upset the normal action of the heart, cause indigestion, make waste accumulate at the nerve centers, interfering with communication between the brain and the various parts of the body, and dry up the tissues of the physical organism instead of permitting nature to throw them off and build new ones. He shows specifically the effect of various modes of thinking on temperature, moisture, vitality and other bodily conditions.

The Health Reporter, a leading magazine devoted to health and hygiene, says: "Anger, anxiety or fear will poison the secretions of the body. Anger or fright promote the secretion of poison in the sacs of a venomous snake, and this is where he is ahead of man. We have no organs in which we may store the toxins which we develop for the same purpose and consequently we poison ourselves with the material which was meant for our enemies".

The fact that thought can change the expression of the face is known to everybody. That it can send blood to the face, as in blushing and in moments of anger, is universally understood. That it can take blood away from the face, as when one turns pale, is just as well known. That it can turn the hair white in a few hours, through fear, is also known, this phenomena having frequently happened. That it can cause unconsciousness, as in fainting, is a fact which nobody in his right mind will question. And that thought can kill, as when one drops dead through fear, is a declaration easily confirmed. That specialists in the medical profession, frequently die of the very diseases they specialize in, is a striking fact which speaks for itself.

Everything in our experiences and those of others, is in absolute confirmation of the fact that the more we think of disease, the more disease there is in the world, and the more we think of health, the more health in the world.

No natural force can be used for ill more than for good, and if wrong thinking can make people unconscious, turn the hair white and even cause sudden death, right thinking can heal disease, preserve youth and strength, and lengthen human life.

As a matter of logic, there is not getting away from this. The mind can cause disease and can increase disease. The mind can also prevent disease and can heal disease.

But it is not necessary to depend on logic. Demonstration is even better and the power of the mind to keep the body in perfect health, can be actually demonstrated by any who will obey these other laws of nature which most people habitually disobey. Believers in New Thought and allied philosophies are the best proof of their own beliefs, for they fairly radiate health and vitality from their bodies. They have learned the higher laws and they comply with them so well that sickness is almost unknown among them and when it appears, is quickly banished.

One of the most striking proofs of the limitless power of Mind over body, when exercised to the fullest extent, is afforded in the case of a woman in Spokane, Wash., who showed that teeth could be filled by concentrated thought. Her method was by prayer. The method does not matter, so long as the principle of concentration is complied with. Thousands are healed every year at the Cathedral of the Lady of Lourdes in France, and at various meccas of the Catholic church, where bones of saints and sacred relics are kept. The Catholic thinks the relic heals him. As a matter of fact, his own mind heals him. He has perfect faith that he will recover and he does. The same is often true of medicine. Most doctors have a harmless medicine, which has no effect whatever on the body, one way or the other, and which they often give, curing patients just as well as if regular medicine had been given. Even the strongest medicine can be neutralized by lack of faith in it.

Concluding, it must be said:

The Mind can and does heal all diseases. There are plenty of other cases at hand or nearby, which can be investigated as thoroughly as is desired, and which will afford complete, undeniable proof of this assertion. The honest doubter owes it to himself and to humanity to look into the cases, as a matter of fairness. And after he has done so, if he is fair and impartial in his investigations, he must be convinced.

Without going into the underlying philosophy of mental healing at this time, it may be said that every cell, tissue and corpuscle in the physical organism is a point of consciousness and, therefore, under the control of the central consciousness, the Mind, which acts through the brain. This central consciousness can transform and renew any part of the body, which is but the visible and external crystallization of this internal, invisible reality.

Any person can prove this to his own satisfaction if he will practice right thinking and right living. Try it. Think health, youth, strength, vitality, constantly. Know that you are making yourself well and keeping yourself so. Shut out of your mind every thought of fear, worry and pessimism. Do not mention disease. Act as if it did not exist and the time will soon come, so far as you are concerned, when it won't exist. The beliefs in your own mind will crystallize into visible expression in your own body, always and invariably,—sometimes, not as quickly as other times, but always if you are consistently obedient to the laws of life.

If it be said that right thinking would do no good if one continually violated the laws of sanitation and hygiene, the reply is that nobody can break laws very long, if he thinks right thoughts. He simply can't do it.

Thought is forever proceeding out of the invisible realms of Mind into the visible realm of physical appearances and physical conduct. He who thinks scientifically, who proclaims his own mastery of himself and drives out of himself every belief in the power of disease over him, will instinctively conform with every physical law that is conducive to his well-being, and will send currents of thought into his whole body that will make it practically immune to the contagions and epidemics created by the uncleanliness of others.

"We ourselves are the makers of ourselves".

A majority of cases that are brought to mental healers are cases which have been given up by physicians, as "incurable".

He shows how fear, worry, expectancy of sickness, and evil passions poison the blood, upset the normal action of the heart, cause indigestion, make waste accumulate at the nerve centers, interfering with communication between the brain and the various parts of the body. . . .

The mind can cause disease and can increase disease. The mind can also prevent disease and can heal disease.

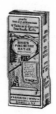
Advertisement for Bing's Pine Needle Baths.

Those Immutable Laws
Benedict Lust

What Have We, Nature Cure Or A Bag Of Tricks?
Herbert M. Shelton, D.P., N.D.

Pain And Disease
Carlos Brandt, N.D.

Dr. B. LUST'S RECREATION RESORT
"YUNGBORN" BUTLER, N. J.
IN THE RAMAPO MOUNTAINS

Natural Life and Rational Cure Health Home for Dietetic-Physical-Atmospheric Regeneration Treatment. Fount of Youth, and New Life School for those in need of Cure and Rest, for the physically and spiritually weakened, for those overworked and for the convalescent.

OPEN ALL THE YEAR
Winter Branch: *Florida Yungborn, Tangerine, Florida*

IN the vicinity of the beautiful country town of Butler, N. J., there spreads, in incomparably ideal beauty, surrounded by majestic pine forests, orchards and parks, the Health Resort of YUNGBORN. The establishment was called a *Yungborn* by reason of the rejuvenating and strength-endowing effects of its Regeneration Cures. And indeed, these extensively known Yungborn-Regeneration Cures are not only health-restoring, but also Rejuvenating and Strength-giving Cures. Already during, and particularly after the treatments are completed, the strength and vitality, formerly low and broken, rise with astonishing assurance. Vital energy and vital strength return; increased nerve-elasticity and an undreamed-of sensation of powerful health make themselves felt. And with the new creative power there asserts iself a feeling of spiritual and physical rejuvenation and unlimited efficiency.

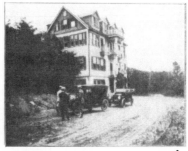

Yungborn Regeneration Cures—The dietetical Regeneration Cures which are applied in their particular gradations as required for the various diseases and conditions of weakness, are fully adapted to the case in hand and modified correspondingly.

The most peculiar and most intense forms of these Cures are the *Schroth Treatment*, so called after its founder, the genial Johann Schroth, and the combined *Diet, Light-Air and Water Treatments* in which the experiences of *Schroth, Kneipp, Rickli, Lahmann, Ehret, Just, Engelhardt, etc.*, are resorted to individually. Furthermore, Fruit Cures, Herb Cures, Vegetal and Mixed Diet, Fasting Diet Cures in combination with Fruit Diets, and so forth. Diet requires individually adapted physical treatment, such as *packings*, bandaging, baths and gushes of various descriptions, barefoot walking, light, sun and air baths, steam, electricity, massaging, Osteopathy, Chiropractic, Mechanotherapy, Neuropathy, etc. Special attention is given to the development of humid warmth treatment as one of the most important curative factors.

Aid in Obsolete, Inveterate Cases—The Yungborn Regeneration Cures will help even in the most deep-rooted and superannuated sufferings and conditions of weakness, where other cures failed, except in cases of organic new growth and destructions (like cancer and consumption) or marasmus.

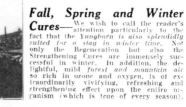

It need hardly be mentioned that not only those requiring cure, but also those *in need of rest*, the *weakened* and *convalescing* derive the best possible benefits of lasting effect from a sojourn at the Yungborn.

Fall, Spring and Winter
Cures—We wish to call the reader's attention particularly to the fact that the *Yungborn is also splendidly suited for a stay in winter time*. Not only the *Regeneration* but also the Strengthening Cures are immensely successful in winter. In addition, the delightful, mild *forest and mountain* air so rich in ozone and oxygen, is of extraordinarily vivifying, refreshing and strengthening effect upon the entire organism (which is true of every season).

The Yungborn located in Butler, N.J. was a haven for those in search of Regenerative Treatment.

THOSE IMMUTABLE LAWS

by Benedict Lust

Herald of Health and Naturopath, XXVI (4), 161-163. (1921)

In the February medical *Review of Reviews* the editor froths a bit over "a class of speakers and writers who love to descant upon the Immutable Laws of Nature (capitalized of course), and to predict the penalties for all such 'violations' of the laws." After giving an example taken from another journal he comments in part: "Somehow the 'violation' of these 'immutable laws of nature' impresses me as something extraordinary. How can one, for instance, violate the law of gravitation, or the law of falling bodies, or Kepler's laws of motion? It is to laugh... Where are these immutable laws of nature recorded, and in what consists the violation, and who administers the penalty?

"The fact is, what we call the 'laws of nature' are merely our formulas for the way we conceive nature to work. These so-called laws are subject to modification from time to time as we learn more about nature's ways. That does not mean that nature works haphazardly without any orderly method. So far as we know, nature works in uniform and orderly manner and 'effect' follows 'cause' with unerring precision. But what we call 'laws' of nature are not laws at all in the legal sense, or in the sense of enactments, but are generalizations, i.e., the sum total of our observations of how nature works."

We admit that this loose talk about the immutable laws of nature without giving any concrete, specific examples used to make us [froth] a bit too. This was largely due to the fact that in school and college there was no relationship shown between physics and physiology. Nor were we given any definite picture of what constituted a normal state. We were given to understand that what the majority did was normal, natural, and what was not commonly done was unnatural, abnormal.

What we call laws in a legal sense, are not laws at all but merely rules and regulations, largely of conduct, enacted with the idea of keeping order in a state. These are timely and subject to change in accordance to necessity.

But who can say that the laws of matter and of motion are whimsical and unchangeable? Man has learned these laws through observation and has discovered that while they govern changes in matter, they themselves do not change.

These laws are applicable to all material operations. Does not the editor we have quoted admit that "effect follows cause with unerring precision?" Does not this suggest to us that there is a law behind every cause, or is it too big for our minds to conceive?

The question is, are natural (physical) laws inviolable? Does a flying machine violate the law of gravitation? Of course not; the law is still operative. The flying machine temporarily overcomes the force of gravitation exerted upon it by the earth.

Every proposition of physics is demonstrated in the human economy. The laws of physics are operative there for a purpose—to preserve, to maintain in manifested form that which we call the life principle. The process through which this is done we call physiology. Now then, can we interfere with normal physiological processes? If we can and do, then we are violating the laws of nature. We are preventing the fulfillment of the law.

The laws of life are the laws of necessity, the laws of supply and demand. If we were asked to put into words what we consider to be the primary law of life we would give it thus: "Every created thing will continue to perform the function for which it was designed, throughout its entire life cycle, provided its environment remains congenial to it." The law says it will (or shall, if you like that form better) do so and so. Why? Who knows? But observation has proven that it will, if not interfered with. If it can draw the proper support from its environment it will fulfill its design. If its environment changes to the extent of becoming uncongenial, then the thing changes its activity. Has a law been violated?

Let's particularize a bit; bring the proposition down to the concrete. Take the human body, or more specifically, the cells of the human body. Can we apply our law to them? Let us see. Suppose we particularized our law to read this way: "Every cell in the human body will function perfectly (according to its design) provided its environment remains congenial to it; i.e., provided it receives the proper quantity and quality of food material and oxygen, has its waste products removed promptly, is not injured by exposure to extremes of temperature, or by violence." That is what we would call a state of health, because the body as a whole will function according to design if every cell in it is in good working order.

Can this law be violated? If so who violates it and what are the consequences? In other words what penalty does the law carry for the violation of it? The Prohibition enforcement act, for example, carries with it a penalty of fine and imprisonment for its violation. The one who breaks man-made laws must suffer some hardship, his freedom is curtailed, his function is altered. All the provisions of the "law of the cell" can be violated. The quantity and quality of blood can be altered, waste products can accumulate, the cell can be injured by violence or exposure to extremes of temperature. Who violates the "law of the cell"? Let us see. Violence and extremes of temperature we can account for. The difficulty is in placing responsibility for an alteration of the cell's environment.

Before we proceed suppose we determine what constitutes the environment of the cell. We are all agreed that cells live in a fluid medium, which fluid is derived from the blood. In other words it is the substance which leaks out from the walls of the capillary blood vessels, flows through the spaces between the cells and on into the lymphatic vessels. Then, it is this fluid medium which must be congenial to the cells. It must contain all the physical requirements of that cell, as well as to afford the cell an opportunity to empty waste into it. If the cell discharges its waste into the fluid surrounding it, and this waste would react on the cell if the cell should happen to take it back into its body, then this fluid must promptly move on to make way for new. Therefore, the normal cell environment is a constantly flowing stream bringing nutrient material to the cell and carrying off waste.

The law is violated if the cell is not supplied with proper nutrition and oxygen, for, under those circumstances it cannot function according to design. But who is responsible? The stomach? The liver? The lungs? The heart? No person possessing a grain of common sense would ask me to go further. The custodian of the cell is responsible. He is the one who determines what goes into the body. It is for him to say how that body shall be cared for. He may abuse it or preserve it. If he feeds it improperly, interferes with its oxygen supply, allows the waste channels to become clogged, deprives it of rest, exhausts its vitality or in any way places too great a handicap upon it, he violates the law.

And what is the penalty for violating this law of nature—the law of the cell? Does it not carry with it the penalty? Is not disease the effect of the violation of this law? The very interference with the normal function of the cells, preventing them from fulfilling their design and thus, interfering with the design of the whole organism, is punishment enough.

But, unfortunately, it does not stop there. Because the sick man will not acknowledge his fault, he looks for some cause outside of himself, on which to blame his infirmity. The physician encourages him to believe he is "more sinned against than sinning". He holds out the hope of vicarious atonement—science will shoulder the burden and relieve him of all his iniquities. Medicine will subdue the naughty germ and the man will be well. But why continue? We know that the last state of this man shall be worse than the first unless—he falls into the hands of a Naturopath.

And what is the penalty for violating this law of nature—the law of the cell? Does it not carry with it the penalty? Is not disease the effect of the violation of this law?

WHAT HAVE WE, NATURE CURE OR A BAG OF TRICKS?

by Herbert M. Shelton, D.P., N.D.

Herald of Health and Naturopath, XXVI(6), 283-287. (1921)

> In modern times, and more remarkably in Great Britain, no one thinks of proposing a new mode of practice without supporting it by the results of practical experience. The disease exists, the remedy is prescribed and the disease is removed. We have no reason to doubt the veracity or the ability of the narrator and his favorable report induces his contemporaries to pursue the same means of cure. The same favorable result is obtained and it appears impossible for any fact to be supported by more decisive testimony. Yet in the space of a few short years the boasted remedy has lost its virtue; the disease no longer yields to its power while its place is supplied by some new remedy, which, like its predecessor, runs through the same career of expectation, success and disappointment.

The above quotation from *Bostock's History of Medicine* is as true today as when he wrote it many years ago. It is as true of the drugless as of the drugging profession. At what period of the world's history was the sick person confronted with such a "conglomeration of therapeutic measures", or the student with such a "hodge-podge of un-unified principles and hypotheses" as are in vogue today?

In whatever direction one turns he is met by a number of little two-by-four "healing systems," each clamoring for recognition, each claiming superior merit, while a part of them are clamoring for an exclusive place in the sun. Then we have the mixers.* These are they who use all methods and are as proud of the fact that they have swallowed all the rubbish as are the single-trackers of their self-imposed obscurity.

Once we had the Nature Curist or Naturopath. We still retain terms but no longer do we have a "Nature Cure". We came out boldly with our "Back to Nature" slogan, but this battle cry that could, and would, have carried us on to victory, has long since been forgotten. We were stung by the progressive bee and went after strange gods. No longer have we a consistent philosophy of disease and cure, of health and its preservation. Where once was unity and consistency, chaos now reigns. Let us inquire why this is true.

And I believe the true answer will be found in our desire to be broad minded and progressive. We wanted all that was valuable for our patients. We started out preaching the simple life but when that progressive bug

---

*Term used by straight Chiropractors (those who do nothing for their patients but adjust vertebrae by hand) to designate Chiropractors who use other therapeutic methods.

got into our gray matter and we became so broad minded we declared: "There is good in all systems, we'll take all that is good and reject the chaff." The result has been an ever increasing complexity of measures and methods for treating human ailments. We have lost sight of those great laws of Nature upon which we first builded, we have turned away from our unifying principles. We have invaded the realm of the artificial and mysterious. Nature Cure is passing and in its stead we are using everything in the universe of art and invention to promote human health and cure disease.

Our offices bid fair to develop into ware rooms or junk shops. In fact, many of them are that already. We have many "essentials" of the physician's equipment—vibrators, dilators, therapeutic lamps of every conceivable size, style and cost; electrical apparatus galore, adjustment tables, traction tables, vacuum apparatus, etc. Then we have the various bath equipment, dry air, steam, cabinet, sits, tub, shower, douche, etc. And George Starr White gave us another lot of pretty things to play with in his bio-dynamo chromatic diagnosis and treatment. Dr. Abrams gave us a few little play pretties with which to tickle the spine. And we have a whole lumber room full of other apparatus, too numerous to mention.

Some one defined medicine as "the art of entertaining the patient while Nature restored him to health." And surely, if we can't find amidst all these new needs of the human body, anything that will entertain a patient he is an incorrigible cuss and deserves to die. We started out to get the "good in all" and got instead, a junk shop.

And what excuse have we to offer for the continued use of all these novelties? Only this, "Experience has demonstrated their practical value." Experience! Have we forgotten the words of that grand old pioneer of Natural therapeutics, R. T. Trall, M. D., when he exclaimed: "Experience! What is experience? It is merely the record of what has happened. It only tells what has been done, not what should be. I would not give a green cucumber for all the experience of all the medical men of all the earth in all the ages, unless predicated on some recognized law of Nature, and interpreted by some demonstrable rule in philosophy. Medical men have been curing (killing) folks for three thousand years with drug medicines, and their experience has led them away from truth and nature continually." Listen, again, "ye mixers" to these words of wisdom from the same source: "Without some fixed and unalterable and demonstrable rule of judgement, all our reasoning may be in vain; facts may be misapplied; experience misinterpreted; observation deceptive; and logic perverted."

"Though an angel speak to us in the voices of the rolling thunders; though God send instruction in the red lightings flash; yet, without a principle of interpretation, without the recognition of some law by which to explain the phenomena, we only know that it thunders, and that the sky is ablaze. But with the knowledge of the law which determines the results, we may rightly apply all the data of science and misapply none; we may use all things and abuse nothing."

But by what rule of interpretation do we interpret experience? It's just a case of "The disease exists, the remedy is prescribed and the disease is removed." We never stop to ask ourselves what our remedy had to do with the removal of the disease.

Years ago Dr. Trall wrote: "But unfortunately the guide (experience) points all ways at the same time." How true it is as one must see if he but thinks a moment.

There are to day in the United States not less than five large divisions of the drugging system—allopathic, homeopathic, eclectic, physio-medical and bio-chemic. Their theories are different, their practice differs, their results differ but slightly. Yet the experience of the men in each of these schools of drugging has been that his methods cure. Only a few years since it was good allopathic practice to confine fever patients in a hermetically sealed room, allow no water, smother them in blankets, bleed and leech them and purge them with calomel. And the experience of those who treated fever in this manner pointed to this method as the best.

Our grandfathers used to carry potatoes or horse chestnuts in their pockets to cure rheumatism. And experience proved their value. They got well of the rheumatism. The experience of the Indian medicine man with his tom-tom and that of the Chinese doctors with his red-hot poker, point as strongly to the healing power of these "valuable aids to Nature". If an Indian medicine man or a Chinese healer ever meets a "mixer," he bids fair to lose his tom-tom or poker.

But we moderns have a more refined way of entertaining our patients. While attending a class in psychotherapy in Chicago during the past summer we were told by the teacher that if we could only imbue our patient with enough faith in our ability to cure him he would get well, it matters not how we treat him, nor how much or little the treatment. Upon being asked, by the writer, if a sufficient amount of faith would convert green paint into good food, or compensate for the deficiency of organic salts that would result in Beri-beri, she admitted that we would have to use common sense in the latter case, even admitted that it is was necessary to feed the proper food.

Psychotherapy has its uses (as well as its abuses) but I could never find any reason for such absurd statements as the one mentioned above.

This same lecturer said: "Suggestion is mostly lie." Then added: "We must never let our conscience stand in our way for everybody's life is a living lie." And it must be recognized by every intelligent man or woman that she told a truth when she asserted that suggestion is mostly lie. Take this advice recently given to the patients in a certain Sanitarium here in

New York State: "Think of yourself as perfect, as perfect beings, as perfect health. Now why do we want to hold these thoughts? Because" etc. The true explanation was given by Barnum but he neglected to say that the same average individual is as fond of humbugging himself as of having someone else do it for him.

I once listened to Dr. Lindlahr tell in a lecture of one of our long range mental healers, who used a "sun phone" or something similar, being in his institution in Chicago for treatment by natural methods. He had to be pushed around in a wheel chair by an attendant. In spite of this, however, he continued the good work of healing others and almost every mail brought him money and testimonials from all parts of the world.

We can transfer our thought to the back of our brain but this only proves that Barnum was right. We "enter the silence" only to hear Puck exclaim: "What fools these mortals be."

Then we have electricity. This is an interesting toy and furnishes us with much amusement as well as the patient. See the operator point with unfeigned delight at the contraction of a muscle in a paralyzed limb from electrical irritation of the part. The same can be accomplished by laying bare the muscle and sprinkling common table salt on it, and this would do as much good. Electricity is just another toy to play with.

The muscle has not lost the ability to contract. This is proven by the fact that it does contract when external stimulas is applied. But the nerves or nerve centres are "down and out". The cure of paralysis is a thing of nerve regeneration and can't be accomplished by tickling the muscles with the slow sinusoidal. If the principle that something cannot come out of nothing be a correct one, where is the sense of attempting to force into renewed activity a paralyzed or dead nerve? The cure, if it be possible, is one of regeneration, and only the power that built the nerve in the beginning can accomplish this. It is a vital process and can be done only by life or vital power, not by electrical stimulation.

The head of an institution where I was employed, said to me once in conversation: "Now there's electricity," pointing to his machine, "it may not do any good. I don't know. Anyway it works on the mind." And this, I think accounts for its popularity. "It works on the mind." It furnishes an excellent means of entertaining the patient.

We have many varieties of baths, to entertain our patients. Oh, I beg your pardon, I intended to say "to build vital power." We increase vital power with water only we can't agree among ourselves just how we do it. Some of us use only cold water because warm or hot water is so enervating. Others of us use only hot because cold is such a vital depressant, while others use only warm or natural because extremes of temperature are so stimulating and only serve to weaken our patient. Then there are those who use all temperatures from very hot to very cold but who profess to adopt the temperature to the condition of the patient. And each points to his experience; the guide points in all directions at once. What is such experience worth? Yet was ever a theological battle waged with more dogmatism? How the gods must laugh as they watch the comedy from their box seats on Mt. Olympus!

Then we have Chiropractic with no less than four schools of thought. By a lavish misuse of printers ink, Chiropractic has become very popular. It is, however, gratifying to see its height has been reached and it is now on the decline.

The Chiropractor "needs to know but a bit about the manifestation of God's will and desire; its absorption into a unit; its transportation to all parts through nerves; learn about twenty four places where there may be obstruction and how to adjust them if such exists. More than this is superfluous." They know that all disease is caused by impingement upon the nerve trunks where they leave the spine, from subluxated vertebrae. The fact that it has been demonstrated over and over again that a mere subluxation can cause no impingement of the nerve does not bother them. Their experience has shown them that Chiropractic is the panacea for all our ills. There is only one violation of natural law that their little punch on the spine won't atone for and that is the taking of drugs.

You may smoke and chew and drink, you may eat and dance and sing, if you only get your punch on the spine. No longer can these harm us. For now we have the spine puncher. B.J. Palmer has found that a man can digest leather if he only gets his punch in the back. One need give no attention to diet. To abuse the stomach is impossible while we have Chiropractic. One Carver has found that that same little punch will answer for a bath. And B.J. has again discovered that by this same means the "cooties" can be made to scamper. Then there is another who has "cured" many cases of morphinism and nicotinism by the punch alone.

It is very amusing to hear one of these Chiro's explain that a subluxation can be caused by a cough, a sneeze, a slight mis-step in the dark, or by merely reaching across the desk for a blotter, etc., and then explain to us that our heart or stomach or liver or kidneys or skin can withstand all manner of abuse if we only keep the "kinks" out of our spines. It is a very strange thing that while such little things as a sneeze or cough can cause a subluxation, that the kiddies, puppies, kittens, colts and calves can roll and tumble without filling their spines with kinks. And the wrestlers, contortionists, weight lifters, gymnasts and acrobats are a constant source of bewilderment. One wonders how they ever survive.

But the Chiro has made one real discovery; there are only two diseases, "plus" and "minus." The "minus" is the vacuum in the public's cranial cavity, while this same public carries its "plus" in its purse. The patient is "minus" part of his "plus" after visiting a Chiro. This explains why so much attention is given by them to the "psychology of salesmanship" and why B.J.P. says: "If you have thirty minutes to spend with a patient give him adjustment for one minute and spend the other twenty nine explaining why you adjusted him as you did and why you didn't adjust more."

But the band plays on, the end is not yet. We have other ways of entertaining our patients. We have a whole library full of metaphysical formulas which we sell at so much per, and each one guaranteed to get results. We have Iridiagnosis, basic diagnosis, and some of us have adopted astrology, also. We need only to add palmistry and fortune telling by cards to these to have a complete system of diagnosis.

The "mixers" have truly mixed it. And they are also, mixed. Take the milk diet as an instance. Milk contains a magic principle that seems to go to the very root of a disease and eradicate it. And one can be a milk glutton without harm. Anywhere from four to fourteen quarts per day will work wonders. It won't even hurt one if he eats three good meals per day and absorbs milk between meals. He should also, take a glass before retiring at night and one before breakfast next morning. No two are agreed on just how it should be given but that is of no consequence. Each fellow is convinced that his method is best, but the main thing is take milk. The diarrhea, constipation and nausea that are so common on a milk diet should be ignored. For we are to remember that milk is baby food and the sick man is a baby. Yes the sick man is a baby but not an infant. He has the digestion of maturity, not of infancy.

As Dr. Trall so appropriately remarked: "These facts are enough to show the utter fallacy of medical experience, and the unsatisfactory nature of medical testimony unless based upon some intelligible principle to which we can refer the phenomena they present."

Deluged as we are with a multitude of theories and "curative" measures it behooves us to "prove all things" and "hold fast that which is good". It is time we begun to pick the beam from our own eyes. After this is done there will be left plenty of time to get the mote from the eyes of the medical man. A lady said to me recently: "I am able metaphysically to correct actual anatomical lesion of the spine." She was once an Osteopath. Another "mixer" from a drug school remarked to me: "We often speak of Nature curing, but Nature never cures anything unless we help her. Otherwise there would be no need for doctors." Strange were his ways of aiding Nature. I had just witnessed him administering one of these "aids" in the form of a sub-cutaneous injection of strychnin to "sustain the heart".

It is time to turn our minds from our junk shops and ware rooms and go once again to "the very agencies by which the whole vegetable and animal creation are developed and sustained" for our "aids" to Nature.

We need to come to a realization of the fact that the body restores itself to normal by identically the same process by which it was first built and maintained, that regeneration and healing takes place in the cells and that these cells are constantly and ceaselessly striving with might and main, night and day, asleep or awake, every minute of our lives, to restore and maintain the normal. We need to realize that health is normal and that disease is the result of some disturbance of nutrition, drainage and inner-vation—one or all three.

Dr. John W. Sargent of the International College once told the follow-ing story to his class. He had a man under his care in the Health Resort, who being of the wealthy class and being used to pampering, was a bit fussy. He complained that he wasn't getting enough treatment. To this Dr. Sargent replied: "Treatment won't cure you. If it would we would hire three shifts and give you twenty four hours per day of it. The man understood, became contented, and soon recovered. The "mixer" needs to come to a realization of the fact that treatment won't cure.

Having become mixers we are mixed. Having gone after "strange flesh" we are now in bondage to a lot of harlot "systems". It is time Nature Cure became divorced from these recently acquired concubines and returned to its first love. Stop this making "your patients believe you are going to do something new for him," and assert your loyalty to correct principles. When told: "experience has demonstrated" etc., find out whose experience and by what law the experience was interpreted. For as Darwin said of analogy, so we can safely say of experience: it "may be a very deceitful guide".

Some one defined medicine as "the art of entertaining the patient while Nature restored him to health."

"Experience! What is experience? It is merely the record of what has happened. It only tells what has been done, not what should be. I would not give a green cucumber for all the experience of all the medical men of all the earth in all the ages, unless predicated on some recognized law of Nature, and interpreted by some demonstrable rule in philosophy.

Pain And Disease

by Carlos Brandt, N.D.

Herald of Health and Naturopath, XXVI(8), 373-376. (1921)

> *In order to strengthen the body and make it grow, nature has means which we should never oppose.*
> —Rousseau

Pain is an admirable warning of nature; a means to preserve life. Without it, we can say, that neither man nor animal would exist. Pain is not only the source of human progress, but is also the cause of the development of the greater part of the biological world. If we stumble against something, pain tells us that we have hurt ourselves, our cellular web, and that therefore we must be more careful. The reason we try to protect ourselves from blows and wounds, is not because we care so much for our cellular web and our organs, but simply to avoid pain. Like pain, sickness is another means to preserve life; it is a warning against some deep state of degeneration in the organism. We are so careless in regard to our body that no one would think of protecting himself against blows, wounds and diseases if these did not produce pain and discomfort. Like physical pain and sickness, moral pain and remorse are also warnings, to make us preserve life. Sickness, the same as pain, is disagreeable, but at the same time useful, necessary, for it serves to avoid a greater danger, and therefore to protect life. Sickness and pain are vital imperatives, whose aim is to protect the law of the conservation of life.

It is unnecessary to say that the ideal state of man is health. In the rest of the biological world sickness is the exception, and health is the rule, but in the human race sickness is the rule and health the exception; and what an exception!! . . . Wild animals do not suffer diseases. The latter is a product of civilized man, and of the animals subject to him.

All disease have a common origin. This statement, uttered by Louis Kuhne, is the most scientific and fundamental principle of medicine. Everything tends toward monism,—not only in philosophy, but also in science. Instead of there being several diseases, there is only one disease, although that one disease manifests itself in different forms or symptoms. Disease is like a tree; the leaves are all as different as its manifestations, but they all combine to form one thing—a tree. To try to destroy the tree by means of plucking its leaves, would be the same as to try and fill the Danaides barrel. It is foolish to think that the symptoms are the disease. If you want to eradicate the tree of evil, do not lop off its leaves, but destroy its roots.

Chronic diseases are the result of a deep state of degeneration in the system, an over-clogging of foreign matter, a predisposition, an anormal condition, which we acquire and then transmit to our descendants through inheritance which they are burdened with for a long time—often without even knowing it—until finally it appears in one form or another (cancer, diabetes, insanity, heart disease, etc.). The aim of acute diseases (curative crisis), is to destroy and cure chronic diseases, or to kill those individuals who are not able, fit or strong enough to survive through the curative process. In other words, the aim of sickness is either to cure or to rid the world of those so degenerate who might perpetuate degeneracy.

So we see that sickness is a warning, and therefore that it is useful and of great advantage to our nature. When man begins to detach himself from his natural environments, that is when he begins to transgress the law of the conservation of life (morals), he begins to clog his body with foreign matter. In order to get rid of the latter, acute diseases (fevers, etc.) appear, whose aim is to free the body of foreign matter, which, as we have seen before, is the primordial cause of all chronic diseases. Still if after we are cured (i.e. after the foreign matter is eliminated from our system), we continue to live wrongly, again clogging up our body with foreign matter; or if the cure is not real, but irrational, as are all so called cures through drugs, serums, etc., then, there appears in us a deeper form of degeneration, which manifest itself by means of chronic diseases (cancer, diabetes, insanity, heart diseases, etc.). It seems to be an undeniable fact that the purpose of these chronic diseases is to eliminate all the persistent sinners, in order that they do not breed transgressors like themselves, who might continue to further degenerate the species.

Disease, like pain, is undoubtedly unpleasant, but its aim is to avoid a greater evil and so we must consider it as a gift from nature, as beneficial to us. The aim of disease is to promote the law of the conservation of life, curing by means of acute diseases those who are in good condition, that is, the more fitted in the Darwinian sense, and eliminating by means of chronic diseases those who are in bad condition, who are less fitted. He who sins against the law of the conservation of life, does not only injure his own nature, but also his offspring, transmitting diseases to them in the inheritance. So we see not only in the spiritual, but also in the physical sense, that saying: "The sins of the fathers will be visited on their children, even to the seventh generation." It is not nature which punishes human race but it is human race which eliminates itself by means of its sins and wrong living. On the other hand, we should not believe that if a person is vicious, he becomes diseased, and dies on account of his vice, but we must turn to the axiom to read in this manner: When a person is vicious, it is because his nature and faculties are already perverted, being therefore and unfavorable factor for the human race, it is right and just that he should succumb.

When I speak of nature, do not think that I believe that there are several natures and that the nature of man and that of his environment are two different things. In nature there is not You and I. If I say that nature reacts to cure us, that nature protects us by furnishing us with this and that, that nature sends us light, water, food, etc., I only do that to avoid a long dissertation, just as we simply say that the sun rises and sets, instead of having to explain that the earth moves around the sun.

Nature is not an individual, a person who sends us the environment (water, food, etc.) in order to help man, but on the contrary, man exists because there is the environment: foods, adequate conditions of living, etc. We can hardly consider that the woods are obliged to nature because the latter sends tempests which purify the air, irrigate the soil, and violently waves the trees, leaving the staunch ones and destroying those which are old and decayed. The fact is that the woods exist because the tempests exist. In the same way, mankind exists because acute diseases exist, which are our tempests. What nature really seems to want is life on the surface of our planet. The form of that life is conditioned by the element and circumstances.

As already stated, acute diseases are a **curative crisis**, by means of which foreign matter, clogging the body, is removed. As Wigelsworth says, these crises appear every time nature has to resort to its valve of safety. We must recognize that nature never does anything that is not good, that is not reasonable, although we, in our ignorance may not see the reason why. Acute diseases are neither degenerative nor incurable, but are easily cured by means of any rational method (naturopathy, etc.). They are therefore, as beneficial to us, as our persistence is stupid in trying to prevent their good work abortively, by means of drugs, serums and other poisons of regular medicine.

The ultimate cause of disease is something which science has not yet been able to explain. It is something indefinite (predisposition, degeneration, clogging of foreign matter), which is in our body, generally without our knowing it, and which develops little by little until it suddenly appears in the form of symptom, and then we term it disease.

Man is not perverted (wicked) because he does evil, but he does evil because his nature is already perverted (wicked). This philosophical axiom can be applied to pathology in the following form: Man is not sick because he has symptoms, but he has symptoms because he is sick. So we see that the original cause of disease is something so deep that it constitutes a mystery for science and its study belongs rather to philosophy. On the other hand, symptoms (disease) are only of secondary importance. The simpleton says, "You are wicked because you practice evil", but the thinker says, "You practice evil because you are wicked." In the same way regular medicine says, "You are sick because you have symptoms;

let me cure the latter and you will be well"; but any rational or drugless medicine will say: "You have symptoms because you are already sick; do not mind the symptoms, but try to cure your whole system, in which lies the root of the disease. In doing this, the symptoms will disappear spontaneously." When we remove symptoms, we do not cure the disease, but we simply help to prolong or to change it into another and more dangerous form which appears later on.

It is a matter of fact that some serums, quinine and other drugs occasionally succeed in reducing fever, but this is simply because they weaken the body. If, as Dr. Rizquez says: "Generalized febrile infections are more dangerous when they develop themselves apyretically", it is because the sick person is so weak, that his system is no longer able to produce fever (curative crisis). Thus, in this lies the secret of the apparent success of quinine, serums, vaccines, etc. Namely, they weaken the body of the sick person to such an extent that make it impossible for him to have a curative crisis (fever, acute disease). It is quite obvious that this success is most dangerous for the life of the patient. It is very interesting to notice that the most malignant, degenerative and incurable diseases, such as cancer, diabetes, insanity, heart disease, etc., generally are not accompanied by pain or by fever.

Acute disease, like tempests, and pain, are a necessary evil, whose aim is to remove a greater evil. Without the tempest, which purifies the air, the forests could not exist. This shows us that diseases are convenient and necessary. It would certainly be better if disease were not necessary, but that can not be, unless man were perfectly healthy, which is very far from being the fact.

The scientific principle of Kuhne regarding the unity of disease; that all diseases have only one cause, and that they exist in our body long before they appear, has been corroborated by the vegetarian philosophy. The principle of disease exists in our system, and even in that of our ancestors, long before it manifests itself. Logically, all diseases can have only one method of cure. This principle of Kuhne has also been corroborated by philosophy, as we will see later on in the chapter "Common Origin of Diseases".

In regard to the primordial cause of disease (predisposition, degeneration, clogging of foreign matter, etc.), if we have been unlucky enough to acquire it, or to have inherited it, when the time comes for it to appear (acute diseases, fever), let it go through its natural process, or as Hippocrates says, "let us help this natural process by natural means" (naturopathy), but never try to dull, to damp it by means of drugs, serums, vaccines and other poisons. If for instance we catch a cold, a fever, etc., let the disease accomplish its natural development, and avoid taking quinine and other drugs, which disturb this natural development. If we try to oppose nature, we will become weak and endanger our health. Remember that nature never fails to punish us for our transgressing of its laws.

All acute diseases (fever, etc.) are, as already stated, curative crisis. They are like the tempests which purify the air and causes the plants to grow, but which at the same time destroys old and gnawed trees which are not fit, not staunch enough to resist the tempests. On account of their diseased state, these trees are a breeding place for worms and disease; their existence is dangerous for other trees and a menace to the purpose of the law of the conservation of life.

As forests exist because tempests exist, which purifies the air and destroys old and unfit trees, so does mankind exist because there are small-pox, fevers, Spanish Influenza and other acute diseases. If in order to preserve old, diseased and unfit trees, we would endeavor to bridle the tempests, the consequence would be the slow but sure destruction of the forests. Still man is so stupid, that in order to try to preserve (only for a short time!) the life of some persons who do not consider themselves strong enough to undergo a curative crisis, he tries to stop the latter. If this practice is continued, in the long run it will bring about the extinction of the whole human race.

Sickness is an evil, the aim of which is to avoid a greater evil. Dandruff is perhaps the reason why everyone is not bald. The small insects which compel us to scratch our head, makes us perform a constant and beneficial massage to our scalp. It would be surely much better if it were not necessary to have dandruff, small-pox, fevers, etc., but in order not to need these diseases we would have to possess perfect health, which is so far from fact, that we do not even dream of possessing it.

Curative crisis, or acute diseases, are favorable, but they should be spontaneous, natural, since to try and incite them artificially, as in the case of vaccination, is so absurd as it would be to spread chronic and incurable disease in order to destroy the degenerates. Our mission is not to suppress the degenerates, but to try and cure the human race in order that neither acute nor chronic diseases will be necessary.

We must respect the lofty designs of nature, even if we can not understand them. Every drug, every serum which we discover to cure syphilis, is immoral, since by means of that medicine we would remove the punishment due, and therefore encourage prostitution. Besides that, syphilis is a reaction by means of which human nature frees itself of the venereal disease... or of the individual who is not for nor strong enough to stand the reaction.

As Indian philosophy tells us, everything that nature does, is good, even if we do not think this it to be so; that is to say, even if the ignorance of man does not allow him to understand the reason why. So we see that in his persistence to correct nature, man has done nothing else but harm himself. If there were not pain and disease (symptoms) mankind would have disappeared long ago. Therefore pain and disease are beneficial, as they are a form, a manifestation of nature, whose aim is to preserve life. In other words, pain and disease exist in order to promote the law of conservation of life (morals).

. . . acute diseases are a **curative crisis**, by means of which foreign matter, clogging the body, is removed.

When we remove symptoms, we do not cure the disease, but we simply help to prolong or to change it into another and more dangerous form which appears later on. . .

The scientific principle of Kuhne regarding the unity of disease; that all diseases have only one cause, and that they exist in our body long before they appear.

We see that in his persistence to correct nature, man has done nothing else but harm himself.

MEDICINES
BENEDICT LUST

PROCLAMATION
BENEDICT LUST

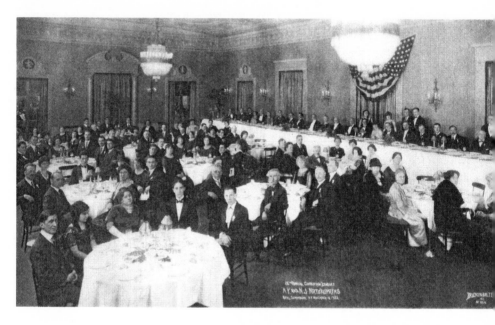

The 26th Annual Convention of the A.N.A. of the New York and New Jersey State Societies of Naturopaths held at the Hotel Commodore [NYC] on November 17th and 18th, 1922.

MEDICINES

by Benedict Lust, N.D., D.O., M.D.

Herald of Health and Naturopath, XXVII(1), 5-6. (1922)

The delusion that health can be restored by swallowing drugs is so widely spread that one doubts the sanity of people who spend large amounts of money for medicines, inasmuch as their experience gives them usually, if not always, unsatisfactory and often fatal results. The whole tendency of popular pharmacy, has been in the direction of introducing to the public a great variety of powerful medicines put up in convenient form and advertised in such a manner as to produce in the unthinking a belief that they may be safely and rightly administered at all times and seasons for some real or supposed malady.

These medicines have been extensively advertised in the newspapers; but the medical profession must admit that it cannot be held free from some amount of blame in the matter, or from some responsibility for the way drugs have been popularized and brought into common use, as articles of domestic consumption.

Medical men have failed sufficiently to impress upon the public and upon patients that their aim should be to keep themselves in health, rather than to be always seeking assistance from drugs.

The over-eating, the lack of exercise, the excessive use of tobacco, excessive eating of meat and starchy foods, are the producers of uric acid, which seems to be one of the underlying troubles the drugs are supposed to cure, but, which at the very best, only temporarily relieve or suppress the disease and gradually lead to the degeneration of the tissue and to premature death.

The various alkaline solutions which are given for gout or rheumatism cannot be taken very long without serious disturbances of nutrition; but the aim of treatment in cases of all derangements should be to cure them by changing the condition under which they arise, not to palliate them for a time by the neutralization of acid which may give temporary relief, but which leaves the original diseased condition unaltered.

Among the most pernicious and dangerous of all the drugs and patent medicines are the so-called "headache powders," the almost instantaneous effects testify to the potency of the drugs they contain. Such powerful agents are dangerous to health for they cannot remove the cause of the pain. Hence their action is limited to narcotize the nerves. The disease continues and the damage is done. Headache powders increase deaths by heart failure, therefore it is necessary to warn the public against them.

Medicines used for children are detrimental to their health. Mothers very often use cooling medicines for their babies when a little feverish.

Many of the best doctors believe that no medicines can cool fever. Common sense however can surely tell anyone that cold water will cool. Doctors know this, and cold baths are daily used in the great fever hospitals throughout the world. Rheumatic fever, typhoid fever and small pox have been found to yield to cold baths when no other treatment would save life. Cold water is only dangerous when the body is cold, always remember that. Also remember that unless the body warms up well after a cold bath it must not be repeated; but when the body is hot, cold water can only do good; and when very hot and feverish often nothing else will save life.

After taking a cold bath be careful that the feet get warm. Warm feet always relieve headache, if they should remain cold too long after the bath put a warm bottle to them well wrapped in flannel. Cool abdominal packs give excellent results in fever. With weak people frequent washing of the whole body is best after the bath; or if they are afraid of a cold bath then start with a warm bath and gradually cool it off. With very weak children who are often hot and cold by turns, a better plan is to use a handful of salt in a warm bath and afterwards wash the body with cool water. I advise mothers and nurses not to use fever drops for babies and growing children, but regulate the diet and use water. Microbes cannot breed if the nest in which they incubate is cooled down below the breeding heat.

Pure water to drink, pure water to cool the surface (hot or cool as vitality calls for), no foods that induce fever, pure non uric acid making foods, afterwards, pure air through the house and fever will be no longer regarded as a plague but as a beneficent servant to remind us of neglected duty and self-indulgent greed.

The delusion that health can be restored by swallowing drugs is so widely spread that one doubts the sanity of people who spend large amounts of money for medicines, inasmuch as their experience gives them usually, if not always, unsatisfactory and often fatal results.

Cold water is only dangerous when the body is cold, always remember that.

PROCLAMATION

For the Twenty-sixth Annual Convention of the N.Y. and N.J. State Societies of Naturopaths, Accredited Sections of The American Naturopathic Association.

by Benedict Lust, N.D., M.D.
President, American Naturopathic Association
Herald of Health and Naturopath, XXVII(12), 583-584. (1922)

NATUROPATHY

Today we look back with pride over the twenty-six years' record of the American Naturopathic Association. Our object is to help mankind by teaching and practicing the natural method of living, which is the basic plank of all rational methods of healing, constituting the great art and science of naturology and naturopathy. This science is not a cult idea, the egotistical aim of an autocrat or leader, nor the product of the mercenary ambitions of a group of exploiters or imposters.

The American Naturopathic Association is a union for the mutual advancement of non-drug physicians and other progressive men and women of the United States and Canada who not only lead the natural life themselves but who employ and teach non-drug methods of therapeutics and disease prevention.

The six majors of Naturopathy are the agents which make for life and form the congenial environment under which each normal life can express itself. These essentials are air, light, water, food, physical culture and mind. That which preserves health and life in its normal function and expression is also the cure. Therefore, naturopaths use the *atmospheric* cure, the *light* cure, the *water* cure, the *diet* cure, the *earth* (clay) cure, the *work* cure, and the *mind* cure. These six are majors, not adjuncts. They are not immaterial side issues. They precede and must underlie any method of specific treatment that may be employed in the healing art, rational chiropractic not excepted.

Minors of the healing art which can be combined and used as adjuncts to the six majors are:

Mechano-therapy, which covers massage and its sub-headings, such as productive physical work, exercise, curative gymnastics, osteopathy, spinotherapy, neuropathy, naprapathy, etc.

Psychotherapy in its different presentations and applications such as psychoanalysis, suggestive therapeutics, magnetism, mental science, new thought, music therapy, personal and vocational efficiency, divine healing, etc.

Electrotherapy in all its branches, such as the use of different currents, mechanical vibration, X-rays, hydro-electrotherapy, high frequency, heliotherapy, phototherapy, etc.

Physiotherapy a la Priessnitz, Ehret, Platen, Engelhardt, Kuhne, Kneipp, Bilz and Just systems of hydrotherapy and nature cure in over one thousand different ways of applying water, such as ablutions, baths, douches, sprays, packs, bandages, compresses, herb baths, fomentations, vapor and steam, dry heat, etc.

Phytotherapy. The use of plants, herbal juices, botanic home-remedies, specific, approved and harmless vegetable compounds.

Biochemistry. Supplying to the body what it lacks in organic and inorganic constitutional elements. Nutritive salt therapy, a la Schuessler, Lahmann, Hensel, Cargrie, etc.

Orificial and bloodless *Orthopedic Surgery.* Obstetrics practiced in the natural way. Accidental and Unavoidable Surgery.

Natural Living

Natural life is the first requisite of all rational therapies and must be the outstanding feature of all there is to human wholeness, such as eugenics, pre-natal culture, the natural way of raising children, an educational system, elementary, advanced and professional, which must never be in the way, or given at the expense of health and general welfare.

Reform of Agriculture, Horticulture and Forestry, in which the welfare of the human family as a whole must be strictly employed. In conformity with the laws of nature, we must raise food for man and animals on a soil which has the normal proportion of mineral elements, so that instead of disease curing we will have disease prevention, which starts in the plants in the fields, with the fruits on the trees and bushes in the orchard, and the fruits and nuts in the woods.

The utter failure of official medicine to teach natural and rational disease prevention is largely the cause of our social unrest, moral degeneration, war, and is the stumbling block and menace to true science, progress and humanity. The American Medical Association is the arch enemy to the individual and natural freedom of our bodies and our minds. It does not fit in and should never have been permitted to nestle into the fabric of the American Democracy. It is un-American all the way through. It is an imposition in its inception and in its practices. The nefarious work of this autocratic institution and the terrible results of it were brought out by the World War. Its destructive power is exercised in every department of life in the United States, Federal, State, Municipal, Army and Navy, Educational, Church, Home, and finally with the individual. It has prostituted our Public School system, our educational and health boards, and is claiming the right over the child even before it is born. The last convention of the American Medical Association brought out some terrible statement of what they intend to do in the future. It is high time for America to wake up and chop off the heads of this Hydra in Washington, through the elections kill its bills in Congress and in every legislature in the States and block every move it makes in the Aldermanic Chambers of the cities, in the Educational Boards and the Boards of Health. Furthermore, we must wipe from the statutes of every State in the Union the unconstitutional medical laws, none of which were placed there by the people. They were put there by political doctors, graft politicians under the pretense of safeguarding the public health, but in reality for exploitation of the people, for medical graft, and to shut out every new and independent system of practice that might spring up outside of their own making.

Naturopathy, the art and science of natural living and natural cure by all rational methods, which is a word of protest, was coined in the days of persecution when the New York County Medical Association arrested and fined with heavy money sentences and long prison terms the noble pioneers and humanitarian characters that stood up as representatives of the rational healing art and for the rights of the people. Naturopathy and Nature Cure is non-sectarian, is progressive and adjustable to the needs of mankind in our present era, and for ages to come Naturopathy is here and will stay as the true healing art serving mankind in the prevention and cure of physical, mental and spiritual ailments and to work for personal, natural and constitutional rights the separation of politics and medicine.

The American Naturopathic Association stands for medical freedom of the people. In the year 1896 its founders wrote in its constitution that every citizen of the United States must have the choice of his method of healing and the free right of his body and mind and every doctor should have the free exercise of his profession (parity of all methods of healing) as long as he is honest and serves the people in a constructive and legitimate way. We should have no laws except the general penal laws to cover the art of healing. We stand now and for all time for comparity and equality of all systems before the tribunal of the American People. The self-constituted tribunal of the American Medical Society we will not recognize as a legal body. By the actions and deeds of the past, by the attitude of the present and plans for the future, it has forfeited its charter, which was granted to it by the Commonwealth.

The A.N.A. is non-sectarian, its members being both practitioners and laymen. Our doors are open to medical men who have given up the use of poisonous drugs and avoidable surgery. Our society is open to the people at large to get the benefit of the education this Association administers in the science of prevention of disease by natural living. The naturopath or drugless doctor is essentially a teacher in his locality and his mission is rather to prevent than to cure disease.

We welcome all honest truth seekers, people of the larger life, who believe in reforming themselves, and see that a happy future of the human race is only possible if each one of us reforms himself. We cannot reform the people by coercion, we cannot usher in happiness and good health for the American people unless we treat and practice prevention of disease, and by each one of us leading a natural and efficient life. We must prevent the further pollution by vaccination and other superstitious and health undermining practices as they are imposed upon us by the American Medical Association. Let us work for the welfare of all mankind; let us not hate anybody, even our enemies. We do not oppose medical doctors individually, but we oppose the politico-medical machine in its un-American practices and in its harmful results. We stand for better health for the American people, greater harmony and tolerance among Drugless Doctors, co-operation, and the realization of a Federal Association covering all the drugless schools and societies and all rational practitioners in one great power for still more progress in natural therapeutics, protection, defense and for a blessing to all mankind.

The six majors of Naturopathy are the agents which make for life and form the congenial environment under which each normal life can express itself. These essentials are air, light, water, food, physical culture and mind.

Naturopaths use the atmospheric cure, the light cure, the water cure, the diet cure, the earth (clay) cure, the work cure, and the mind cure.

Minors of the healing art which can be combined and used as adjuncts to the six majors are: Mechano-therapy, which covers massage and its sub-headings, such as productive physical work, exercise, curative gymnastics, osteopathy, spinotherapy, neuropathy, naprapathy, etc.

Naturopathy, the art and science of natural living and natural cure by all rational methods, which is a word of protest, was coined in the days of persecution when the New York County Medical Association arrested and fined with heavy money sentences and long prison terms the noble pioneers and humanitarian characters that stood up as representatives of the rational healing art and for the rights of the people.

1923

Doctor And Physician Are Naturopathic Terms
Dr. M. E. Yergin

The Functions Of A Health School
Herbert M. Shelton, D.P., N.D.

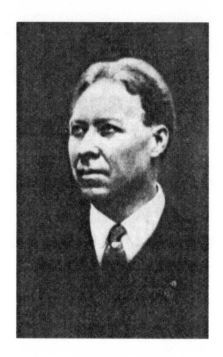

Dr. M. E. Yergin

Doctor And Physician Are Naturopathic Terms

by Dr. M. E. Yergin

Naturopathic Health School, Chicago, Illinois

Herald of Health and Naturopath, XXVIII(5), 227-228. (1923)

Tracing the usage of the terms DOCTOR and PHYSICIAN into the centuries of the past, it is found that both these terms in their original usage and customary application, have nothing specially to do with those who practise medicine and surgery.

Both these terms are of very ancient origin; the exact date of their first usage being unknown.

The word PHYSICIAN is from the Greek *physis*, nature; and the terminal which means a student or philosopher,—one who studies and works according to the laws of nature.

In the earlier uses of this term, it applied to a school of philosophers whose student body went forth with their instructors into the fields, under the skies, by the brooks and rivers and mountains, to observe the workings of the laws of nature by which human life could be brought up to its best in all departments of human capacity.

The laws of nature were studied by this school, for the purpose of correctly ordering social, business, and moral life; and had to do with the ordering of the physical, mental and spiritual life to the best purposes and accomplishments.

In its original meaning and its common usage from the earliest times up to the present, the term DOCTOR means first and over and above all other things,—a TEACHER.

In Webster's International Dictionary, edition A.D. 1912, is given the following definitions of DOCTOR.

These definitions are quoted verbatim herewith,—

Doctor (noun); . . . Latin, **doctor,** teacher; from *docere*, to teach. ...

1—A teacher ; one skilled in a profession, or branch of knowledge; a learned man. . . .

2—An academical title, originally implying that possessor of it is so well versed in a department of knowledge as to be qualified to teach. Hence: One who has taken the highest degree conferred by a university or college, or has received a diploma of the highest degree; as, a **doctor** of divinity, of music, of philosophy, etc. "Such degree may be merely honorary. . . .

3—a) One duly licensed to practice medicine; a member of the medical profession; a physician; a surgeon. . . .

    b) A wizard or medicine man in a savage tribe. . . .

6—A cook, as on shipboard or in a camp. . . .

8—A repairer of anything; as, a chair **doctor**. . . .

Doctor, verb transitive; . . .

2—To treat as a physician does; to apply remedies to ; to repair; as, to doctor a sick man or a broken cart."

Out of eleven distinct definitions under the noun, only one—the third definition is applied to those who use medicine and surgery.

Thus it is seen that both the terms DOCTOR and PHYSICIAN, originated in ancient usage and in our authentic dictionaries to very recent date, have persistently continued to bear meanings strictly of naturopathic character.

And in the instance of the term doctor, referring to those who practise medicine and surgery, the definition holds in the ratio of one out of eleven. All the other definitions applying to natural applications of the term within the field of natural and drugless usage.

And it is notable that in every instance where the medical and surgical profession have endeavored to prosecute the natural and drugless therapists who are using the term doctor and physician, which is entirely within their inherent and lawful rights,—that the courts, even the supreme courts; as, in Illinois and other States, have always rendered the decision in favor of the drugless and natural doctor. Stating that the terms have nothing to do in their essential and natural meaning with the practise of medicine and surgery.

Every naturopathic physician should so understand his or her profession, that he or she shall be a capable teacher; and as such, is therefore fully entitled to use both the terms doctor and physician.

A doctor in the original and constantly and persistently applied meaning of the term is first and over and above all, a TEACHER.

And this is the high calling to which all naturopathic doctors and physicians are called. They should essentially and necessary be teachers originally; and continue to be teachers throughout the term of their active practice.

In the essential underlying principle of the naturopathic profession, each physician of this order has a continual necessity for constant instruction of the patient in natural things.

They recognize that sickness, disease and suffering, are conditions that are brought upon the patient through departure from natural law; and that the only way to fully and practically restore such to perfect health, is to treat them as required, in the natural way; and at the same time impart instruction that will enable them to harmonize their lives with nature and her beneficent laws.

Every naturopathic physician throughout the world, is, both by the character of his or her profession and the original and persistent meanings of the terms doctor and physician, entitled to use these terms openly and freely at all times and in all places.

Both the term DOCTOR and PHYSICIAN should appear on the literature of all naturopathic physicians throughout the world, and on their office signs, and elsewhere before the public.

These terms have been stolen by the medical and surgical profession, and do not originally belong to them at all, as the origin of both these terms show.

It is time the naturopathic profession quit their begging, and take to themselves those things which belong to them inherently and naturally.

> *In its original meaning and its common usage from the earliest times up to the present, the term DOCTOR means first and over and above all other things—a TEACHER.*
>
> *This is the high calling to which all naturopathic doctors and physicians are called. They should essentially and necessary be teachers originally; and continue to be teachers throughout the term of their active practice.*

THE FUNCTIONS OF A HEALTH SCHOOL

by Herbert M. Shelton, D.P., N.D.

Herald of Health and Naturopath, (XXVIII(10), 541-543. (1923)

Dr. H. Lahn says in his work on Iridology that the highest aim of the physician is to make himself dispensable. He explains that by this he means that the physician should so instruct and advise his patient that they reach the point where they are independent of him and can do without a physician. The patient would then be able to help and care for himself.

This same ideal has been held by such pioneers in the Nature Cure movement as Just, Kuhne, Ehret, Kneipp, Lust, Macfadden and others. The founding of the Crandall Health School was an effort to realize this ideal and this school is dedicated to the service of eradicating disease and discomfort by ministering to the patient's intelligence rather than to his stomach or liver. It is our endeavor to teach health, not to impart it, for we hold that health must be built, not bought, and that a plan of life, and not a treatment, is the way to build health. This is the old Nature Cure doctrine of "health by healthful living."

The Health School recognizes that all disease is an outgrowth of a common fundamental cause—toxemia. Toxemia is a state of the body tissues and fluids in which there is an abnormal percentage of toxins or poisons.

Toxins are constantly being formed in the body or are being absorbed from some external source. These are, however, eliminated by the normal body. Elimination is a fundamental function of the living organism just as fundamental as the function of digestion. It is a ceaseless process that never stops as long as life lasts. However, it cannot be maintained at a normal standard without a normal amount of nerve energy or vitality.

Any act, habit, indulgence or influence that uses up an excessive amount of nerve energy or which prevents complete recuperation from the daily expenditures, if habitual, lowers the functional powers of the body, thereby lessening its functional efficiency. The power to consume food is not necessarily decreased.

If this condition is allowed to continue there is a gradual accumulation of poisons within the body, because, due to its lack of power, the body is unable to eliminate the toxins as fast as they are formed. This retention and gradual accumulation of toxins results in toxemia. The body is overcharged with those same poisons that are being thrown off by the healthy body every moment of our lives.

The lowering of digestive efficiency due to the enervation or functional weakness brought on by the excessive expenditure of nerve force allows the food eaten to ferment, forming poisons, which are absorbed to add to the poisons formed within the body itself. When digestion is normal and the body is not overloaded with food fermentation does not take place. If food is taken in excess and fermentation does follow, the digestive juices are capable of neutralizing the poisons formed.

But overeating is a well-nigh universal habit. Not only so, but people eat when there are pain and discomfort, and when these exist digestion is impaired; people eat rapidly and do not thoroughly masticate their food. They also eat unwholesome combinations that do not digest well.

The systemic poisoning (toxemia) thus brought about is the basic cause of all so-called disease. It produces all internal irritation. The irritation produces congestion, the congestion becomes exaggerated into inflammation. The inflammation results in structural changes, suppuration (decomposition of tissues with the formation of pus). The "disease" thus formed is named according to the local seat of the trouble. Thus if the inflammation is in the appendix, the disease is called appendicitis, while if the inflammation is in the ovaries or tonsils it is called ovaritis or tonsilitis. It should be known that inflammation is the same in whatever part of the body it is located.

If the intense irritation produced by these toxins is prolonged, it causes degenerative changes to take place which produce such diseases as Bright's disease, tuberculosis, etc. An organ that is inherently weak or one that is weakened by our mode of life has less resistance than the other organs and is the first to undergo such changes.

It should be known, however, that nature or the organism attempts to free itself of these toxins by means of acute reaction or crises. But as the individual continues to pursue the same habits that built the toxemia at the start a chronic condition is started, crises are less shocking and come less often and the body learns to tolerate more and more of these toxins. It becomes readily apparent from this that chronic and degenerative diseases become possible only where the disease producing habits are continued or where suppressive treatment is employed.

As all diseases have their origin in toxemia it is worse than useless to treat the body for a disease called tuberculosis or one called Bright's disease or another called rheumatism or pneumonia. The thing that must be accomplished, if the disease is ever to be overcome, is the removal of the toxemic condition and its causes. All enervating habits, all excesses, all weakening influences must be corrected.

The employment of various measures to stimulate elimination provides temporary relief—palliation—but since they do not restore the dissipated vital energies nor correct the habits and influences that are responsible for the enervation they are in no sense curative. Indeed, since they accomplish their work by forcing the eliminative organs to do more work and do not cut off the source of toxin supply they further weaken and enervate. By such means of stimulation the organism may be whipped up into a temporary semblance of health and both the patient and doctor may be fooled.

Perhaps the reader is, by this time, better able to understand what we meant when we said in the first part of this article that health is built by a plan of life and not by a treatment.

It is the functions of a HEALTH SCHOOL to teach people how to correct the habits of life that build enervation and toxemia. When this has been accomplished and the patient has lived his knowledge his body will throw off disease and take on health. The patient is then cured by obedience to the laws of his being and is prepared to understand that there are no short cuts to health, no fountains of youth, no philosophers' stones, that will enable him to have health while building disease.

In our HEALTH SCHOOL the patient learns why he was sick, how he got well and how to stay well. When he goes away he is mentally prepared to care for himself in the future.

We place the patients in the most ideal state for the working out of natural law and they recover.

But what is perhaps of greatest value to our patients we teach them self-reliance. They are not taught to rely on the doctors and nurses. No one dances attendance on them and feels sorry for them.

People have become so accustomed to depend on the doctors that they are no longer able to depend on themselves. The average person is helpless in the absence of the physician. He is dependent upon some physician and gives up one school of healing only to transfer his allegiance to another. The HEALTH SCHOOL teaches people how to care for themselves and requires that they do it. It is interesting to note the decided change in the psychology of a patient as he gradually learns to depend on himself and ceases to feel sorry for himself. As he learns that he and not Providence, Adam or a germ is responsible for his trouble, he begins to realize that health and disease are individual matters. This is why we minister to the patient's intelligence instead of to his stomach, liver or spine.

> *Elimination is a fundamental function of the living organism just as fundamental as the function of digestion . . . . In our HEALTH SCHOOL the patient learns why he was sick, how he got well and how to stay well.*

REFERENCES

Bilz, F. E. (1901). The natural method healing, how to protect oneself against disease and illness. *The Kneipp Water Cure Monthly*, II(5), 131-134.

Bloch, S. (1906). Vital force in man. *The Naturopath and Herald of Health*, VII(7), 255-258.

Brandt, C. (1921). Pain and disease. *Herald of Health and Naturopath*, XXVI(8), 373-376.

Buell, C. J. (1910). Social health and personal health. *The Naturopath and Herald of Health*, XV(8), 454-457.

Carr, C. S. (1908). Nature as doctor. *The Naturopath and Herald of Health*, IX(6), 180-181.

Corbin, C. M. (1909). A suggestion. *The Naturopath and Herald of Health*, XVI(12), 769.

Dickenson, E. (1920). Can the mind heal all diseases? *Herald of Health and Naturopath*, XXV(3), 419-420.

Ehret, A. (1912). Sick people. *The Naturopath and Herald of Health*, XVII(3), 166-170.

Erieg, S. T. (1908). Doctors and their exorbitant fees. *The Naturopath and Herald of Health*, IX(1), 14-15.

Erz, A. A. (1912). Help to abolish an unhuman industry. *The Naturopath and Herald of Health*, XVII(7), 423-425.

Erz, A. A. (1913). Medicine and psychology. *The Naturopath and Herald of Health*, XVIII(2), 81-84.

Gray, H. S. (1912). In justice to Thomas and Tabby. *The Naturopath and Herald of Health*, XVII(8), 501-506.

White, E. G., Gulick, Dubois, P., Saleeby, C. W., James, W., Hunter, J (1909). The effect of the mind on the body. *The Naturopath and Herald of Health*, XIV(11), 697.

Havard, W. F. (1915). An answer to Mr. Purinton's article in March *Naturopath*. *The Naturopath and Herald of Health*, XX(4), 211-215.

Havard, W. F. (1915). Eclecticism in drugless healing. *The Naturopath and Herald of Health*, XX(4), 253-254.

Havard, W. F. (1918). Editorial, the point of view. *Herald of Health and Naturopath*, XXIII(5), 419-420.

Havard, W. F. (1919). Stenographic report of the 22nd annual convention of the ANA. *Herald of Health and Naturopath*, XXIV(6), 272-274.

Havard, W. F. (1919). Stenographic report of the 22nd annual convention of the ANA. *Herald of Health and Naturopath*, XXIV(9), 427-431.

Hodge, J. W. (1911). Preventative medicine. *The Naturopath and Herald of Health*, XVI(3), 166-170.

Hotz, W. (1900). Cleanliness, the first principle of hygiene. *The Kneipp Water Cure Monthly*, I(6), 89-90.

Just, A. (1901). Return to nature, the voices of nature. *The Kneipp Water Cure Monthly*, II(10), 264-267.

Just, A. (1910). The new paradise of health, the only true natural method. *The Naturopath and Herald of Health*, XV(12), 711-721.

Kaessmann, F. (1913). Remove the cause. *The Naturopath and Herald of Health*, XVIII(3), 158-159.

Kuhne, L. (1917). The new science of healing, disease a transmission of morbid matter. *Herald of Health and Naturopath*, XXII(6), 337-342.

Kuhne, L. (1917). The new science of healing, cold hands and feet, hot head: their cause and cure. *Herald of Health and Naturopath*, XXII(6), 354-355.

Lindlahr, H. (1910). Three great methods of cure. *The Naturopath and Herald of Health*, XV(1), 31.

Lindlahr, H. (1910). Catechism of Nature Cure. *The Naturopath and Herald of Health*, XV(1), 32-35.

Lindlahr, H. (1918). How I became acquainted with Nature Cure. *Herald of Health and Naturopath*, XXIII(2), 122-130.

Lust, B. (1900). The natural treatment and medicine. *The Kneipp Water Cure Monthly*, I(2), 17-18.

Lust, B. (1900). Just and his method. *The Kneipp Water Cure Monthly*, I(8), 127-131.

Lust, B. (1900). The Kneipp cure. *The Kneipp Water Cure Monthly*, I(9), 148-149.

Lust, B. (1903). Naturopathy, what hinders the propagation of Naturopathy? *The Naturopath and Herald of Health*, IV(7), 194-195.

Lust, B. (1903). Return to nature. *The Naturopath and Herald of Health*, IV(7), Advertisement.

Lust, B. (1904). Naturopathy. *The Naturopath and Herald of Health*, V(1), 1-3.

Lust, B. (1905). The natural method of healing. *The Naturopath and Herald of Health*, VI(7), 175-177.

Lust, B. (1906). Ten commandments. *The Naturopath and Herald of Health*, VII(1), 7.

Lust, B. (1907). The purpose and method of nature-cure. *The Naturopath and Herald of Health*, VIII(3), 68-70.

Lust, B. (1913). Principles of ethics. *The Naturopath and Herald of Health*, XVIII(6), 376-379.

Lust, B. (1915). The editor again differs with Mr. Purinton. *The Naturopath and Herald of Health*, XX(7), 538.

Lust, B. (1921). Editorials, those immutable laws. *Herald of Health and Naturopath*, XXVI(4), 161-162.

Lust, B. (1922). Medicines. *Herald of Health and Naturopath*, XXVII(1), 5-6.

Lust, B. (1922). Proclamation. *Herald of Health and Naturopath*, XXVI(12), 583-584.

Muckley, F. (1917). The poison of Lake Erie water. *Herald of Health and Naturopath*, XXII(12), 335.

Nelson, P. (1920). Naturopathy versus medicine. *Herald of Health and Naturopath*, XXV(2), 78-82.

Purinton, E. E. (1915). Efficiency in drugless healing, standardizing the Nature Cure. *The Naturopath and Herald of Health*, XX(3), 141-147.

Purinton, E. E. (1918). Affirmations. *Herald of Health and Naturopath*, XXIII(1), 33..

Staden, L. (1900). The causation of diseases. *The Kneipp Water Cure Monthly*, I(6), 100.

Staden, L. (1902). What is Naturopathy? *The Naturopath and Herald of Health*, III(1), 15-18.

Schultz, C. (1905). Naturopathy, what it is, what it does, and why it is opposed by the medical trust? *The Naturopath and Herald of Health*, VI(8), 216-219.

Shelton, H. M. (1921). What have we, nature cure or a bag of tricks? *Herald of Health and Naturopath*, XXVI(6), 283-287.

Shelton, H. M. (1923). The functions of a health school. *Herald of Health and Naturopath*, XXVIII(10), 541-543.

Strueh, C. (1913). Symptomatic treatment a waste of effort and time. *The Naturopath and Herald of Health*, XVIII(3), 170-171.

Strueh, C. (1914). Brief 7, Naturopathy. *The Naturopath and Herald of Health*, XIX(4), 253-258.

Tunison, E. H. (1916). Drugless healing. *Herald of Health and Naturopath*, XXI(6), 3371-373.

Wallace, C. L. H. (1902). General rules for the physical regeneration of man. *The Naturopath and Herald of Health*, III(10), 403-405.

White, E. G. (1909). The effect of the mind on the body. *The Naturopath and Herald of Health*, XVI(11), 697.

Wigelsworth, J. W. (1918). Nature's safety valve. *Herald of Health and Naturopath*, XXIII(8), 731-732.

Wilmans, H. (1918). Omnipresent life. *Herald of Health and Naturopath*, XXIII(2), 168-171.

Yergin, M. E. (1923). Doctor and physician are naturopathic terms. *Herald of Health and Naturopath*, XXVIII(5), 227-228.

Zeff, J. (2013). Reference taken from a personal communication.

INDEX

A

About the Editor, NCNM, NCNM Press

Sᴜssᴀɴɴᴀ Cᴢᴇʀᴀɴᴋᴏ, ND, BBE, is a 1994 graduate of CCNM (Toronto). She is a licensed ND in Ontario and in Oregon. In the last twenty years, she has developed an extensive armamentarium of nature-cure tools and techniques for her patients. Especially interested in balneotherapy, botanical medicine, breathing and nutrition, she is a frequent international presenter and workshop leader. She is a monthly Contributing Editor (Nature Cure —Past Pearls) for NDNR and a Contributing Writer for the Foundations of Naturopathic Medicine Project. Dr. Czeranko founded The Breathing Academy, a training institute for naturopaths to incorporate the scientific model of Butyeko breathing therapy into their practice. Her next large project is to complete the development of her new medical spa in Manitou Beach, Saskatchewan, on the shores of a pristine medical waters lake.

NCNM (National College of Natural Medicine, Portland, Oregon) was founded in 1956. It is the longest serving, accredited naturopathic college in North America and home to one of the two U.S. accredited graduate research programs in Integrative Medicine. NCNM is also home to one of North America's most unique classical Chinese medicine programs, embracing lineage and a powerful mentoring model for future practitioners.

NCNM Pʀᴇss, an ancillary venture of NCNM, publishes distinctive titles that enrich the history, clinical practice, and contemporary significance of natural medicine traditions. The rare book collection on natural medicine at NCNM is the largest and most complete of its kind in North America and is the primary source for this landmark series—*In Their Own Words*—which brings to life and timely relevance the very best of early naturopathic literature.

The Hevert Collection: *In Their Own Words*

A Twelve-book Series

Origins of Naturopathic Medicine

Philosophy of Naturopathic Medicine

Principles of Naturopathic Medicine

Dietetics of Naturopathic Medicine

Practice of Naturopathic Medicine

Physical Culture in Naturopathic Medicine

Herbs in Naturopathic Medicine

Hydrotherapy in Naturopathic Medicine

Mental Culture in Naturopathic Medicine

Vaccination in Naturopathic Medicine

Clinical Pearls of Naturopathic Medicine, Vol. I

Clinical Pearls of Naturopathic Medicine, Vol. II

From The NCNM Rare Book Collection On Natural Medicine.
Published By NCNM Press, Portland, Oregon.

Lightning Source UK Ltd.
Milton Keynes UK
UKOW01f2203210916

283526UK00001B/204/P